The Gender Politics of HIV/AIDS
in Women

The Gender Politics of HIV/AIDS in Women

Perspectives on the Pandemic in the United States

Edited by

Nancy Goldstein and
Jennifer L. Manlowe

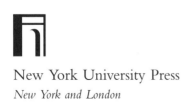

New York University Press
New York and London

New York University Press
New York and London

© 1997 by New York University
All Rights Reserved

Library of Congress Cataloging-in-Publication Data
The gender politics of HIV/AIDS in women : perspectives on the
pandemic in the United States / edited by Nancy Goldstein and
Jennifer L. Manlowe.
p.   cm.
Includes bibliographical references (p.   ) and index.
ISBN 0-8147-3094-9 (cloth : alk. paper). — ISBN 0-8147-3093-0
(paper : alk. paper)
 1. AIDS (Disease)—Social aspects—United States.   2. Women—
Health and hygiene—United States.   3. AIDS (Disease)—Government
policy—United States.   4. Women's rights—United States.
 I. Goldstein, Nancy, 1961–   .   II. Manlowe, Jennifer L., 1963–   .
RA644.A25G466 1997
362.1′969792′0082—dc21   96-45877
CIP

New York University Press books are printed on acid-free paper,
and their binding materials are chosen for strength and durability.

Manufactured in the United States of America

10   9   8   7   6   5   4   3   2   1

Contents

Part III. Working (through) Solutions

Part IV. Women with AIDS Speak Out

Acknowledgments

Nancy Goldstein: I'd like to thank Julie Rivkin for her steadfast friendship and her wholehearted endorsement of the Gender Politics of HIV conference that inspired this volume. The conference, which took place at Connecticut College in September 1994, was generously supported by the Steering Committee of the Program in Gender and Women's Studies, Unity House, and the Everywomen's Center. It was there that Jennifer Manlowe and I met in person for the first time (we'd initially made contact on the internet some weeks before) and began thinking in ways that eventually led to this volume. Thanks to Paul Morrison and Sally Zierler for their incredibly helpful critiques of my work, their wisdom, their kindness, and their invaluable time. In addition to being fine scholars, patient teachers, and thorough readers, Paul proved fearless in the face of my awful first drafts; Sally shared her vision of a better and more equitable world with me. Thanks to Nina DeLuca and Rosa V. DeLuca for their constant faith and love. My immense gratitude to Jennifer Hammer, our editor at NYU Press, for her lucidity, her guidance, her patience, and her unwavering support for this project.

Jennifer Manlowe: To the 100-plus women I interviewed on the HIV Epidemiological Research Study (HERS) who inspired me to offer a more nuanced version of their lives than a statistical or quantitative, CDC-sponsored study would allow, I am deeply grateful. To the contributors who dared to tell their version of living and working with HIV/AIDS in a climate that would prefer they fall in line, accept the status quo, and keep quiet, I commend you all and am truly honored to have your stories told in this volume. My thanks go out to my coworkers Dennis Thomas and Naomi Sachs at the Brown University AIDS Program who encouraged me to have faith in the worthiness of this project. To my coeditor, Nancy Goldstein, I offer much appreciation for your tireless effort in editing this volume and creatively collaborating every step of the way. Christian Couto, you are in a league of your own when it comes to nurturing me and helping me think constructively. Finally, to Jennifer Hammer, our editor at NYU Press, thank you for your ongoing belief in this project and enthusiasm in facilitating writing that we all hope will be part of transforming how females are treated and represented by health researchers and providers.

Introduction

Our understanding of the AIDS epidemic requires us to sort out an extraordinary number of difficulties about identity. These have serious implications for women: perhaps no area of AIDS commentary has been more consistently confusing and problematic as gender—for AIDS experts, AIDS educators, clinicians, and media commentators as well as for women themselves.

> Paula A. Treichler, "Beyond Cosmo: AIDS, Identity, and Inscriptions of Gender"

The assumptions of the biomedical model as embodied in the paradigms of gay plague and chronic disease have shaped scientific knowledge about AIDS as well as the medical and public health responses to this epidemic. The biomedical orientation has led to an almost exclusive focus on HIV and the mechanisms—as opposed to the social determinants—of its transmission. As methodology, biomedical individualism has resulted in data being collected chiefly on individuals with or at risk of AIDS, and rarely on the social context of their lives. Working under the rubric of "objectivity" as defined by the biomedical model, scientists have failed to see how social biases affect the type of research questions they ask. Physicians and other health care workers have failed to see how similar assumptions shape the medical care they provide. And these assumptions, if not addressed, threaten to vitiate our still-inadequate response to the epidemic.

> Elizabeth Fee and Nancy Krieger, "Understanding AIDS: Historical Interpretations and the Limits of Biomedical Individualism"

The human immunodeficiency virus (HIV) has been studied primarily as a biological rather than a social or cultural phenomenon in the United States, and as a male virus in female bodies. This should come as no surprise given the history of twentieth-century U.S. medicine, health care, research, and biomedical education. In the thirties and forties, popular opinion tended to place an enormous amount of confidence in what was commonly thought to be the ultimate tendency of science and medicine to liberate humanity from ignorance and illness. This faith in the ability of biomedicine and epidemiology to discern, define, and address disease ran strong until around 1960; it was only then, according to historian Charles E. Rosenberg, that "medicine's conceptual foundations . . . [came] under increasing attack" as a result of what he calls "the marriage of cultural criticism and antipositivism":

> Critics [have] turned the delegitimating tools of cultural relativism on medicine as they have on so many other areas in which knowledge and power are closely linked. For such scholars, Michel Foucault, not Robert Merton, has become the sociologist of choice.[1] . . . Medical knowledge is not value-free to such skeptics, but is at least in part a socially constructed and determined belief system, a reflection of arbitrary social arrangements, social need, and the distribution of power. . . . This relativist point of view has sought to undermine not only the apparent objectivity of particular disease entities but also, by implication, the legitimacy of social authority wielded by the medical profession, which has traditionally articulated and administered diagnostic categories. The physician is not above social interest, but is a social actor whose mission of defining and treating disease can express and legitimate professional, class, or gender interests.[2]

The union of cultural criticism and antipositivism that encouraged greater scrutiny of, and skepticism about, the alleged efficacy, objectivity, omniscience, and neutrality of biomedicine during the 1960s and early 1970s has come apart significantly since 1981. Ironically, HIV/AIDS has, to a considerable extent, forced those branches of Euro-American culture most likely to question and oppose the medical establishment—sexual, racial, and economic minorities—back into the position of relying upon science and its "experts" for legitimation, definitions, explanations, information, and cures. The past fifteen years have seen the return of science as king: "Gay leaders who had for decades urged the demedicalization of homosexuality now find their community anxiously attuned to the findings of virologists and immunologists."[3]

From the beginning of the pandemic there has been a tug of war for the role of determining paradigm between immunology and virology—two different forms of inquiry that represent two primary, separate, and often opposed ways of understanding, defining, and responding to HIV/AIDS.[4] Although there are immunologists who work on vaccines, and virologists who support preventative programs such as needle exchange, the difference between them, crudely put, is that immunology upholds an idea of health based on the body as an ecosystem; in this model, health is balanced and sustained by careful management of the individual human body. By contrast, virology typically seeks to restore the individual human body to health by embarking on a mission to stop killer cells from replicating inside it.

For the disciples of immunology, AIDS is a syndrome, not a disease; the goal is to prevent people from contracting HIV in the first place or to help HIV-infected people maintain health. Virology, on the other hand, takes a microscopic view of AIDS in which "HIV disease" begins the moment a person is infected with HIV. In this paradigm, the search for HIV's origins and the search for a cure both take place in the human body, and the goal is to stop the virus from replicating there. For the immunologically inclined, methods for intervening successfully in the pandemic include implementing programs designed to educate people behaviorally, attending to the lives of people living with HIV, and trying to strengthen their immune systems; for the virologically inclined, they include contact tracing, mass testing, and searching for a cure in the form of a vaccine. Hence, one's choice of paradigm is no small matter, affecting as it does one's governing conception of HIV/AIDS, its manifestations, and the path oneself and one's culture should take in combatting it. Cindy Patton notes: "The two names—AIDS and HIV disease—represent in relief the differences in thinking about the two subdisciplines, differences duplicated in education strategies, treatment trials, and public policy."[5]

But both of these models for understanding, categorizing, and addressing HIV/AIDS have their limits—specifically, their reliance upon individualistic models that presuppose agency and free will for subjects while failing to consider the subjects' social context. And neither is inherently culturally sensitive. Simply put, virologic/immunologic models that limit the study of HIV to the workings of the virus/immune system within the individual body tell us absolutely nothing about the social circumstances that render certain bodies particularly vulnerable to infection. The best-intentioned prevention campaigns are bound to fail if they assume that education combined with free condoms and clean "works"[6] are all that is needed to prevent the spread of HIV. Since there is more to risk than microbes, there must be more to preventing people from contracting HIV than telling them to "just say no" to exchanging bodily fluids or sharing needles.

As the epigraphs that head this introduction suggest, this volume is founded on a dual premise: first, that HIV and AIDS are best understood as socially, culturally, and ideologically—as well as biologically—determined phenomena; and secondly, that gender, especially as it intersects with race, class, and sexuality, plays a significant role in the way in which women have been infected and affected, and alternately singled out and ignored, in relation to HIV/AIDS in the U.S. This is not to suggest that there is such a thing as generic *woman,* or that we consider gender *the* primary difference/similarity among and between people. Individually and collectively, our contributors acknowledge the importance and the specificity of race, class, and sexuality in their work; at the same time they argue that it is vital for those who address HIV infection in women, regardless of their discipline, their methodology, or their goal, to begin taking into account the social contexts in which femaleness and femininity are constructed and lived when formulating their responses to the pandemic.

Safer sex campaigns that urge women to "just say no" to sex without a condom presume not only heterosexuality, but a degree of physical, cultural, and economic parity that simply does not characterize the majority of women who are having heterosexual sex, whether as a form of pleasure, work, or cultural expectation—or under the threat of violence. Historically specific socioeconomic factors such as the continued relative poverty of women compared to men and the absence of universal health care in the U.S. has limited women's access to standard, let alone expensive, medical procedures. Health centers that have no facilities for child care, that force their clients to travel long distances to get there, or to travel between distant locations to see a variety of different practitioners ultimately cannot support many of their female clients' struggles to maintain their own health as yet one more item on an agenda where a variety of other needs—food, children, work, drugs and alcohol, a partner, a place to sleep, money, safety—clamor for precedence. Prisons that do not provide their inmates with the kinds of education and self/family support that might make it possible for them to live crime-free lives upon release insure skyrocketing rates of recidivism. Drug and alcohol treatment centers that cannot accommodate children and teens, and "safe homes" for abused women that cannot accommodate children and teens, let alone women still struggling with their addictions, force women to make impossible choices. Once infected, women become sicker faster and die sooner than men with AIDS, but studies addressing this disparity point to differences between women and men that are not biological: once a study controls for social class and access to/use of prophylactic medications (like antibiotics and AZT), there's little, if any, difference between women and men in this regard. Apparently those that do exist reflect differences in access to and utilization of care.[7]

Women's risks for HIV infection include poverty, racism, classism, sexism, incarceration, isolation, lack of access to health insurance or medical care, illiteracy, homophobia, sex work, sexual abuse, domestic violence, alcohol and drug addiction, and an ideology of heterosexual romance that demands that women never question the fidelity of their male, presumably monogamous, sexual partners or put any "demands" on men (like condom usage) that might interfere with the male prerogative to enjoy sex. In short, women's risks for HIV infection are not limited solely to physiological conditions, like the amount of HIV concentrated in seminal fluid or the vulnerability of vaginal mucosa, although those factors are very real;[8] nor are they best addressed by forms of education and prevention that direct themselves to individuals without regard for the relations of power that underscore their lives. By producing critiques of existing biomedical methodologies, accounts of risk factors in women's lives that fall outside of current institutional definitions, descriptions of successful public health interventions, and the stories of some HIV affected and/or infected women, this anthology suggests the very real impact of the social determinants that expose women to HIV and the very real power of responses to the pandemic that take this knowledge into account.

In addition, many of the volume's contributors encourage readers to consider the ways in which popular definitions and understandings of HIV/ AIDS are shaped by the discursive operations of contemporary Euro-American culture—in particular, the ways in which culture itself determines the very definition of the "natural" and the biologically "true." From the perspective of social construction, the human body is not a singular, historically stable, uncontested site of meaning with its essence encoded on its surface in script that all well-educated professionals have read unproblematically and in complete accord with one another.[9] On the contrary, as a good deal of contemporary scholarship in the humanities and social sciences has argued, the body's shape, its content, and its meanings are all defined by the ruling paradigms of its observers, their prejudices, preferences, and assumptions: It is the product of culture and of cultural ideologies, the site of innumerable battles couched in the lexicons of law, religion, medicine, and science.

Nor does the definition of AIDS constitute a single, uncontested, historically stable site of meaning. On the contrary, it has changed three different times since the Centers for Disease Control (CDC) first reported the deaths of five urban homosexual men from *Pneumocystis carinii* pneumonia in June

1981. For AIDS is a syndrome, not a disease; HIV is a virus, not a disease. AIDS manifests itself in countless diseases that the CDC then decides it will or will not count, and the issues of when the CDC recognizes discrete diseases as having a similar underlying cause in the syndrome, or what the CDC will recognize, are very thorny ones indeed. In examining cultural constructions of HIV/AIDS it is particularly important that we pay close attention to the ways in which certain biomedical and epidemiological "observations" of the "natural" literally come to embody previously held values, assumptions, and prejudices regarding race, class, gender, ethnicity, and sexuality.

Long before 1981 the human body had already served simultaneously as weapon, ammunition, and battlefield for innumerable skirmishes in which various relations of power vied to situate their ideologies within its skeleton, its organs, its skull, its blood. A retelling of some of these historical narratives provides a useful framework for considering contemporary framings of HIV. Consider this: Thomas Laqueur has argued that Enlightenment-era reinterpretations of the body, from a hierarchical perspective that viewed women's bodies as inverted and inferior versions of men's to a new model of incommensurability, were based in newly created political needs rather than any real discoveries in anatomy or advances in reproductive biology.[10] The origins of the problem? Political theories that claimed there was no basis in nature for the domination of one being over another—in other words, the very logic that fueled and justified the dismantling of the monarchy—had other, more troubling implications for the men of that time. For if this was indeed true, "there seemed no reason why the universalistic claims for human liberty and equality during the Enlightenment should exclude half of humanity."[11] It was then, in response to the "woman" question, that "a biology of hierarchy grounded in a metaphysically prior 'great chain of being' gave way to a biology of incommensurability in which the relationship of men to women, like that of apples to oranges, was not given as one of equality or inequality but rather as a *difference* whose meaning required interpretation and struggle."[12]

Racism also submerges to the level of skin and bones, deploying itself from within the human body as "scientific" knowledge. As Evelynn Hammonds writes:[13]

> One of the first things that white southern doctors noticed about blacks imported from Africa as slaves, was that they seemed to respond differently than whites to certain diseases. Primarily they observed that some of the

diseases that were epidemic in the south seemed to affect blacks less severely than whites—specifically, fevers (e.g. yellow fever). Since in the eighteenth and nineteenth centuries there was little agreement about the nature of various illnesses and the causes of many common diseases were unknown, physicians tended to attribute the differences they noted simply to race.

In the nineteenth century when challenges were made to the institution of slavery, white southern physicians were all too willing to provide medical evidence to justify slavery.

Here Hammonds quotes from James H. Jones's book on the Tuskegee syphilis experiment:

They justified slavery and, after its abolition, second-class citizenship, by insisting that blacks were incapable of assuming any higher station in life. . . . Thus, medical discourses on the peculiarities of blacks offered, among other things, a pseudoscientific rationale for keeping blacks in their places.[14]

Hammonds continues:

If, as these physicians maintained, blacks were less susceptible to fevers than whites, than it seemed fitting that they and not whites should provide most of the labor in the hot, swampy lowlands where southern agriculture was centered. Southern physicians marshalled other "scientific" evidence, such as measurement of brain sizes and other body organs to prove that blacks constituted an inferior race. For many whites these arguments were persuasive because "objective" science offered validity to their personal "observations," prejudices and fears.

The history of the HIV/AIDS pandemic can be read as yet another narrative about the workings of determinist ideology embedded in the allegedly dispassionate discourse of biomedicine: In short, it reads as a virtual textbook of the ways in which prejudice becomes naturalized as biological fact. The history of early AIDS research and epidemiology, the "discovery" of HIV, and the course and current direction of scientific inquiry, while it may not tell us as much about preventing HIV as we would like, has much to tell us about how available epistemologies of knowledge determine the ways in which a public health crisis is characterized, responded to, and classified. For many years, the only stories that could be told, as directed by the CDC's definition, were ones in which demonized identities gave proof of their own promiscuity, profligacy, and dereliction by falling prey to a disease that told the truth of their sins as marked on their bodies.

Looking back to the early eighties, when HIV and AIDS were in their first stages of construction, it is now apparent that an impressive multiplicity of prejudices, "isms," and acts of denial coincided to deem the new epidemic the "gay plague" or gay-related-immune-deficiency (GRID)—all this despite evidence, from within months of the first reported cases, that it was affecting people whose identities or behaviors were other than those ascribed to urban, gay men. The isolation of the human retrovirus HIV in 1983 and the formation of the "4–H Club" that same year—so called because the four "risk groups" determined by CDC epidemiologists to be at highest risk for the virus were homosexuals, Haitians, heroin (and other injection drug) users, and hemophiliacs ("hookers" were later added to the list)—did little to dispel the linkage of HIV with "bizarre," "immoral," and "foreign" behavior. This tendency to attribute HIV/AIDS to identity rather than behavior, and to "others" as opposed to ourselves—specifically, to attribute the presence of HIV in the U.S. to the sexual "promiscuity" of urban gay men, the fetishized foreignness of Haitian immigrants, and the moral and psychic bankruptcy of sex workers and the drug-addicted—has everything to do with ideology and little to do with some unidentifiable entity called "pure science."

Part of that ideology was that women did not contract HIV. For the first thirteen years of the pandemic, the CDC failed to alter its AIDS definition to include a single female-specific HIV-related condition. In January 1993, under intense pressure from feminist health activists, the definition finally expanded to include cervical cancer (a preventable/treatable disease if caught early), which had gone unrecognized in positive women since 1981.[15] True, the U.S.'s unpreparedness to deal with a health crisis as it affects women has in part to do with the general tendency of biomedical research to presume the universality of the white, Euro-American, heterosexual male body and use it as the standard model for teaching and research. Biomedical accounts, which often serve as the basis for education, outreach, and treatment programs for specific populations and "risk groups" routinely fail to take into account the specific manifestations and implications of HIV (or, for that matter, cancer, heart disease, or stroke) in women's bodies and women's lives. But this inability to recognize "women's" diseases, such as vaginal yeast infections, as AIDS-related is an example of biomedical ideology's hold on "knowledge": specifically, the homophobic ideology of AIDS as a gay men's disease prevents members of the biomedical community from deeming discrete diseases as AIDS-related in women.

Despite this important and shockingly recent single recognition—that the diagnosis and interpretation of HIV may be different in some regards in anatomically female bodies—women still only account for only 5,091 of the 37,146 adult participants in the AIDS Clinical Trial Group (ACTG) study entries, or 14 percent.[16] And these numbers represent a vast improvement since 1993 when the Food and Drug Administration (FDA) officially lifted its ban on women participating in early experimental drug trials.

Given that CDC statistics, if anything, *underreport* the extent of HIV in the female population, their figures for 1995 are particularly alarming: In 1981, the first year AIDS was recognized, only five women were reported, accounting for a minority of AIDS cases (3 percent). Since then these proportions have been increasing steadily: They doubled to 6 percent in 1984 and more than tripled to 19 percent in 1995, "the highest proportion yet reported among women."[17] Women of color have routinely accounted for more than three-fourths of all AIDS cases in women: in 1995, 55.8 percent were African-American and 20.7 percent were Latina, although African-American women constitute only 15 percent of the population and Latinas only 7 percent.[18] HIV has become the third leading cause of death for all women age 25 to 44; it is the leading cause of death among African-American women in that age group, whose death rate is nine times higher than that of white women in the same age group.[19]

By the end of 1995, a total of 71,818 women had been reported to the Centers for Disease Control (CDC) with AIDS.[20] According to 1995 CDC reports, the median age of women with AIDS was 36 years, and 90 percent of cases were reported in women 20 to 50 years of age. Twenty-five percent of women were diagnosed with AIDS between the age of 20 and 30 years, indicating that substantial transmission of HIV occurs during adolescence and the early twenties. Women over 50 accounted for 9 percent of reported cases. Women accounted for 83 percent of cases reported among 13–19–year-olds who were infected through heterosexual contact or injection drug use, 66 percent of 20–24–year-olds, and 36 percent of 25–50–year-olds. These data point to young women becoming infected by sexual or needle-sharing partners older than themselves, and are consistent with reported age differences between adolescent mothers and their partners.[21]

Some evidence suggests a possible link between the high incidence of sexual assault in the lives of young girls and women and the high rates of HIV in adolescent girls and women in their twenties. As early as 1992, the national study entitled *Rape in America: A Report to the Nation* found that 61 percent of all rapes occur when females are seventeen years old or younger; 29 percent when they are less than eleven years old; 6 percent when they are older than twenty-nine.[22] And nearly half of the three thousand women surveyed in one college study said they had experienced some form of pressure to have sex since the age of fourteen.[23]

In 1995 injection drug use remains the predominant mode of transmission among women with AIDS in the Northeast, but the number of women with (presumably) heterosexually acquired AIDS exceeds the number infected through injection drug use in the South, the Midwest, and the West.[24] Physically, women are at greater risk than men during heterosexual sex,[25] and the proportion of AIDS cases in women that is attributed to heterosexual transmission has steadily increased from 15 percent in 1983 to 38 percent in 1995.

Our contributors argue that women remain misrepresented and underrepresented by the CDC's definition, in drug trials, and in research. Furthermore, they trace the current androcentrism of medical discourse to a long scientific tradition which regards women merely as reproductive subjects or as potential contaminators of so-called "innocent" populations (fetuses, children, and male sexual partners). Even now, almost two decades into the pandemic, it is rare for clinical trials and scholarly research to focus on women; when they do, the goals and methodologies of these putatively women-focused studies almost invariably reconstitute the traditional female subject who is worthy of attention only insofar as she represents a potential childbearer or a possible vector of disease. Moreover, our contributors share a commitment to making visible the populations and issues that have been marginalized despite their position at the epicenter of the pandemic and their centrality to women's lives. From their own key and disparate positions in the war on HIV/AIDS, they address the homeless, sex workers, youth, the elderly, injection drug users, transgendered people, lesbians, bisexuals, incarcerated women, and victims of sexual abuse and domestic violence.

In addressing a public health crisis that affects and is affected by the multiplicity of roles that women take on in culture, it seems important to us that professionals' understanding of both women and HIV be fluid, multidisciplinary, and as comprehensive as possible. Too often the various actors in HIV/AIDS discourse have been terribly isolated from one another. Listening to the different voices and language of clinicians, M.D.s, epidemiologists, psychologists, community-based organizers, AIDS activists, and people infected with or affected by HIV/AIDS, it sometimes seems as though they were sequestered on separate planets and spoke entirely different languages. With their separate conferences, journals, and foci, members of simultaneously disparate and overlapping fields have faced very real impediments to staying current with one another's findings and developments. But the cost of this kind of ideological, professional, and institutional segregation is very high: ultimately it makes a multifaceted and fully informed response to the pandemic virtually impossible.

Our hope for this volume is that it will make available more nuanced and truly useful information on topics related to women and HIV/AIDS and improve communication throughout different populations about these concerns. In our travels through an array of conferences, clinics, and meetings of activist organizations we have been fortunate to meet people whose work addresses underrepresented and misrepresented issues in a comprehensive, effective, and interdisciplinary manner. Our goal is to bring their work together in one place so it can be made available to the larger community of readers interested and involved with the issues they confront.

Part I of this volume, "Critiques of Biomedical Discourse," acquaints readers with the assumptions and methods that govern the biomedical community's examination of HIV/AIDS in women and of foregrounding problems endemic to this model.[26] Bill Rodriguez opens the section with "Biomedical Models of HIV and Women." His essay reviews the development of biomedical models of infectious diseases and sexually transmitted diseases, and proposes that the relative invisibility of women in epidemiologic and biomedical constructions of HIV derives directly from these historical models. In addition, the reductionist model of retrovirology has emerged as the most potent biomedical characterization of HIV, an approach that has perpetuated the absence of social, political, economic, and gender issues from the biomedical literature.

In "Barriers to the Inclusion of Women in Research and Clinical Trials," Theresa McGovern argues that while the federal government has responded to the requests of gay men living with HIV disease to assume greater risk in the drug development process in the hopes of obtaining effective therapies with the development of a New Drug Application (NDA) process, it has created a double standard when it comes to women: men with AIDS may assume greater risk in the hopes of obtaining effective treatment while women with AIDS continue to be excluded from trials.

Feminists have had an articulate voice in critiquing the method and application of scientific research for many years. Especially eloquent has been the description of the ways in which science has studied the female body, and the ideological results of that study. Michelle Murrain has two goals in "Caught in the Crossfire: Women and the Search for the Magic Bullet." The first is to describe the situation regarding women and AIDS, and to describe a case study of research done on women which is deeply problematic due to the ways in which a combination of social factors have come into play. The second is to use this example to encourage feminists, and other scholars who study science to broaden the perspectives of the ways in which bias—not only by gender, but also by race—and political economy, can influence and determine the path of scientific research.

Kate Barnhart's "Adolescent Underrepresentation in Clinical AIDS Research" explores the gaps in knowledge about adolescent HIV infection that have been created by years of neglect and a profound lack of resources for research in this area and details the implications of this deficit for clinical care of HIV-infected adolescents. Societal stereotypes about adolescents, such as the myth of adolescent noncompliance, and legal complexities around capacity to consent are used by researchers to justify excluding young people from clinical AIDS research. Barnhart addresses several issues that conspire against adolescent access to health care, including concerns about confidentiality, disclosure, and payment. Throughout the article, she offers recommendations for increasing adolescent participation in clinical AIDS research.

In "Lesbians and the Medical Profession: HIV/AIDS and the Pursuit of Visibility," Nancy Goldstein argues that the clean bill of health issued to lesbians (and women who have sex with women) regarding HIV has been issued in a research/statistical vacuum; this in turn has been created by faulty methodology and the misconceptions of the CDC and the larger biomedical community, both of whom have narrowed the lesbians and HIV/AIDS debate to the single issue of female-female transmission. Goldstein maintains that it is only by comprehending and addressing the multitude of ways in which sexual identity and behavior intersect in the lives of women who have sex with women—along with prejudice, poverty, compromised access to health care, isolation, sex work, alcoholism and drug abuse—that researchers and service providers can begin to address HIV issues pertaining to women who have sex with women.

Part 2, "Institutional(ized) Myopia," examines the ways in which a variety of cultural institutions create and sustain marginalized populations through a combination of stigmatization, neglect, and denial.

"As many scholars have noted, representations of AIDS serve to draw the boundaries of risk and construct identities for whom the epidemic is meaningful; however, the complexities of the representations of African-American women and AIDS have not been taken up by cultural studies scholars writing about AIDS." So begins Evelynn Hammonds in "Seeing AIDS: Race, Gender, and Representation," her examination of the ways in which race is depicted or elided in representations and narratives of women and AIDS such that African-American women are simultaneously rendered invisible and exposed. Whether fetishized as the only population at risk for HIV, barred from the category of "women (who count) with HIV/AIDS," or both, African-American women are faced with a crisis of representation in AIDS discourse.

Laura Ramos's " 'Sí tenemos sexo con mujeres, pero no somos marimachas.' (Sure, we have sex with women, but we're not lesbians.): Sexual Diversity in the Los Angeles *Latina* Community—Ethnographic Findings, 1987–95" highlights the advantages of using ethnographic methods in the investigation of sexual risk behaviors for women, particularly for Latina lesbian and bisexual women and Latinas who have sex with women (LSW). Having "met untold numbers of LSW in Los Angeles and elsewhere who are living with STDs/HIV and who are not well served by scientists, clinicians, and educators who refuse to acknowledge their existence," Ramos urges professionals to find ways to minister to the communities with whom they are working, rather than treating them as "subjects" from whom they can gather data if they hope to be effective.

Diane Siegal and Christie Burke inform readers that little attention has been paid to the impact of HIV/AIDS on midlife and older women. In their article entitled, "Midlife and Older Women and HIV/AIDS: "My (Grand)mother Wouldn't Do That," they illustrate how HIV/AIDS has affected an entire population in dire need of reassessing. AIDS has increased 17 percent among people 60 and older, and women over forty-five accounted for close to 9,000 of the cumulative total of AIDS cases reported to the CDC through December 1994.

"HIV and Asian and Pacific Islander Women" is taken from Willy Wilkinson's assessment of HIV prevention and direct services targeting Asian and Pacific Islander women in San Francisco. As the first API community health outreach worker (CHOW) in San Francisco, she conducted street-based AIDS education and ethnographic research in the Tenderloin, Chinatown, and South of Market neighborhoods. Pioneering an outreach model that she developed specifically for API communities, she accessed

API drug users and their sexual partners, API women working in massage parlors, and the general API community.

"Interpersonal Power and Women's HIV Risk" presents the findings of a study conducted for the Women's Health Research Project at the University of Rhode Island by Kathryn Quina, Lisa Harlow, Patricia Morokoff, and Susan Saxon. The authors note that while earlier studies on the negotiation of safer sex often focused on variables which presume personal control (e.g. health belief, self-efficacy) and group peer norms, such as those found in the gay community, applying the same methods and conclusions to heterosexual women fails to take into account social, cultural, and intrapersonal variables which affect their sexual and health-related behavior. By contrast, their feminist model deploys a new data collection and interpretation methodology that takes into account the various factors, both positive and negative, that affect women's ability to negotiate for safer sex in heterosexual situations.

In "Hitting Hard: HIV and Violence," Sally Zierler explores connections between physical and sexual violence by partners of women who are living with HIV infection. Although few empirical data exist to document this link, women with HIV may be at particular risk for partner violence because conditions of poverty, sexual-economic exchange, and drug use affect risk for violence as well as HIV infection. After reviewing related studies, the article concludes with recommendations for research and action to reduce the occurrence of violence in relationships by bridging personal violence that seems to accompany the public injustice of gender authority and social and economic control.

Debi Cuccinelli, a seropositive incarcerated woman, and Anne S. De Groot, her HIV physician, began to write "Put Her in a Cage: Childhood Sexual Abuse, Incarceration, and HIV Infection" after Anne asked—during her first appointment at the prison HIV clinic—if Debi had been forced to have sex against her will when she was still a child. Debi had never been asked that question by a doctor before. This chapter tells Debi's story. Both Anne and Debi believe that there is a link between Debi's HIV infection and her sexual abuse, beginning at age six, by her brother. Debi says that telling this story made her a free woman even though she remains behind bars. This story is also about the special vulnerability of women to HIV infection: "We have written this chapter to speak out about sexual abuse and to give a name to this aspect of women's vulnerability to HIV infection so that we may reduce HIV's impact on women before it is too late."

In "Around Women, Violence, and HIV/AIDS," Diane Monti-Catania explores the interrelated issues of HIV/AIDS, poverty, addiction, women's health, and violence against women and discusses the gender bias inherent in the HIV prevention strategies that have been developed to date. Her article addresses the challenges facing both the advocate community and institutional social service and health organizations to develop services that acknowledge and meet the complex needs of women who have HIV/AIDS and are victims of violence. It calls for an organized and integrated community and institutional response to women that includes universal access to care, recognition of women's commitment to their children, and long-term supportive programming.

In "Social Context and AIDS/HIV: Testing and Treatment Issues among Commercial Street Sex Workers," Kim Blankenship discusses qualitative research (field work, focus groups) with commercial street sex workers that demonstrates some of the social contextual factors that shape the testing behaviors of women at risk for HIV and influence the types of treatment, if any, they receive. She focuses in particular on three aspects of the social context, namely the institutions of HIV-related research, women's economic vulnerability, and their social isolation. Women on the street are well aware of the advantages of early treatment, but struggle against these contextual constraints to take care of themselves. The policy implications of these findings are clear: to take care of themselves, women must have access to resources and power.

Part 3, "Working (through) Solutions," recounts some of the strategies that have been developed for analyzing, addressing, and sometimes stemming the effect of HIV on women's lives. In "Healing from Within: Women, HIV/AIDS, and the African-American Church," Reverend Carol Johnson asserts that while "churches and other religious institutions intending to develop AIDS ministries for African-American women infected/affected by HIV/AIDS need to sensitize themselves to issues around gender, power, and sexuality, . . . ministries are faced with a real dearth of theological reflection on the moral, ethical, and social justice issues which attend to African-American women and HIV/AIDS." Her intention in writing this article "is not only to alert readers to some of these specific issues, but to point out how an AIDS ministry can be developed which takes into account the continuum of experiences and needs of people infected and affected by HIV/AIDS."

In "The Bond Is Called Blackness: Black Women and AIDS" Sheila Battle presents her personal experiences working with a program specifically designed for HIV + African-American pregnant women. This article examines lifestyles, institutionalized racism, discrimination, poverty, political issues, and the attitudes of medical staff and the African-American community towards one another. Finally, it presents her vision of a successful HIV program in the African-American community. She hopes that the experiences and insights she presents will open the eyes of her readers to a growing problem of social, racial, and gender bias.

Nina Brand, the author of "Coming to Their Own Rescue: Teens Teach Teens about HIV," maintains that peer education programs have developed out of a notion that one way in which we learn best is from "our own kind." Age is one of many factors that help us define our peers, and for teens it seems crucial to the process of believing that they can be understood, be respected, and teach others. Teen HIV/AIDS peer education programs offer a sense of control to a group of people who are systemically denied rights and have been, until recently, overlooked throughout the HIV/AIDS pandemic, resulting in a growing number of teens infected with HIV. By looking at the numerous ways in which teen peer education benefits the adolescents of a community and through an informal look at two particular teen peer HIV/AIDS education programs, we can begin to understand the magnitude of opportunity such programs create for all who are working to alleviate the oppression associated with access to HIV/AIDS-related resources.

In "Haitian Teens Confront AIDS: A Partners in Health Program on Social Justice and HIV/AIDS Prevention," Loune Viaud, Paul Farmer, and Guitèle Nicoleau describe Haitian Teens Confront AIDS (HTCA), a peer leadership program for Haitian adolescents sponsored by Partners In Health (PIH), now in its sixth year. PIH established HTCA to create a comfortable environment for adolescents to share feelings and perspectives on appropriate HIV/AIDS prevention, to raise awareness about Haitian culture, and to break down stereotypes. The proliferation of scientific accounts blaming Haitians for the origin and spread of the virus throughout the 1980s resulted in deep mistrust of public health professionals by many in the Haitian-American community. As a result, Haitians in the United States were placed in a defensive posture by these accusations and began to deny the reality of a serious deadly virus. This situation made prevention efforts extremely difficult. In this paper, the authors explain the importance of integrating issues related to discrimination and racism in AIDS education by describing aspects of the HTCA program, specifically why and how it developed into one of the few AIDS-prevention programs explicitly based on a social justice model.

In "HIV Does Not Erase Desire: Addressing the Sexual and Reproductive Concerns of Women with HIV/AIDS," Risa Denenberg describes a paradox that society imposes on those living with HIV/AIDS. People with AIDS are told that they can learn to "live with HIV," and at the same time there is an overt message to abstain from life's normal activities of sex and procreation. Successful adaptation to living with HIV infection requires early diagnosis, concrete support systems, excellent medical care, and self-empowerment. Lamentably, gender bias has rendered a significant information gap that has blinded women at risk, the public at large, and the medical and scientific community to early recognition of HIV infection in women. Late recognition, late diagnosis, and late entry to care all contribute to premature death in women with HIV infection. Thus for women, more so than for men, the diagnosis of AIDS is associated only with illness and death. Denenberg asserts that it is the responsibility of providers to support women and their families to enact their personal hopes and dreams as they concomitantly learn to accept and live with HIV infection. This transition in attitude is required to affect women's survival, and the survival of their communities.

"Native Women Living beyond HIV/AIDS Infection," cowritten by Linda Burhansstipanov, Carole laFavor, Shirley Hoskins, Gloria Bellymule, and Ron Rowell offers a brief overview of the effects of HIV and AIDS on Native American women, their families, and their communities. The data and descriptions included within this chapter are based on ongoing service projects being implemented nationwide through Health Resources and Services Administration (HRSA) Special Initiatives Project of the National Native American AIDS Prevention Center (NNAAPC). The chapter provides a brief overview of the NNAAPC initiatives, a synopsis of how western medicine (e.g., medical doctors) compares with traditional Indian medicine, a brief summary of needs which were identified by Native women infected with HIV or who have AIDS, case management issues, provider issues, Ryan White limitations, and a case study.

In "Can Needle Exchange Better Serve Women?" Kaveh Khoshnood

and P. Clay Stephens recount the origination and operations of the successful New Haven, Connecticut, needle exchange program (NEP). Such
programs warrant particular concern in the late nineties when a growing
proportion of AIDS cases in the United States is made up of injecting drug
users, a group whose primary etiologic cause of HIV transmission is the
sharing of contaminated drug paraphernalia, particularly syringes. Among
women, over 50 percent of AIDS cases can be attributed to intravenous
drug injection either by the woman herself or indirectly through sexual
exposure to an injection drug user.

"Leather, Lace, and Latex: Safer Sex for Women," by Denise Ribble, is
derived from ten years of her experience presenting safer-sex workshops
for women. It is presented in a mixed format to allow her reader to learn
and apply what she has garnered over the past decade.

A key ethical question had been nagging Jennifer Manlowe ever since
she lectured on Ethics and AIDS to international health practitioners from
Indonesia and the Philippines: In an epidemic, are health safety and sexual
freedom mutually exclusive, interdependent, or one and the same if you
come from a country that values collective rights over individual rights?
Because Manlowe was only going to be visiting Cuba for eleven days in
January of 1996, she knew that she would only get a surface impression of
people's feelings about Cuban policies on HIV but, nevertheless, she
thought such an impression was worth acquiring, especially since the U.S.
has much to learn in terms of the value of making operational universal
health care and Cuba's model has managed to keep the virus contained
better than any "Third World" country. The people she was able to
interview for her essay, "Gender, Sexuality, and Safety: Does the U.S. Have
Anything to Learn from Cuban AIDS Policy?" include six men and two
women living with HIV/AIDS at the AIDS sanitorium in Santiago de Las
Vegas on the outskirts of Havana, Cuba.

In Part 4, "Women with AIDS Speak Out," a number of HIV-infected
and affected women share their life stories, describe their current engagement with HIV activism, and discuss strategies for the betterment of HIV
health information and care. We believe that the voices of women infected
with or affected by HIV should get a wider hearing in precisely this kind
of context rather than being relegated to a separate sphere. They are also
experts on HIV, and their stories reflect key issues raised in the formal
articles: The intersection of domestic violence/sexual abuse and HIV, the
failure of health providers to recognize those who fall outside of the

identified "high risk" categories as being at risk, the intersection of poverty, prejudice, and IDU/sex work. We do not, however, intend for this group of contributors or this section to represent the experiences of women with HIV/AIDS in any kind of definitive or totalizing fashion. Part of the work of this anthology is to broaden and complicate definitions of who is at risk, not reinforce traditional stereotypes or create new ones.

Our hope for this collection of essays (some of which are under pseud-onyms at the authors' request) is that it will provide a forum where health service providers and researchers, social workers, community-based organizers, psychologists, HIV-infected people, cultural critics, and public policy makers can be exposed to each other's works and perspectives. We are both honored and pleased to present our contributors' work to you as they begin to bridge practical and theoretical insights for themselves, their coworkers, their students, and the HIV-infected and affected women in their lives. This volume is dedicated to them all.

Nancy Goldstein
Cambridge, MA

NOTES

A title like *The **Gender** Politics of HIV/AIDS* calls for some explanation given that economic status and race play fundamental roles in putting people at risk, and that sexuality, not gender, has defined the paradigm for the population hardest hit by HIV/AIDS in the United States. From the first time that HIV entered public discourse to the present day, HIV and AIDS have routinely, and often homophobically, been identified with gay men and their "immoral" and/or "promiscuous" sexual practices. Conse-quently, predictions like "by the year 2000, more women than men will be infected with HIV," whose primary intent is to raise consciousness about HIV/AIDS among women, have, as an unfortunate side effect, the potential for inciting yet more homo-phobia against gay men by suggesting that they have for too long "enjoyed" some kind of spotlight or received some kind of magnanimous treatment at the hand of the U.S. government and its agencies that they should now be forced to relinquish to genuinely needy women. The risk of calling attention to gender as a defining category is that it will recreate a similarly false, and homophobic, symmetry. That is not our intention here. It should be possible to bring attention to bear on the ways in which aspects of gender, specifically as they affect women in this country, put them at risk for HIV, without doing so at the expense of gay men.

1. Foucault had as his target what D. A. Miller has called, memorably, "various technologies of the self and its sexuality, which administer the subject's own contribu-

tion to the intensive and continuous 'pastoral care' that liberal society proposes to take of each and every one of its charges" (D. A. Miller, *The Novel and the Police* [Berkeley and Los Angeles: University of California Press, 1988], vii). Specifically, Foucault proposed that science and medicine—with their will to power naturalized as forms of knowledge rooted in the human body itself, and with their endless categorizations and classifications of its symptoms, desires, diseases, and ailments—had come to serve as the primary forms of discipline and surveillance in modernity, replacing the machinations of monarchy and overt corporal punishment.

2. Charles E. Rosenberg, "Disease and Social Order in America: Perceptions and Expectations," in *AIDS: The Burdens of History,* ed Elizabeth Fee and Daniel Fox (Berkeley and Los Angeles: University of California Press, 1988), 12–32; 12–13.

3. Rosenberg, 13.

4. This entire paragraph owes a debt to Charles E. Rosenberg and Cindy Patton, the two scholars whose commentary on immunology and virology has most influenced my own thinking. As early as 1988 Rosenberg wrote that AIDS

> reminds us of the way society has always framed illness, finding reasons to exempt and reassure in its agreed-upon etiologies. But it also reminds us that biological mechanisms define and constrain social response. Ironically, this new disease [*sic*] reflects both elements—the biological and cultural—in particularly stark form. Only the sophisticated tools of modern virology and immunology have allowed it to be defined as a clinical entity; yet its presumed mode of transmission and extraordinary fatality levels have mobilized deeply felt social attitudes that relate only tangentially to the virologist's understanding of the syndrome. If diseases [*sic*] can be seen as occupying points along a spectrum, ranging from those most firmly based in a verifiable pathological mechanism, to those, like hysteria or alcoholism, with no well-understood mechanism but with a highly charged social profile— then AIDS occupies a place at both ends of the spectrum. (Rosenberg, 28)

Also see Cindy Patton's section on "Virology and Immunology: Cultural Tropes/ Scientific Pursuits," in *Inventing AIDS* (New York and London: Routledge, 1990), 58– 61.

5. According to Patton,

> AIDS refers to effects observed as dysfunctions of the immune system and evaluates "health" and "disease" in relation to an established norm of immune function. "AIDS" tends to construct diagnosis around symptoms suggestive of serious immune system failure, hence the use of PCP, Kaposi's sarcoma, and other opportunistic infections as the diagnostic markers of AIDS, to be confirmed by HIV testing. HIV disease refers to a causative virus and its sequential effects, regardless of whether these are experienced as harmful or uncomfortable to the individual. Here, presence of the virus is itself diagnostic of "disease," which is defined as the presence of a potentially harmful external agent. "Health" is considered a subjective stage which does not correlate well with the progress of the virus, except in late stages—that is, except in "AIDS." (Patton, 150 n. 20)

6. Jargon for injection equipment.

7. Studies have reported that HIV-infected women already in the medical system received fewer services than men (F. J. Hellinger, "The Use of Health Services by Women with HIV Infection," *Health Services Research* 28 [1993]: 543–61), were less likely to have a primary provider of care (J. Mauskopf, B. Turner, L. E. Markson, R. L. Houchens, and T. R. Fanning, "Patterns of Ambulatory Care for AIDS Patients, and Association with Emergency Room Use," *Health Services Research* 29 [1994]: 489–510), and were more likely to make emergency room visits (V. Mor, J. A. Fleishman, M. Dresser, and J. Piette, "Variation in Health Service Use among HIV-Infected Patients," *Medical Care* 30 [1992]: 17–29).

8. Sally Zierler writes:

It is understandable that women would be more at risk during heterosexual sex. HIV is highly concentrated in seminal fluid, which is packed with lymphocytes and therefore capable of concentrating the virus. Once ejaculated into the vagina, (or, less typically, the rectum), seminal fluid is absorbed through a large mucosal surface and into blood vessels. This route may be one of the ways that intracellular as well as free virus gains access to host cells in women's bodies; or it may be that women's vaginal mucosa or cervix is already hosting inflammatory cells because of local infection or abrasions due to sexual penetration, birth control devices, herbal drying preparations, or tampons. ("Women, Sex and HIV," *Epidemiology* 5 [1994]: 565–67)

9. Elizabeth Fee and Daniel Fox write: "Social constructionists, to oversimplify, hold that historical reality is created by people; that is, it does not exist as a truth waiting to be discovered. Some social constructionists include the data of biological and physical sciences in their analysis, arguing that the institutions and procedures of these disciplines are the result of complex social interactions. The human body, they argue, has no historical existence except in primary sources about how it has been perceived and described by members of different societies at different times" (Elizabeth Fee and Daniel Fox, eds., *AIDS: The Burdens of History* [Berkeley and Los Angeles: University of California Press, 1988], 4).

10. Thomas Laqueur, "Orgasm, Generation, and the Politics of Reproductive Biology," in *The Making of the Modern Body: Sexuality and Society in the Nineteenth Century,* ed. Catherine Gallagher and Thomas Laqueur (Berkeley and Los Angeles: University of California Press, 1987), 1–41.

11. Laqueur, 18.

12. Laqueur, 24.

13. Evelynn Hammonds, "Race, Sex, AIDS: The Construction of 'Other,' " *Radical America* 20, no. 6 (1987): 28–36.

14. James H. Jones, *Bad Blood: The Tuskegee Syphilis Experiment* (New York: Free Press, 1981), 21.

15. This most recent expansion includes all HIV-infected persons with CD4 counts under 200 cells. Three additional clinical conditions associated with HIV were also added: pulmonary tuberculosis (TB), recurrent pneumonia, and cervical cancer. Centers

for Disease Control and Prevention, "1993 Revised Classification System for HIV Infection and Expanded Surveillance Case Definition for AIDS among Adolescents and Adults," *Morbidity and Mortality Weekly Report* 41, RR-17 (1992): 1–19.

16. Centers for Disease Control, *Demographic Summary of ACTG Study Entries from Beginning to 2/23/96.*

17. Centers for Disease Control and Prevention, *HIV/AIDS Surveillance Report* 7, no. 2 (1995): 1–39: 6–7.

18. 22.6 percent were White, 0.3 percent American Indian/Alaska Native, 0.5 percent Asian/Pacific Islander. Centers for Disease Control and Prevention, *HIV/AIDS Surveillance Report* 7, no. 2 (1995): 1–39.

19. Centers for Disease Control and Prevention, "Update: Mortality Attributable to HIV Infection among Persons Aged 25–44 Years—United States, 1994," *Morbidity and Mortality Weekly Report* 45, no. 6 (1996): 121–25.

20. Ibid.

21. Centers for Disease Control and Prevention, *HIV/AIDS Surveillance Report* 7, no. 2 (1995): 1–39. See also M. A. Males, "Adult Involvement in Teenage Childbearing and STD," *Lancet* 340 (1995): 64–65; Alan Guttmacher Institute, *Sex and America's Teenagers* (New York: Alan Guttmacher Institute, 1994); National Center for Health Statistics, *Births to Teen Moms by Age of Mother, by Age of Father and Race of Mother, U.S., 1992* (Washington, D.C.: U.S. Department of Health and Human Services, 1994).

22. *Rape in America: A Report to the Nation,* prepared by the National Victim Center and Crime Victims Research and Treatment Center, 1992.

23. Mary Koss, Christine A. Gidycz, and Nadine Wisniewski, "The Scope of Rape: Incidence and Prevalence of Sexual Aggression and Victimization in a National Sample of Higher Education Students," *Journal of Consulting and Clinical Psychology* 55 (1987): 162–70, cited in *Fraternity Gang Rape: Sex, Brotherhood, and Privilege on Campus,* by Peggy Reeves Sanday (New York: New York University Press, 1990), 26.

24. In 1995, 37 percent of heterosexually acquired AIDS cases were attributed to heterosexual contact with an injection drug user. The remainder of heterosexually acquired AIDS cases were attributed to sex with a partner with HIV infection or AIDS whose risk was unreported or unknown (54 percent), sex with a bisexual man (7 percent), sex with a transfusion recipient (1 percent), and sex with a person with hemophilia (1 percent). The majority of HIV transmission among women remains related to injection drug use either directly, or as a result of sexual transmission from an injection drug-using partner. Centers for Disease Control and Prevention. *HIV/AIDS Surveillance Report* 7, no. 2 (1995): 1–39.

25. Zierler, 565.

26. The following abstracts have been provided by the contributors.

Part I

Critiques of Biomedical Discourse

1

Biomedical Models of HIV and Women

Bill Rodriguez

Bill Rodriguez is a resident in internal medicine at the Brigham and Women's Hospital in Boston, and the former associate director of the Institute for Health and Social Justice.

> We have learned very little that is new about the disease, but much that is old about ourselves.
>
> Frederick C. Tilney, M.D., on the 1916 polio epidemic

Nearly fifteen years into its global pandemic, HIV infection continues to spread rapidly. More than one million cases of AIDS have been reported to the World Health Organization; 14 million people are estimated to be infected with HIV worldwide, including one million in the United States.[1] Women now represent the fastest-growing "risk group" for acquiring HIV infection.[2] Already, more than 50,000 cases of AIDS have been reported in women in the United States.[3] In 1994, more than 14,000 new AIDS cases were diagnosed in women, representing 18 percent of all new cases and a dramatic increase in incidence from the 534 cases and 8 percent of total cases reported nine years earlier.[4] The grim situation in this country shines compared to the devastation HIV has caused among already impoverished, abused, and marginalized women worldwide.

The regular updates on the unfathomable numbers of infected and affected women have become numbing, though after years of neglect the impact of the HIV epidemic among women has finally begun to gain some attention. Nonetheless, research on HIV among women remains underfunded; inclusion of women in clinical trials remains disproportionately low; and women continue to be studied and characterized primarily as prostitutes, or as vectors of HIV infection to their innocent babies and male partners.[5] Moreover, though an understanding of the global pandemic among women requires anthropologic, epidemiologic, political, and feminist as well as biomedical inquiry, the social, economic, gender inequality, and structural issues that have placed women at an ever-growing risk of acquiring HIV garner little attention among Western clinicians and researchers.

Biomedical Models of Infectious Disease

It is useful to underscore the role of the biomedical construction of HIV in the general failure to address the HIV epidemic among women. To do this, we must examine how biomedicine has incorporated HIV into its framework of disease, and then examine how this construction has contributed to the growing burden of HIV among women. First, we must take a distant gaze into the history of human intersection with transmissible diseases.

Historians of science have written eloquently about the impact of infectious diseases on civilizations both before and after the transition to sedentary life.[6] Prehistoric patterns of infectious disease appeared quite different than those that are familiar today. The "zoonotic" infections—those that infect humans only secondarily, such as tularemia, trichinosis, anthrax, gangrene and tetanus—likely had a larger impact on nomadic societies of antiquity than they do today. Although these illnesses were rapidly fatal in the preantibiotic era, their virulence made them ill-suited to cause *epidemics* among human populations; in addition, the low density of early migratory societies was ill-suited to the spread of epidemics.

In the historical era of civilization, much has changed. Several factors independent of the virulence and nature of the infectious organism have become of paramount importance in the spread of infectious disease. On the protective side, access to a stable and adequate food supply and improved nutrition have led to improved resistance to and recovery from illness; herd immunity and adaptation to local organisms have led to fewer sporadic and more endemic infections; and improved cooking and sterilization of foods has decreased the spread of zoonotic illnesses.[7]

On the down side, however, the advances of civilization accompanied human social patterns and collective and individual behaviors that have increased the spread and propagation of infectious epidemics. Migration, urbanization, trade and commerce, and interactions between societies have led to more exchange of organisms; political and economic organization have led to increased gender, class, and racial inequities within societies, and with them unequal protection from and treatment for infections; close contact and crowding have led to increased rates of propagation of infections within communities; and inadequate processing of human wastes has led to local proliferation of disease vectors such as mosquitoes, fleas, rats, and lice, all important hosts for human infectious agents.

Historical perspective tells us that large-scale social, political, and economic forces have had a significant impact on the spread of infectious epidemics prior to HIV, ranging from the "Black Death" bubonic plague in Europe and Asia in the fourteenth and seventeenth centuries, to recurrent epidemics of cholera worldwide, to the appearance of influenza and tuberculosis as major epidemic pathogens today.[8] While the spread of each of these agents has been described retrospectively in terms of the social context in which they arose, contemporaneous views tended to reflect prevailing attitudes on disease causation: bubonic plague was blamed at times on bathing, as well as on Satan, impiety, heresy, and Jews. Cholera was felt to be a vengeance wreaked on the immoral members of society. Tuberculosis was until this century felt to be inherited and the curse of several families. As a general rule, the "otherness" and ostracization of those with infections was emphasized.

These interwoven social and political threads of disease causation are familiar to the medical anthropologist and social scientist. In all likelihood, future historians with a distant lens focused on our century will view the spread of HIV primarily in terms of social, political and economic events, rather than in terms of the emergence of a clever and debilitating virus. And yet, such discussions and the implications for prevention and treatment are largely absent from the prevailing biomedical discourse. How do these concepts remain relevant to HIV infection in the 1990s? Given the explosion of information about this virus, what can we learn from the historical analysis of human interaction with infectious organisms? How has the biomedical discourse about infectious diseases incorporated the human immunodeficiency virus? And in particular, as the disease continues to spread in epidemic proportions along a gradient of inequity that includes women, minorities, homosexuals, and citizens of Third World countries—the marginalized and disenfranchised groups of the world—what has fifteen years of the effort to understand this organism in biomedical terms told us about the disease, and about ourselves?

HIV: An Infectious Disease?

In large part, the failure of biomedicine to broaden its analysis of the HIV epidemic follows directly from the relentless progression of the "infectious disease" model in medicine. As scientific and biomedical knowledge has accumulated, a *macroscopic* view of the nature of infectious diseases has eroded, and given way to a *microscopic* world of viruses, bacteria, T cells and B cells. Disease has become a mechanical process whereby "germs" are "transmitted" between "vectors" and "hosts"; eliminating disease—maintaining public health—has developed into an equally mechanical intervention in this process.

To what do we owe this dissociation? The seeds of the current infectious disease model were sown at the end of the eighteenth century, a full hundred years before the germ theory of disease was widely accepted. As political revolutions took hold in Europe and the United States—with long-term consequences for both the global political economy *and* the spread of infections—the *concept* of disease and its political utility changed. Disease came to be seen as a deviation from normal health, rather than an innate reflection of fixed social or political class. Concurrently, buoyed along the first wave of the scientific revolution, Edward Jenner developed a vaccine for smallpox, ushering in a new understanding of the biology of infection. Within one hundred years, the simultaneous rise of individualism and scientific reductionism in the context of a century remarkable for complicated social transformations, the institutionalization of the industrial economy, and rapid advancements in the technology of science brought to prominence a germ theory of disease.

For a time, the nascent field of epidemiology maintained a broader perspective on disease causality. John Snow's intervention at the Broad Street Pump in London to halt the spread of cholera recognized implicitly what we might now call the political economy of infectious disease. Nonetheless, our own century has seen the progressive development of an increasingly *reductionist* biomedical model of disease causality, prevention, and treatment. Concepts of trade, migration patterns, human waste processing, and political economy have given way to microbes, cell walls, and antibiotics, and ultimately to molecular biology, virology, host defense factors, vaccines, lymphokines, cytokines, and antiretrovirals. A large share of the credit for the significant decline of infectious diseases in developed countries is placed in the hands of biomedicine, antibiotics, and hospital care, and serves to perpetuate the reductionist approach. Nonetheless, despite the obvious accomplishments of scientific inquiry, the now well-worn consensus is that the dramatic decline in death and disease from infections correlates directly with water purification, efficient sewage systems, milk sterilization, and improved nutrition, and not with the advent of antibiotics.[9]

Retrovirology

Before turning to examine how the infectious disease model has been applied to HIV among women, it is important to note how, over the past decade, the focus of biomedical inquiry into infectious disease has reduced even further, from the microscopic to the ultrascopic. The subdiscipline of retrovirology represents perhaps the final evolution of the reductionist approach to infectious diseases. Although first discovered in birds in 1911,[10] retroviruses—viruses that flaunt the "central dogma" of modern molecular biology through the relatively simple process of retroforming DNA from RNA—remained relatively obscure in the biomedical literature for sixty years, and were studied only in the margins of cancer medicine. At the time of the initial reports of *Pneumocystis* pneumonia in homosexual men in June, 1981, the study of retroviruses remained confined primarily to birds, cats and mice. Only a handful of retroviruses had been found in non-human primates, and definitive identification of the first human retrovirus, HTLV-1, occurred almost simultaneously with the initial CDC reports of a new immunodeficiency disease in gay men.[11]

Thus, although retroviruses had been in the biomedical discourse for more than sixty years, the advent of powerful reductionist molecular techniques and the discovery of human retroviruses coincided with the onset of the HIV epidemic. Within a decade, the field of retrovirology exploded, and became definitively established as an academically supported, clinically relevant and economically powerful branch of the biomedical enterprise. For most HIV biologists, clinicians, and researchers trained in the era of molecular biology, retrovirology represents the standard model for understanding the transmission, pathogenesis and treatment of HIV and AIDS. It has its own language—the language of reverse transcriptase, *tat, env, pol,* CD4 cells, gp120, proteases, polymerases, receptors, and PCR; it has an extensive communication network and dozens of regular journals and programs; [12] and it has an extensive economic and social structure, in the form of an academic and pharmaceutical research complex with literally billions of dollars at stake in the development of vaccines, antibiotics, and antiviral agents. [13]

The reductionist approach has also been extended to epidemiologic construction of HIV disease. Several epidemiologic studies focus on the "molecular epidemiology" of HIV, examining genetic variation of individual HIV strains, mutation rates in HIV regulatory proteins, or geographic variation of HIV envelope proteins. [14] While such an approach promises important insights into the pathogenesis of HIV infection, it is important to note how far removed it is from classic epidemiology. Molecular epidemiology is about the virus, but not about human society.

HIV: A Sexually Transmitted Disease?

Although the current biomedical understanding of HIV derives more directly from this infectious disease model, the development of a sexually transmitted disease model in this country—which differs in meaningful ways from the infectious disease model—also has important implications for the way HIV has been perceived among women. The most useful analogies for HIV among the history of sexually transmitted diseases can be seen in the historical constructions of syphilis and gonorrhea.

As Allan Brandt has described in *No Magic Bullet,* [15] the discourse on the major sexually transmitted diseases of the early twentieth century was intimately connected with the political and social milieu of the day, rather than with the emerging germ theory. While germ theorists strove to characterize the infectious nature of the venereal diseases, biomedical construction of syphilis and gonorrhea fell under the rubric of "social hygiene." In the early years of this century, the biomedical profession was largely allied with the leading social reformers of the day. Control of sexually-transmitted diseases was thus inseparable from issues of women's rights, sexual education, antiprostitution efforts, and Prohibition, as well as America's military strength and global geopolitical stance.

Not surprisingly, the reductionist model of infectious diseases was rapidly applied to non—sexually acquired infections such as polio, tuberculosis and influenza, but was less quickly adopted in the control of venereal diseases. Polio and diphtheria could be unapologetically eradicated through vaccination and antibiotic therapy, but the use of antibiotics for the treatment of sexually transmitted diseases carried the promise—and fear—of a previously unknown sexual freedom. In the logic of early twentieth century American society, this equated with a breakdown of moral fabric.

Rather than rely on antibiotic therapy for STDs, public health officials and the U.S. military pursued a vigorous campaign against prostitution and prostitutes. As late as World War II, leading public health authorities would write that

> routine dissemination of prophylactic advice and material [antibiotics] carries with it an inherent contradiction, in that it automatically suggests and sanctions promiscuity. . . . The horns of this dilemma cannot be evaded: venereal disease control must be planned as behavior control.[16]

As Brandt notes, despite an aggressive militaristic campaign aimed at behavior control—a campaign which stigmatized and forcibly detained women and portrayed them generically as prostitutes, while equating all men with the patriotic virtues of the male soldier—behavior control was an utter failure. Reluctantly, public health officials turned to antibiotics and venereal disease clinics to stop the epidemic of sexually transmitted diseases. As Elizabeth Fee has noted in the case of syphilis, with the advent of penicillin therapy in 1943, sexually transmitted diseases slowly became incorporated into the infectious disease model.[17]

Despite the sublimation of the sexually transmitted disease model in biomedicine, strains of the early biomedical characterization of STDs persist today, particularly in the stigmatization of women. For instance, when funding for research and treatment of STDs was scaled back dramatically, the venereal diseases reemerged as significant pathogens in the 1970s. Women again became the target of blame, this time under the guise of "promiscuity" and "Pill-use" rather than prostitution. Promiscuity and "natural immoral proclivities" were also used to explain the high rates of syphilis in Africa, despite the obvious impact of socioeconomic factors such as colonization, overcrowding, poverty, and poor sanitation.[18]

In Brandt's summary, three recurrent themes in the biomedical conception of venereal disease emerge: first, that STDs are diseases of individual behaviors, and therefore a punishment for those who "take risks"; second, that potential spread of venereal disease is often made the explicit basis for legislating behaviors and restricting sexuality; and third, as Prince Morrow noted eighty years ago,[19] that venereal diseases are construed as symptoms of larger problems in society that fall to rest on the backs of women.

The parallels between the biomedical construction of the venereal diseases in the early twentieth century and of HIV in its first decade are, perhaps, obvious. Once HIV transmission was linked to sexual practices among homosexual men, the stigmata of venereal diseases were applied to them, and to sexual freedom in general. As the disease spread to women, they were invariably characterized in both popular and medical literature as prostitutes, hookers, and whores.[20] Promiscuity became the focal point of both epidemiologic construction and health policy interventions to control the disease, and behavior control once again appeared as the dominant public health initiative. As with syphilis and gonorrhea sixty years earlier, the impact of HIV *on* women was largely ignored.

Historical Snapshots of HIV and Women

> Everyone knows that pestilences have a way of recurring in the world; yet somehow we find it hard to believe in ones that crash down on our heads from a blue sky.   Albert Camus, *The Plague*, 1948

To understand the impact of the biomedical construction of HIV among women, it will be useful to apply this historical lens to a few selected time points in the HIV epidemic. Predictably, we will see how women were ignored in the earliest months of the epidemic as scientists (and the general public) cast a wide net of blame on marginalized groups and behaviors. When the sexually transmissible nature of the disease became evident, traditional stereotypes were applied to both gay men and women, along familiar lines of the sexually transmitted disease model outlined by Brandt. As the reductionist scope of retrovirology emerged, large-scale political and social forces disappeared even further from the biomedical gaze, replaced by viral proteins, T cell receptors, and antiretrovirals.

June 5, 1981: Entering the Discourse

On June 5, 1981, HIV entered the biomedical discourse when the CDC's *Morbidity and Mortality Weekly Report* published a report of five homosexual men from Los Angeles, all of whom had developed unexplained *Pneumocystis carinii* pneumonia and evidence for severe immune deficiency.[21] The CDC, in fact, acted relatively quickly in tracking this emerging syndrome, and within a month published a second report linking

Pneumocystis, the unusual cancer Kaposi's sarcoma, and immune suppression in twenty-six young, gay men in New York and California.[22] By the end of the year, the constellation of findings had been diagnosed in more than two hundred Americans and a similar number of Europeans and Africans, most of whom were gay men. Additional cases were described in heterosexuals within the first year of the recognized epidemic. The first case at Mt. Sinai Hospital in New York was a Dominican housewife with a single lifetime sexual partner; five of the first thirty-seven cases reported from New York City were heterosexual injection drug-users; and by the end of the year, several Haitian citizens living in Miami had been diagnosed with the syndrome.[23]

Here then was Camus' pestilence, fallen from the blue sky. Resonance with past plagues in initial analyses of HIV in both the popular imagination and the biomedical literature were quite loud.[24] The earliest biomedical constructions on causality sound eerily familiar to the epidemiologic construction of early twentieth-century sexually transmitted disease. The leading theory linked the syndrome to a modern conception of immorality, the homosexual lifestyle: the use of amyl nitrite "poppers," a sexual stimulant; weakened defenses due to "promiscuity"; and unusual "immoral proclivities" such as fisting. All were felt to be likely explanations for the disease, despite the fact that within a year of the initial CDC report, the syndrome had been clearly identified in several groups of people who fell well outside this construction. When nonhomosexuals were acknowledged, it was often to cast aspersions and perpetuate gross asymptotes. One 1983 editorial in a leading medical journal speculated that AIDS in Haitian Americans was due to "use of drugs; malnutrition; promiscuity; homosexuality; and, perhaps, voodoo."[25]

The general perception both within and outside the biomedical community, however, was of a gay male scourge. Popular descriptions referred to the "gay plague," with little protest, and even some support, from the biomedical community. As Gerald Oppenheimer notes in his review of the epidemiologic construction of AIDS, the CDC itself doggedly focused on the "immoral" behaviors of homosexual men, echoing its counterparts of seventy years earlier, and was "unwilling to dismiss the life-style hypothesis and commit itself completely to a microbe theory."[26]

Alongside this initial epidemiologic construction, many biomedical researchers began pursuing an infectious etiology. One prominent early theory proposed cytomegalovirus as a candidate culprit—though in the context of "unprecedented promiscuity arising in the late 1960's," presumably among gay men.[27] Thus, even in a reductionist construction, the "promiscuous" gay man became a paradigm for understanding the disease.

Where did women begin to fit in the initial biomedical model? The authors cited above went on to conclude that "[w]e cannot, at this time, explain why AIDS is *thought to be occurring* in Haitians, hemophiliacs, and *others*" (italics added). It was a widely held perspective: even researchers who pursued a viral etiology refused to recognize the spread of the disease to women, or its implications. Thus, from the time of the initial case reports, women as victims of this disease were largely ignored in the biomedical and epidemiologic constructions, entering the discourse characterized facelessly as "others."

March 4, 1983: No Room for Women in the 4–H Club

In 1983, HIV was isolated and characterized as a human retrovirus. HIV infection was spreading rapidly in the United States to several groups outside the male homosexual community; in Africa, AIDS had been identified at epidemic levels in equal proportions among men and women. Two complementary models of HIV began to solidify: the epidemiologic model of a sexually transmitted infection, and the new biomedical model of retrovirology. While both provided important insights into HIV transmission and pathogenesis, both held an equal disregard for larger social and political forces that were contributing to the emerging pandemic. The focus instead was on epidemiologic "risk groups," which largely stereotyped and misrepresented women at risk, and a reductionist analysis of the novel retrovirus, which largely ignored them.

Two years into the epidemic, women gained official recognition, albeit along predictable lines. On March 4, 1983, the CDC published a review of the epidemiologic pathways along which HIV was spreading, identifying specifically homosexual men, hemophiliacs, Haitians, and intravenous drug users as the groups at risk for contracting HIV.[28] The CDC also included "female sexual partners of bisexual or intravenous drug-using men, and their children" in their listing of at-risk groups; nonetheless, this description became known and written about in the popular scientific literature as the "4–H club": homosexuals, heroin users, hemophiliacs, and Haitians.

Women remained relatively invisible, although they were beginning to enter the discourse as potential "vectors" and "reservoirs" for infection, as "sexual partners of men," and as being "of reproductive age," able to transmit disease to innocent babies. Such a characterization, as Allan Brandt noted for STDs, allowed for an association of the disease with individual behaviors, and thereby a certain degree of blame on the victim, and ignored the larger social forces that may have driven the epidemic into these "vectors." As with gonorrhea and syphilis, women with HIV became particularly victimized and stigmatized by the risk classification system. When recognized as anything beyond "female sexual partners" of men, it was generally as a fifth H: hookers. One of the first medical textbooks devoted to AIDS, published in 1984, covered women in a single chapter devoted to prostitutes and children.[29] Nowhere were men described as "vectors," "johns," or "sexual partners of women."

Increasingly, clinicians and researchers refused to link poverty, economic hardship, or sexual oppression to the now rapidly emerging epidemiologic patterns of spread to minorities, drug users, and women. Rather than pursue the social, political and economic forces that drove the spread of the epidemic, the biomedical and epidemiological constructions narrowed. Studies focused on how much virus was present in different bodily secretions, and whether or not mosquitoes, toothbrushing, casual contact, or contact sports could lead to transmission of the disease. A significant amount of energy was also spent in trying to identify where the virus came from, although the utility of this information other than to place blame remained unclear.

A few scientists speculated about the human, social, and economic *consequences* of HIV; none speculated about the human, social, and economic *causes,* except to place blame on homosexuals, Haitians, or the entire African continent. Leading popular science journals continued to refer to AIDS as a gay disease, despite the overwhelming evidence to the contrary; the December 1985 issue of *Discover* magazine profiled AIDS as the price gay men paid for anal intercourse. As late as 1988, leading biomedical research journals attributed the African pandemic to unspoken and widespread homosexuality; anal intercourse as a means of birth control; repetitive use of unsterile needles for routine shots and immunizations; frequent sex during menses; ritual sexual mutilations; frequent contact with monkeys; and even a transcontinental, primary deficiency of the immune system throughout Africa.[30]

January 1, 1993: Women at Risk

By 1992, a global pandemic among women could no longer be denied. Public health officials mobilized to combat HIV through behavior control, a familiar method from the sexually transmitted disease era. The male condom became a panacea against the spread of HIV, a fallout from the epidemiologic construction of HIV. Condom promotion, however, largely ignored social, economic, and gender inequality issues that made condoms irrelevant to the lives of millions of women at risk both in the United States and worldwide.

Women finally emerged in the biomedical discourse as victims of the disease in the late 1980s, although official recognition by the CDC did not come until January 1, 1993, when a revised classification system recognizing clinical manifestations of HIV disease unique to women went into effect.[31] The acknowledged heterosexual transmission of HIV to women, however, remained in the biomedical interpretation a consequence of individual behaviors (the sexually transmitted disease model) or biologic differences at a cellular level (the infectious disease model). Epidemiologists continued to invoke concurrent infections, genital ulcerations, unusual sexual practices, and promiscuity as the most likely explanations for the spread of HIV to women in epidemic proportions.[32] Molecular biologists paid significant attention to the differences between vaginal mucosa, rectal mucosa, and the male urethra to explain why women appeared to be at higher risk in sexual encounters with men, and retrovirologists hypothesized that molecular distinctions among individual viral strains accounted for the rapid increase in risk among women.[33]

Current Understandings of HIV among Women

Several key elements can be discerned from the biomedical construction of HIV among women. First, the history of infectious diseases tells us that epidemic diseases arise along complex paths that are intimately connected to structures of human society such as trade patterns, urbanization, migration, and in particular class and gender inequalities and the perpetuation of poverty. The biomedical concept of infectious disease has changed over time, however, as the role of health and disease in society has come to take on new meanings. Thus, the structural nature of the HIV epidemic among women was not part of the biomedical conception of disease when the virus emerged in the 1980s, and continues to be underrecognized and underexamined today.

Second, epidemiologic construction of the disease has continued to characterize women in the context of male risk behaviors, and perpetuated traditional constructions that characterize women as victimizers rather than victims. The initial descriptions of HIV ignored the impact of the disease on women, and initial constructions that included women perpetuated earlier constructions of women as immoral sexual "vectors" of disease. Moreover, within epidemiology there has been an increasingly reductionist approach to understanding the nature of epidemics, with an attendant disregard for large-scale or even local social, economic, and gender issues.

Finally, the emergence of retrovirology allowed emphasis to be placed on understanding the molecular biology of the virus, rather than the social welfare of its victims. Women in this construction became equated with their vaginal epithelium and their CD4 cells, and the ability of the virus to infect them was felt to be an immutable facet of their biology and gender, and of the virus' genetic make-up.

Only recently have the large-scale forces involved in perpetuating the epidemic among women begun to appear in biomedical constructions. Virologist Stephen Morse has written about the "viral traffic" patterns that shaped the emergence of HIV and other viruses,[34] although even his description stops short of a political economy of viral spread. Mary T. Bassett and Marvellous Mhloyi have examined the structural roots of the epidemic among women in Africa.[35] Nancy Krieger and Elizabeth Fee have reviewed how class, gender, and ethnicity issues are systematically excluded from biomedical models of women's health, including AIDS.[36] But despite this beginning, the powerful lens of the biomedical construction of HIV is all too evident in its inability to account for the social, political, and economic issues that affect the lives of so many women at risk, and its inability to stop the spread of HIV among them. Thus, the emergence of HIV from within the narrow confines of the infectious disease model is not without irony: while from a social science perspective HIV may come to epitomize the paramount importance of political economy in the spread of an infectious disease, it simultaneously represents the zenith of the infectious disease model's reductionist analysis. Put simply, HIV may soon prove to be a disease carried primarily by social and political forces, along fault lines of racism, gender inequality, classism, and economic oppression. Nonetheless, for biologists and clinicians, HIV is simply a bloodborne, sexually-transmitted, retroviral illness that attacks T cells and depletes immune function in individuals. The dissociation between the microscopic world of molecular medicine and the macroscopic world of human society has perhaps never been more crystallized than in the bio-medical approach to this epidemic.

NOTES

1. Thierry E. Mertens, Anthony Burton, Rand Stoneburner, Paul Sato, Michel Carael, and Elizabeth Belsey, "Global Estimates and Epidemiology of HIV Infection and AIDS," *AIDS* 8, Suppl. 1 (1994): S361–72.

2. D. Rebecca Prevots, Rosemary A. Ancelle-Park, Joyce J. Neal, and Robert S. Remis, "The Epidemiology of Heterosexually Acquired HIV Infection and AIDS in Western Industrialized Countries," *AIDS* 8, Suppl. 1 (1994): S109–17; Arlene Bardeguez and Margaret A. Johnson, "Women and HIV-1 Infection," *AIDS* 8, Suppl. 1 (1994): S261–73.

3. Centers for Disease Control, "US Public Health Service Recommendations for Human Immunodeficiency Virus Counseling and Voluntary Testing in Pregnant Women," *Morbidity and Mortality Weekly Report* 44 (1995): 1–15.

4. Centers for Disease Control, "Update: AIDS among Women—United States, 1994," *Morbidity and Mortality Weekly Report* 44 (1995): 81–84.

5. Kathryn Carovano, "More than Mothers and Whores: Redefining the AIDS Prevention Needs of Women," *International Journal of Health Services* 21 (1991): 131–42.

6. See for instance Aidan Cockburn, *The Evolution and Eradication of Infectious Diseases* (Baltimore: Johns Hopkins University Press, 1963); William H. McNeill, *Plagues and Peoples* (New York: Anchor Books, 1976); Thomas McKeown, *The Role of Medicine* (Princeton: Princeton University Press, 1979); and Mark Nathan Cohen, *Health and the Rise of Civilization* (New Haven: Yale University Press, 1989).

7. Cohen, *Health and the Rise of Civilization,* 32–74.

8. While a comprehensive treatment of the political economy of infectious disease is lacking in the literature, the political economy of health is the subject of wide-ranging texts such as Vicente Navarro, ed., *Imperialism, Health and Medicine* (Farmington: Baywood Publishing, 1981) or David Sanders, *The Struggle for Health: Medicine and the Politics of Underdevelopment* (London: Macmillan, 1985). Analyses of specific infectious diseases include Rene Dubos, *The White Plague: Tuberculosis, Man and Society* (New Brunswick: Rutgers University Press, 1952); Paul Farmer, *AIDS and Accusation: Haiti and the Geography of Blame* (Berkeley: University of California Press, 1992), and Richard Levins, Paul R. Epstein, Mary E. Wilson, Stephen S. Morse, Rudi Slooff, and Irina Eckardt, "Hantavirus Disease Emerging," *Lancet* 342 (1993): 1292. The impact of

global environmental change on emerging diseases has gained recent attention; see Richard Levins, Tamara Awerbuch, Uwe Brinkmann, Irina Eckardt, Paul Epstein, Najwa Makhoul, Cristina Albuquerque de Possas, Charles Puccia, Andrew Spielman, and Mary E. Wilson, "The Emergence of New Diseases," *American Scientist* 82 (1994): 52–60. The political economy of HIV has only recently appeared in the general biomedical literature; see Peter Lurie, Percy Hintzen and Robert A. Lowe, "Socioeconomic Obstacles to HIV Prevention and Treatment in Developing Countries: The Roles of the International Monetary Fund and the World Bank," *AIDS* 9 (1995): 539–46.

9. Sanders, *The Struggle for Health,* 14–44.

10. Peyton Rous, "A Sarcoma of the Fowl Transmissible by an Agent Separate from the Tumor Cells," *Journal of Experimental Medicine* 13 (1911): 397–411.

11. Biologists began searching intently for human retroviruses in the 1970s, in an effort to demonstrate a role for viruses in the pathogenesis of certain cancers. Before 1980, however, only a handful of viruses in the primate family had been discovered, with the zoonotic names of Baboon Endogenous Virus, Gibbon Ape Leukemia Virus, and Simian Sarcoma Virus. The first definitive evidence for a human infectious retrovirus, HTLV-1, derived from work in Robert Gallo's laboratory, and was published in Marvin S. Reitz, Jr., Bernard J. Poiesz, Francis W. Ruscetti, and Robert C. Gallo, "Characterization and Distribution of Nucleic Acid Sequences of a Novel Type C Retrovirus from Neoplastic Human T Lymphocytes," *Proceedings of the National Academy of Science (USA)* 78 (1981): 1887–91. Gallo later gained notoriety as the codiscoverer with Luc Montaigner of HTLV-III, later renamed the Human Immunodeficiency Virus.

12. Perhaps the leading journal of retrovirology is the *Journal of the Acquired Immune Deficiency Syndromes,* a publication of the International Retrovirology Association. While this journal publishes epidemiologic, clinical and public policy articles, the editors recognized the implicit transformation through which HIV became conceived solely as a retroviral illness, and in 1995, the journal was renamed *Journal of the Acquired Immune Deficiency Syndromes and Human Retrovirology.* Similarly, in 1987, the journal *AIDS Research* had been renamed *AIDS Research and Human Retroviruses.*

13. It also has a steady supply of young disciples. I went to medical school from 1989 to 1993, a time of heightened consciousness towards AIDS and HIV. In that time, I learned in minute detail the structure of the HIV genome; the names and functions of the important viral-specific proteins, *tat, env, pol,* and *rev*; the molecular interactions between the gp120 and CD4 proteins at the level of specific electrons; and the molecular machinery of reverse transcription, differential splicing, protein translation and post-translational processing. As future clinicians and researchers, my classmates and I were taught nothing about the basic epidemiology of HIV, nor about social and political forces that may have contributed to its emergence and spread.

14. There are hundreds of published studies on the molecular epidemiology of HIV. For a recent review, see Carla L. Kuiken and Bette T. M. Korber, "Epidemiological Significance of Intra- and Inter-person Variation of HIV-1," *AIDS* 8, Suppl. 1 (1994): S73–83.

15. Allan M. Brandt, *No Magic Bullet: A Social History of Venereal Diseases in the United States since 1880* (Cambridge: Harvard University Press, 1985).

16. Quoted in Brandt, *No Magic Bullet,* 117.

17. Elizabeth Fee, "Sin versus Science," in *AIDS: The Burdens of History,* ed. Elizabeth Fee and Daniel M. Fox (Berkeley: University of California Press, 1988).

18. Randall M. Packard and Paul Epstein, "Medical Research on AIDS in Africa," in *AIDS: The Making of a Chronic Disease,* ed. Elizabeth Fee and Daniel M. Fox (Berkeley: University of California Press, 1992).

19. "The fatal defect of every sanitary scheme to control venereal disease has been that the masculine spreader of contagion has been entirely ignored as mythical or practically non-existent; the woman has been regarded not only as the chief offender against morality, but the responsible cause of disease; all repressive measures to stamp out the diseases of vice have been directed against the woman alone" (Prince A. Morrow, 1910, quoted in Brandt, *No Magic Bullet,* 155).

20. Kathryn Carovano, "More than Mothers and Whores: Redefining the AIDS Prevention Needs of Women," *International Journal of Health Services* 21 (1991): 131–42.

21. Centers for Disease Control, "*Pneumocystis* Pneumonia—Los Angeles," *Morbidity and Mortality Weekly Report* 30 (1981): 250–52.

22. Centers for Disease Control, "Kaposi's Sarcoma and *Pneumocystis* Pneumonia Among Homosexual Men—New York City and California," *Morbidity and Mortality Weekly Report* 30 (1981): 305–8.

23. Centers for Disease Control, "Update on Acquired Immune Deficiency Syndrome (AIDS)—United States," *Morbidity and Mortality Weekly Report* 31 (1982): 507–14.

24. Several authors have covered the fertile ground of comparing cultural responses to AIDS with plagues from antiquity to the present; for example Mary Catherine Bateson and Richard Goldsby, *Thinking AIDS* (New York: Addison-Wesley, 1988); Susan Sontag, *AIDS and Its Metaphors* (New York: Farrar, Straus and Giroux, 1989); and Richard Goldstein, "The Implicated and the Immune: Responses to AIDS in the Arts and Popular Culture," in *A Disease of Society: Cultural and Institutional Responses to AIDS,* ed. Dorothy Nelkin, David P. Willis, and Scott V. Parris (New York: Cambridge University Press, 1991).

25. Jean-Robert Leonidas and Nicole Hyppolite, "Haitians and the Acquired Immunodeficiency Syndrome," *Annals of Internal Medicine* 98 (1983): 1020–21.

26. Gerald M. Oppenheimer, "Causes, Cases and Cohorts," in *AIDS: The Making of a Chronic Disease,* ed. Elizabeth Fee and Daniel M. Fox (Berkeley: University of California Press, 1992).

27. Joseph Sonnabend, Steven S. Witkin, and David T. Portilo, "Acquired Immunodeficiency Syndrome, Opportunistic Infections and Malignancies in Male Homosexuals," *Journal of the American Medical Association* 249 (1983): 2370–74.

28. Centers for Disease Control, "Prevention of Acquired Immune Deficiency Syndrome: Report of Inter-Agency Recommendations," *Morbidity and Mortality Weekly Report* 32 (1983): 101–3.

29. Pearl Ma and David Armstrong, *The Acquired Immune Deficiency Syndrome and Infections in Homosexuals* (New York: Yorke Medical Books, 1984).

30. As Paula Treichler has noted in "AIDS and HIV Infection in the Third World," in *AIDS: The Making of a Chronic Disease,* ed. Elizabeth Fee and Daniel M. Fox (Berkeley: University of California Press, 1992), one influential article perpetuating these stereotypes was Daniel B. Hrdy, "Cultural Practices Contributing to the Transmission of Human Immunodeficiency Virus in Africa," *Reviews of Infectious Disease* 9 (1987): 1109–19. Although Hrdy conceded that there was little evidence to support these modes of transmission, his article perpetuated African stereotypes and was oblivious to the social and economic factors driving the epidemic in Africa. The abstract from Hrdy's article reads as follows:

> Differences between the epidemiology of AIDS cases in Africa and that in Western societies have prompted speculation regarding risk factors that may be unique to Africa. Because of the age and sex distribution of AIDS cases in Africa, emphasis has been placed on sexual transmission of human immunodeficiency virus (HIV).
>
> Factors thought to influence this sexual transmission include (1) promiscuity, with a high prevalence of sexually transmitted disease; (2) sexual practices that have been associated with increased risk of transmission of AIDS virus (homosexuality and anal intercourse); and (3) cultural practices that are possibly connected with increased viral transmission (female "circumcision" and infibulation). Other nonsexual cultural practices that do not fit the age distribution pattern of AIDS but may expose individuals to HIV include (1) practices resulting in exposure to blood (medicinal bloodletting, rituals establishing "blood brotherhood," and possibly ritual and medicinal enemas); (2) practices involving the use of shared instruments (injection of medicines, ritual scarification, group circumcision, genital tattooing, and shaving of body hair); and (3) contact with nonhuman primates. At the current time promiscuity seems to be the most important cultural factor contributing to the transmission of HIV in Africa.

31. Centers for Disease Control, "1993 Revised Classification System for HIV Infection and Expanded Surveillance Case Definition for AIDS Among Adolescents and Adults," *Morbidity and Mortality Weekly Report* 41, RR17 (1992): 1–19.

32. Nancy S. Padian, "Heterosexual Transmission of Acquired Immunodeficiency Syndrome: International Perspectives and National Projections," *Reviews of Infectious Disease* 9 (1987): 947–60.

33. Scott D. Holmberg, C. Robert Horsburgh, Jr., John W. Ward, and Harold W. Jaffe, "Biologic Factors in the Sexual Transmission of Human Immunodeficiency Virus," *Journal of Infectious Diseases* 160 (1989): 116–25.

34. Stephen S. Morse, "AIDS and Beyond: Defining the Rules of Viral Traffic," in *AIDS: The Making of a Chronic Disease,* ed. Elizabeth Fee and Daniel M. Fox (Berkeley: University of California Press, 1992); Stephen S. Morse and Ann Schluederberg,

"Emerging Viruses: The Evolution of Viruses and Viral Diseases," *Journal of Infectious Diseases* 162 (1990): 1–7.

35. Mary T. Bassett and Marvellous Mhloyi, "Women and AIDS in Zimbabwe: The Making of an Epidemic," *International Journal of Health Services* 21 (1991): 143–56.

36. Nancy Krieger and Elizabeth Fee, "Man-Made Medicine and Women's Health: The Biopolitics of Sex/Gender and Race/Ethnicity," *International Journal of Health Services* 24 (1994): 265–83.

2

Barriers to the Inclusion of Women in Research and Clinical Trials

Theresa McGovern

Theresa McGovern is the founder and Executive Director of the HIV Law Project, a nonprofit organization that provides civil legal and advocacy services to low-income women, communities of color, and lesbians and gay men affected with HIV. The Project works on several levels, providing legal representation to individuals, advocacy for client groups, and public policy leadership through large-scale litigation. It has successfully challenged the definition of AIDS developed by the Centers for Disease Control (CDC) as underinclusive of the illnesses experienced by women and other underrepresented populations. The Project has also successfully challenged the criteria used by the Social Security Administration to evaluate HIV-related disability and the Food and Drug Administration guidelines barring women of childbearing potential from participating in clinical trials. Ms. McGovern is a *summa cum laude* graduate of the State University of New York at Albany and holds the J.D. from Georgetown University Law Center.

Federal Regulations: Mixed Messages

The federal government has a history of promulgating various policies and procedures which have resulted in the exclusion of fertile women from clinical trials. To the extent that the government has attempted to change these policies and encourage the inclusion of women, the federal government has chosen to promulgate policy changes in the form of guidelines, which have no binding effect, rather than as regulations, which would require compliance.[1] This is indicative of the government's ambivalence regarding remedying this long history of discrimination. Guidelines suggesting inclusion are not enforced, leaving trial sponsors free to exclude or limit the participation of women.

National Institutes of Health

In 1986, the National Institutes of Health (NIH) developed and published a policy statement urging applicants to include women in clinical studies.[2] However, in 1987, an inventory conducted of the research activities supported by the NIH found that the NIH spent approximately only 13.5 percent of the budget on women's health issues.[3] Additionally, subsequent investigations by the General Accounting Office (GAO) found a nonuniform implementation of the NIH's stated policy throughout the agency.[4] Although the NIH announced its policy encouraging the inclusion of women in research study populations in 1986, with further published guidance for implementation in 1989, the policies were not applied consistently. Further, NIH officials had taken little action to encourage researchers to analyze study results by gender.[5] Subsequent GAO investigations confirmed earlier findings that women were generally underrepresented in the trials surveyed, and although there were enough women enrolled in some trials to detect gender-related differences in response, the data were not analyzed to determine if women's responses to the investigational drug were different from men's responses.[6]

In March 1994, the NIH established guidelines on the inclusion of women and minorities and their subpopulations in research involving human subjects, including clinical trials. The NIH's 1994 guideline contains three major additions to previous NIH policy: (1) the NIH must ensure that women, minorities and subpopulations are included in all human subject research; (2) the NIH must ensure that women and minorities and their subpopulations be included in the appropriate phase of clinical trials such that valid analyses of differences in intervention effect can be accomplished; (3) the NIH must not allow cost as an acceptable reason for excluding these groups. In addition, the NIH must initiate programs and outreach efforts to recruit these groups into clinical studies. However, there are exceptions to this recommendation which, in effect, render the recommendations quite weak.[7]

Department of Health and Human Services

Since the mid-1970's, the exclusion of pregnant women from clinical trials was codified in a regulation entitled "Additional Protections Pertaining to

Research, Development, and Related Activities Involving Fetuses, Pregnant Women, and Human in Vitro Fertilization."[8] The purpose of this regulation—evidenced in the title by placement of the fetus first—is to put the fetus at minimal risk. In fact, risk to the fetus is to be kept to the lowest minimum while trying to meet the women's health needs. The regulation further requires that the "father of the fetus" give his consent to the pregnant women's participation in research. In this case, the fetus, not the woman, is treated as the trial participant.

The Food and Drug Administration

Although its legislative mandate is to protect all consumers, the Food and Drug Administration (FDA) has also encouraged the exclusion of women from clinical trials. In the past, the FDA has stated a concern not only for the welfare of consumers but also for the welfare of the fetus.[9] Despite this concern, the FDA has played an active role in reducing information about the reproductive effects of drugs on men and women and the different effects of such drugs when used by women. The FDA has purportedly provided protection to the fetus by restricting the access of women of childbearing potential to clinical trials rather than by mandating an adequate analysis of a drug's reproductive effects prior to human testing. Thus, the FDA has played a major role in encouraging and reinforcing discrimination against women.

1977 FDA Guideline

A 1977 FDA guideline barred women of childbearing potential from early phases of clinical trials or until certain segments of animal reproduction studies were completed.[10] Although, according to the 1977 guideline, women with life-threatening diseases (applicable to HIV/AIDS) were an exception to the exclusion, drug companies routinely excluded women with AIDS from their experimental research due to the FDA's failure to monitor the process.

As a direct result of the FDA's failure to monitor the drug development process adequately, trial sponsors have been able to exclude women on the purported basis of fetal toxicity where in fact no evidence of such toxicity exists. Thus, the animal studies which the FDA required as a precursor to women's participation in clinical trials may never have been conducted or may be conducted parallel to, not in advance of, clinical trials. The regulations describing what a new drug application must contain require inclusion of the results of "nonclinical studies *as appropriate,* of the effects of the drug on reproduction and the developing fetus" (emphasis added).[11] This does not require the inclusion of the results of animal studies nor do the regulations require sponsors to elicit those reproductive effects mediated through the male animal. In addition, the FDA is silent on how the results of such studies ought to affect the inclusion or exclusion of women.

This implicit and explicit exclusion of women from early phases of clinical trials has had devastating repercussions. First, as these exclusions are based on scientifically (and legally) unsound principles, the integrity of the entire clinical trials process is called into question. Medically, the 1977 guideline denied treatment to women, ignored the potential reproductive effects a given drug may have on men, ignored the importance of gender differences in drug research, and failed to mandate the completion of important animal studies before human testing begins. Because clinical trials constitute both a procedure for testing new drugs and, particularly in the context of life-threatening illnesses (such as HIV disease), a method of treatment, these exclusions may be a matter of life or death for women whose only hope of treatment may be enrollment in a clinical trial.[12]

Another result of the 1977 guideline is that drugs can be marketed without being tested on women—testing on women before a drug is approved is not mandated by the FDA. Thus, the adverse effects of a given drug will sometimes be discovered only after the drug has been marketed for the general public (including women of childbearing potential) and administered to large numbers of people, exposing drug companies to an even greater potential for liability.[13] By discouraging drugs from being adequately tested on women, the 1977 guideline insures that when such drugs are later approved, the warning for women will not be adequate.[14]

1993 FDA Guideline

On December 15, 1992, the HIV Law Project, the NOW Legal Defense and Education Fund, and the American Civil Liberties Union AIDS Project submitted a citizen petition requesting the Commissioner of the FDA amend the 1977 FDA guideline as discriminatory.[15] The citizen petition suggested alternative regulations which would have removed any gender-based restrictions on access to clinical trials.

On July 22, 1993, the FDA published a proposed new guideline entitled "Guideline for the Study and Evaluation of Gender Differences in the Clinical Evaluation of Drugs" (1993 guideline), which revises the 1977 FDA guideline.[16] The 1993 guideline's stated purpose is to set out the FDA's expectations regarding the inclusion of women in drug development, analyses of clinical data by gender, assessment of potential pharmacokinetic differences between genders, and the conduct of specific additional studies in women where indicated. Despite the FDA's much-publicized claim that it was taking action to eradicate discrimination against women in the drug development process, the 1993 guideline still allows trial sponsors to exclude women of childbearing potential whether or not there is evidence of fetal toxicity. Under the 1993 guideline, human testing may still begin prior to the completion of animal reproduction studies, undermining both men's and women's right to be fully informed of potential reproductive risks. The 1993 guideline does not address the FDA's overall failure to monitor the conduct or results of animal reproduction studies or to halt trials which unnecessarily restrict women of childbearing potential.[17]

Gender-Related Drug Response Differences

Analysis of gender-related drug response differences is necessary if the FDA is to fulfill its mandate regarding approval of safe and effective drugs for consumer use. As noted by the General Accounting Office in its report, "FDA Needs to Ensure More Study of Gender Differences in Prescription Drug Testing," evidence of the importance of gender-related analyses in drug testing is mounting.[18] As the FDA acknowledges, sound drug development requires the study of sex-specific issues in drug response. Doctors and researchers have often complained of a general lack of understanding as to how a drug will affect women and an unawareness of a drug's side effects in women.[19] In addition, the lack of information on teratogenicity and generational effects in men and women often leaves physicians in a quandary as to what to prescribe to persons of child-producing potential.

The FDA's 1993 Guideline Does Not Mandate Any Change in the Treatment of Women

The 1993 guideline does not mandate the inclusion of women in clinical trials, nor does it eliminate gender-based restrictions on access to clinical trials or require an analysis of drug responses in light of potential gender differences. The 1993 guideline merely *suggests* certain by-gender analyses while stating that its recommendations need not always be followed. Unfortunately, the language of the 1993 guideline invariably provides a retreat for the reluctant trial sponsor who is unwilling to analyze gender differences. Given the FDA's history of discouraging the inclusion of women, this approach is likely to result in no change of behavior in trial sponsors.

The closest the FDA comes to requiring that women be included in clinical trials is in a vague passage which states that "in some cases, there may be a basis for requiring participation of women in early studies." The disease under study must be "serious and affect women" and "especially when a promising drug for the disease is being developed and made available rapidly under the FDA's accelerated approval or early access procedures, a case can be made for requiring that women participate in clinical trials at early stages.[20] The 1993 guideline does not define these provisions and it does not commit the FDA to monitoring the drug development process to ensure that trials meeting the vague criteria enumerated will include women.

A 1988 FDA guideline, also not a regulation as in the case of the 1993 FDA guideline, requests a by-gender analysis, but the analysis suggested by this 1988 guideline will detect only relatively large gender-related differences which are not likely to be clinically important. In addition, the trial sponsors are not required to undertake the analyses suggested in the 1988 guideline. If the sponsor happens to comply with the 1988 guideline's suggested by-gender analysis and pharmacodynamic differences are indicated, a sponsor could conduct additional studies.

The FDA Has Not Required an Adequate Analysis of Teratogenicity and Mutagenicity

Animal reproduction studies provide information as to whether a drug is teratogenic as well as information on potential long-term reproductive effects.[21] The results of these studies would help the FDA to determine whether women who wish to participate in a clinical trial were at risk of experiencing reproductive effects. The 1993 guideline does not require the completion of animal reproduction studies prior to beginning testing in human subjects, nor does the 1993 guideline mention the monitoring of the results of such studies (including whether male-mediated effects are observed). The 1993 guideline contains generalized expectations regarding these studies while offering no clear guidance as to when the studies must be conducted.[22] In fact, neither the 1993 guideline nor any of the regulations governing the clinical drug testing process explicitly require that animal reproduction tests be conducted at all. The 1993 guideline does not define the criteria used in determining whether a significant risk to the fetus exists nor does it discuss how the existence of such a risk will be determined.[23] There is *no* discussion of the standards for determining reproductive risk.

In the past, the FDA has stated a concern that mandating animal reproduction studies prior to human testing would delay the clinical trial process as well as serve as a financial disincentive for pharmaceutical companies to test new drugs.[24] An informal survey of two independent laboratories reveals that the range of time for conducting all three recommended segments of the animal reproduction studies can be as short as forty-one weeks to over one year and the range of cost from $150,000 to $295,000. Given the profit range of the pharmaceutical industry and the FDA's stated commitment to fetal protection, these costs are not prohibitive.

Interestingly, in response to these objectives the FDA has stated that the completion of the animal reproduction studies should not be emphasized as these studies are not necessarily predictive of teratogenicity. If this is the case, one must ask why the participation of women of childbearing potential in clinical trials has been predicated on the completion of such studies.

Moreover, the 1993 guideline also fails to discuss the need to monitor male-mediated effects in animal reproduction studies, and it seems that current animal reproduction studies are looking at male animals for fertility effects rather than mutagenesis or generational effects.[25] There is significant evidence that generational male-mediated effects occur.[26]

The FDA Urges the Imposition of Restrictions on the Participation of Women of Childbearing Potential without Placing Similar Restrictions on the Participation of Men of Child-Producing Potential

The FDA refuses to treat men and women similarly situated in the same manner.[27] Although the 1993 Guideline begins by proclaiming that there should not be unwarranted restrictions on the participation of women, it recommends restrictions on women's access even where there is no fetal toxicity at issue. The 1993 guideline states:

> Except in the case of trials intended for the study of drug effects during pregnancy, clinical protocols should include measures that will minimize the possibility of fetal exposure to the investigational drug. These would ordinarily include providing for the use of a reliable method of contraception (or abstinence) for the duration of drug exposure (which may exceed the length of the study), use of pregnancy testing (beta HCG) to detect unsuspected pregnancy prior to initiation of study treatment, and timing of studies (easier with studies of short duration) to coincide with, or immediately follow, menstruation.[28]

This policy is overinclusive as it restricts the access of all women of childbearing potential regardless of their sexual orientation, celibacy, or agreement to refrain from sexual activity. By refusing to mandate the completion of animal reproduction studies prior to human testing, the FDA is guaranteeing the unnecessary restriction of women. According to the 1993 guideline, if a drug is not fetally toxic or does not have reproductive effects, but the animal reproduction studies have not been completed or even undertaken, a woman will be asked to utilize contraception or be tested for pregnancy.

Currently, regardless of whether a drug is fetally toxic or has reproductive effects (usually unknown since no mandate exists for completion of animal studies which would yield this result), a woman will be asked to utilize hormonal contraception and/or detectable barriers and pregnancy testing. Historically, pharmaceutical companies have been overzealous in their application of this proviso to require "detectable" birth control and have required intrauterine devices. For many women fighting severe HIV-related gynecological infections, the requirement of "detectable" birth control has prevented their enrollment in trials. Pursuant to the 1993 guideline, this policy will continue.

While recommending mandatory birth control and/or pregnancy testing for all women of childbearing potential, the FDA does not recommend restricting men of child-producing capacity in the same manner.[29] The FDA simply suggests a risk-benefit analysis for men of child-producing capacity. Moreover, the risk-benefit analysis only needs to occur if reproductive studies have shown abnormalities of reproductive organs or their functions—(i.e., if abnormal sperm production has been observed in experimental animals). In considering whether or not females should be treated differently from males in regard to reproductive outcomes and clinical trials, it is important to note that, at least in some cases, teratogenicity can be traced to alterations in the male gamete.[30] Mutagenic effects of a drug are likely to be more intensified in men because male germ cells, due to their rapid multiplication, are more susceptible to the effects of mutagens are female germ cells.[31] These findings have been interpreted to mean that males of reproductive potential might also cause harm to their potential offspring by participating in clinical trails.[32] However, it is more logical and efficient to inform both men and women about known risks to offspring than to exclude all people of reproductive potential from clinical trials.

The FDA Has Weakened Informed Consent by Refusing to Require Sponsors to Undertake Animal Reproduction Studies Prior to Human Testing and by Telling Sponsors to Assume Fetal Risk

In 1981, the FDA issued regulations to ensure that subjects in clinical trials are fully informed in an unbiased manner about the findings from animal studies of an experimental drug. However, in current practice the purpose of informed consent in clinical research—to educate participants about potential risks and benefits and allow for informed decisions concerning participation—is never truly realized. In short, effective informed consent does not yet exist in the United States, despite its importance when considering the inclusion of women in clinical trials and in respecting the autonomy and decision-making ability of women.

A review of the informed consent documents of thirty-six AIDS clinical trials from a major medical research center shows that the quality and amount of information given to the potential female trial participant is alarmingly insufficient.[33] For example, only 17 percent of the documents reviewed offered information concerning a specific teratogenic risk. Specific risks, when identified, were either scantily described or described in prohibitively technical language, thus precluding genuine informed consent.

The 1993 guideline emphasizes that women, not men, should be fully informed of the status of the animal reproduction studies and of any other information about the teratogenic potential of the drug. If the animal reproduction studies are not complete, the 1993 guideline states that other pertinent information should be provided, such as a general assessment of fetal toxicity in drugs with related properties. The 1993 guideline goes on to state that "if no relevant information is available, the informed consent should specifically note the potential for fetal risk."[34] Thus, the FDA is telling sponsors that they can simply assume fetal risk and place special conditions on the participation of women rather than spend the money on testing the drug to ensure that its effects are known. Again, the FDA is taking an approach to fetal protection that most restricts women's access to clinical trials. By encouraging trial sponsors to place special conditions on the enrollment of women when no analysis of reproductive effects has been undertaken, the FDA has substantially weakened the informed consent process. The FDA is, in effect, in violation of its own duty to investigate the risk of adverse reproductive effects and has substituted restrictions on women for an adequate analysis of reproductive effects and adequate informed consent. Male-mediated reproductive effects have been completely ignored, and the FDA has shifted the responsibility for avoiding fetal toxicity or generational effects exclusively to women.[35] Informed consents also often exclude pregnant women with life-threatening illnesses.[36] The specifics of what is known and unknown about the potential benefits and risks do not seem to be a standard part of the informed consent.

Avoid Liability, Exclude Women?

Many pharmaceutical trial sponsors assert that the risk of future liability for the teratogenic effects of drugs tested on fertile women is great enough to justify a blanket exclusion of women of childbearing potential from the early phases of clinical trials. Pharmaceutical sponsors present, as an example, the following scenario: twenty years after an experimental drug trial is completed, the adult child of a female trial participant sues the pharmaceutical company due to medical complications allegedly caused by the experimental drug taken by the mother who was, at the time of the trial, in the early stages of pregnancy. Notwithstanding a woman's agreement to refrain from sexual activity during a trial, the availability and use of detectable birth control methods, continual pregnancy testing during the trial, and a decade of federal regulations urging the inclusion of women, drug sponsors often use the above hypothetical scenario to support the argument that a blanket exclusion of women is appropriate. Pharmaceutical trial sponsors consistently assert that the exclusion of women based on a fear of liability is justifiable since any question of the adequacy of the informed consent *could* conceivably end up before a jury, and even though a plaintiff might never prevail, it could end up costing a lot of money to defend such a lawsuit. Federal policymakers assert that they are powerless to correct such beliefs and that, in fact, a mandate to include women would result in a disincentive for industry drug development.

It seems, however, that this logic is not consistently applied and is conveniently disregarded whenever government and industry want to test a certain substance on fertile women. Some of the very same NIH and FDA staff members, as well as pharmaceutical sponsors, who speak of the great disincentive of liability and the hypothetical fetus who could become the costly plaintiff, are extolling the virtues of the results of ACTG 076, a clinical trial designed to evaluate the efficacy, safety, and tolerance of Zidovudine (ZDV), commonly called AZT, for the prevention of maternal fetal transmission. ZDV was administered to a large percentage of infants who would probably not have been born infected with HIV and could have caused long term developmental defects to those infants. However, the industry does not seem to be concerned although it seems more likely that a trial sponsor who knowingly administered a toxic agent to an infant would be more liable than the hypothetical adult child of a woman who managed to circumvent birth control requirements and participate in a clinical trial.

In reality, the unjustified exclusion of women may in fact result in greater and more immediate liability for trial sponsors than careful, informed inclusion. Under the equal protection clause's standard for review of government action that discriminates against women, such a policy can only be sustained if the party seeking to uphold the policy shows by "exceedingly persuasive justification" that the classification serves "important governmental objectives and that the discriminatory means employed are substantially related to the achievement of those objectives."[37] Wholesale exclusion of women from the early phases of drug trials cannot be used as a proxy for an analysis of reproductive effects; the Supreme Court has held time and again that "administrative convenience" cannot serve as a rationale to justify sex discrimination.[38] FDA policies regulating experimental drug trials must, therefore, meet constitutional equal protection requirements. This is particularly true where, as in the HIV and AIDS context, access to the experiment may itself be a significant benefit.

In addition to the equal protection clause, the 1977 FDA guideline also violates women's constitutional right to privacy. Particularly for nonpregnant women of childbearing potential and women in the early stages of pregnancy, the constitutional right to privacy and autonomy outweighs any generalized governmental interest in avoiding fetal toxicity.[39] By supporting the exclusion of women of childbearing potential from all drug trials—an exclusion that, in practice, extends to women with life-threatening diseases in search of or seeking treatment—the 1977 guideline places an undue burden on these women's exercise of reproductive choice.[40]

The FDA has allowed the pharmaceutical industry's assumption that the exclusion of women minimizes the potential liability of drug manufacturers to drive federal policy.[41] However, this fear of liability does not justify differential treatment based on sex, particularly in an experimental setting.[42] Since the drugs tested in clinical trials are, by definition, experimental and are not being marketed to the general public, strict liability does not apply. Manufacturers can guard against potential liability in negligence by scrupulous use of adequate warnings and informed consent.

FDA Wrongly Claims That It Lacks the Regulatory Capacity to Mandate the Inclusion of Women in Clinical Trials and a By-Gender Analysis of Results

Claiming that there is no regulatory basis for the inclusion of women and no requirement that various gender analyses and animal reproduction studies be completed and recognizing that the "change will not, by itself, cause drug companies . . . to alter restrictions that they might impose on the participation of women of childbearing potential," the FDA has failed to ensure the inclusion of women in clinical trials and has failed to require a by-gender analysis of clinical data.

In fact, the FDA does have the regulatory authority to both mandate the inclusion of women of childbearing potential in drug trials and to require that such trials employ a by-gender analysis. Title 20 U.S.C. 371 provides that the secretary of the FDA has authority to "promulgate regulations for the efficient enforcement" of the Food, Drug and Cosmetic Act. Among other things, that Act provides specific procedures and reporting requirements applicable to applications for approval of new drugs.[43] The FDA has already promulgated regulations pursuant to this section regulating the content and format of new drug applications.[44] Given the scientific considerations discussed at length above, the "efficient enforcement" of the FDA's statutory mandate would also clearly encompass a requirement concerning nondiscriminatory testing of experimental drugs and appropriate analysis of the drugs' effects on potential consumers of both sexes.[45]

A close analysis of the language of the 1993 guideline indicates that the FDA has done little more than recommend some minor by-gender analysis, reemphasize the need to restrict the access of women of childbearing potential to clinical trials, and place special conditions on the access of women to clinical trials. The 1993 guideline suggests such restrictions even where there is no evidence of fetal toxicity.

Despite the FDA's much-publicized claim that it would take steps to eradicate discrimination against women in the drug development process, the 1993 guideline, in the end, does very little to ensure female inclusion in clinical research. Under this guideline the FDA will not adequately monitor the inclusion/exclusion criteria for women in clinical trials.[46]

Conclusion

Existing FDA regulations must be amended to mandate a by-gender analysis of all drug responses, and to eliminate gender-based restrictions on trial participation.[47] Formal acknowledgment of discrimination is merely the first step towards eradicating it. The FDA must go beyond acknowledging the problem created in part by its 1977 guideline and take an active role in eliminating gender discrimination in the drug testing process.

Because, as the FDA notes, the 1993 guideline has no binding effect, and previous guidelines suggesting by-gender analysis have been largely ignored by trial sponsors, the FDA should amend existing regulations to require that the results of by-gender analyses and animal reproduction studies be filed

with the investigational new drug (IND) applications and new drug applications (NDA).[48] The FDA should not approve any protocol which contains unwarranted restrictions on women of childbearing potential or any
protocol which fails to address the reality of male-mediated reproductive
effects. All protocol criteria must be gender neutral and all reports mandated by the IND process should include a by-gender analysis of all of the
drug's effects.[49] Also, the regulation which requires that the "father of the
fetus" give his consent to the pregnant women's participation in research
must be eliminated.

In addition, the FDA should issue a "clinical hold" pursuant to existing
regulations if a sponsor is violating this mandate. If the unwarranted discrimination continues, the FDA should terminate the IND. The FDA
should also publish a regulation defining the criteria used by the agency to
determine fetal toxicity and should regulate the creation of a databank,
accessible to the trial sponsors and the public, containing information on
the known teratogenicity and mutagenicity of various drugs. This would
help to eliminate unnecessary restrictions where drugs had already been
thoroughly investigated for mutagenic and teratogenic effect.

NOTES

This chapter is based, in part, on the comments on the 1993 Guideline filed by the HIV
Law Project, students of the Rutgers University Women's Rights Clinic, and Martha
Davis of NOWLDF. Thanks, also, to Berna Lee for significant editorial assistance.

   1. *21 Code of Federal Regulations,* 10.90(b), sets forth the definition and legal status of
a Food and Drug Administration guideline.
   2. *NIH Guide to Grants and Contracts,* vol. 15 (November 28, 1986).
   3. R. L. Kirschenstein, "Research on Women's Health," *American Journal of Public
Health* 81, no. 3 (1991): 291–93.
   4. United States General Accounting Office, *National Institutes of Health: Problems in
Implementing Policy on Women in Study Populations* (GAO/T-HRD 90–38, June 18, 1990).
   5. *Id.*
   6. *Id.*
   7. "NIH Guidelines on the Inclusion of Women and Minorities as Subjects in
Clinical Research," *Federal Register* 59, no. 46 (March 9 1994). Exclusions to the
requirement for inclusion of women and minorities include: (1) if the clinical research
is inappropriate with respect to the health of the participants; (2) if inclusion is inappropriate with respect to the purpose of the research; (3) if exclusion is inappropriate under
such other circumstances as the director of the NIH may designate; or (4) in the case of

a clinical trial, the guidelines may provide that such inclusion in the trial is not required if there is substantial scientific data demonstrating that there is a significant difference between the effects that the variables to be studied in the trial have on women or members of minority groups respectively; and the effects that variables have on individuals who would serve as subjects in the trial in the event such inclusion were required. In addition, as is true of all other guidelines, these guidelines contain no effective enforcement mechanism.

8. *45 Code of Federal Regulations* (C.F.R.)(1975) 46.207.

9. *1977 FDA Guideline* 77–3040 barred women of childbearing potential from phase 1 and early phase 2 of the clinical trials and/or until certain segments of animal reproduction studies had been completed to avoid exposing a fetus to a drug that might be teratogenic.

10. U.S. Food and Drug Administration, *General Guidelines for the Clinical Evaluation of Drugs* (FDA 1977), 77–3040.

11. See 21 C.F.R. 314.

12. See *Eighth International Conference on AIDS,* Abstract #MOCOO34 (Amsterdam, July 1992). *See also:* Kenneth Mayer and Charles Carpenter, "Women and AIDS," *Scientific American* 266 (March 1992): 118.

13. See *infra,* p.20, n. 18 (discussing DES cases).

14. See, e.g., Jones et al., "Pattern of Malformations in the Children of Women Treated With Carbamazepine During Pregnancy," *New England Journal of Medicine* 320 (1989): 1661.

15. The citizen petition was filed on behalf of Mary Lucey, an HIV-positive woman who was denied access to clinical trials; ACT UP Women's FDA Working Group, the AIDS Counseling and Education for Women in Transition from Correctional Facilities (ACE OUT); the New Jersey Women and AIDS Network; and Housing Works.

16. *Federal Register 58. Federal Regulations* 139.

17. Petitioners consider the 1993 guideline to be an inadequate response to the citizen petition as it fails to redress, and in fact, encourages, discrimination against women of childbearing potential.

18. Henry A. Waxman et al., *supra,* 5.

19. See Barbara A. Levey, "Bridging the Gender Gap in Research," *Clinical Pharmacology and Therapeutics* 50 (December 1991): 641. See also Jean Hamilton and Barbara Parry, "Sex Related Differences in Clinical Drug Response: Implications for Women's Health," *Journal of American Medicine, Women's Association,* 38 (September/October 1983): 129.

20. 1993 guideline at 39409. It is unclear from the 1993 guideline what the criteria are for determining if a disease is serious and affects women. The Public Health Service has issued a report which listed five criteria to determine whether a particular disease was a "woman's disease": (1) the condition must be unique to women or some subgroup of women; (2) it must be more prevalent in women or some subgroup of women than in men; (3) it must be more serious in women or in some subgroup of women than in men; (4) the condition must be one for which risk factors are different for women or some subgroup of women than in men; (5) it must be one for which treatment

interventions are different for women or some subgroup of women than in men. See U.S. General Accounting Office, GAO/T-HRD-90–38 (1990), Mark V. Nadel, "Summary of GAO Testimony by Mark V. Nadel," *On Problems in Implementing the National Institutes of Health Policy on Women in Study Populations* 2 (1990): 1.

The National Institutes of Health Revitalization Act of 1993, Pub. L. No. 103–43 (to be codified in scattered sections of 42 U.S.C.), also defines "women's health conditions" as all diseases, disorders, and conditions (including with respect to mental health): (1) unique to, more serious or more prevalent in women; (2) for which the factors of medical risks or types of medical intervention are different for women, or for which it is unknown whether such factors or types are different for women; or (3) with respect to which there has been insufficient clinical research involving women as subjects or insufficient clinical data on women.

21. While animal reproduction studies are not always predictive of outcome in humans, the FDA has always relied on such tests as a precursor to the inclusion of women.

22. For example, the 1993 guideline states (in the abstract of section A) that "where animal studies suggest possible effects on fertility, . . . special studies in humans may be needed to evaluate this potential toxicity." (1993 guideline at 39409.) In section G, "Precautions in Clinical Trials Including Women of Childbearing Potential": "in general, it is expected that reproductive toxicity studies be completed before there is large scale exposure of women of childbearing potential." (*Id.* at 39411.) This section later states, "[i]f these studies have not been completed, other pertinent information should be provided. . ." (*Id.*) Finally, in section H, "Potential Effects on Fertility," the 1993 guideline recommends that "where abnormalities of reproductive organs or their functions have been observed in experimental animals, the decision to include patients . . . should be based on a careful risk-benefit analysis . . . [and] should include appropriate monitoring and/or laboratory studies. . . ." (*Id.*)

23. Numerous representatives from pharmaceutical companies and independent laboratories, who do not wish to be identified, have confirmed that the FDA is not monitoring this process.

24. Conversations between FDA officials, who did not wish to be identified, and Theresa M. McGovern.

25. In response to our inquiry, a physician at the FDA recently explained that initial scrutiny of male fertility occurs during general toxicity studies in animals conducted prior to human testing. If effects on spermatogenesis are observed, further studies may be conducted. When asked whether observed effects on spermatogenesis might lead to intergenerational studies, this doctor explained that few male-mediated effects have been found and that fertility represents the focus of study of reproductive effects in males.

26. See, e.g., B. Tobaire and B. Hales, "Paternal Exposure to Chemicals Before Conception," *British Medical Journal* 307 (1993): 341. See also S. Blakeslee, "Research on Birth Defects Shifts to Flaws in Sperm," *New York Times*, 1 March 1991, 27. J. Brody, "Possible Links Between Babies' Health and Fathers' Habits and Working Conditions," *New York Times*, 25 December 1991, 64.

27. It should be noted that the FDA carefully utilizes gender-neutral language in the section of the 1993 guideline titled "Potential Effects on Fertility." The avoidance of gender-specific language in this section cannot disguise the fact that the FDA has recommended the restriction of all women of childbearing potential and has not treated similarly situated men in the same manner.

28. 1993 guideline at 39411.

29. According to the FDA, the decision to include men of reproductive age should be based upon a risk-benefit analysis of the nature of the abnormalities, the dosage needed to induce them, the consistency of findings in different species, the severity of the illness being treated, the potential importance of the drug, the availability of alternative treatment and the duration of treatment (1993 guideline at 39411). Where patients of reproductive potential are included in studies of drugs showing reproductive toxicity in animals, the 1993 guideline states that long-term follow-up will be needed to evaluate side effects in humans (1993 guideline at 39411).

30. Male toxic exposures ranging from lead and other heavy metals to dibromochloropropane (DBCP) and chlordecone (Kepone) also have been demonstrated to affect the likelihood both of conception and of spontaneous abortion. See M. Castleman, "Toxics and Male Infertility," *Sierra Club Bulletin* 70, no. 4 (March/April 1985): 49–52. See also K. Hemminki et al., "Spontaneous Abortion in an Industrialized Community in Finland," *American Journal of Public Health* 73, no. 1 (January 1983): 32–37. See also M. D. Whorton, "Editorial: Adverse Reproductive Outcomes: the Occupational Health Issue of the 1980's," *American Journal of Public Health* 73, no. 1 (January 1983): 15–16.

31. L. Uzych, "Teratogenesis and Mutagenesis Associated with the Exposure of Human Males to Lead: A Review," *Yale Journal of Biological Medicine* 58 (1985): 9–17. L. F. Soyka and J. M. Joffe, "Male Mediated Drug Effects on Offspring," *Progressive Clinical Biological Research* 36 (1980): 49–66.

32. Howard Minkoff et al., "Fetal Protection and Women's Access to Clinical Trails," *Journal of Women's Health* 1 (1992): 137–40.

33. M. B. Caschetta, W. Chavkin, and T. McGovern, "Women and Clinical Trials," *New England Journal of Medicine* (December 9, 1993).

34. 1993 guideline at 39411. *Federal Register:* In the introductory section, "C. Current FDA Position on Participation of Women of Childbearing Potential in Clinical Trials," it states, "it is expected that . . . the woman participant is fully informed about the current state of the animal reproduction studies and any other information about the teratogenic potential of the drug" (1993 guideline at 39408). In section G, "Precautions in Clinical Trials Including Women," the 1993 guideline discusses informed consent as stated above.

35. 21 C.F.R. 50.25(2) requires a description of any reasonably foreseeable risks or discomforts to the subject. 21 C.F.R. 50.25(b)(1) requires a statement that the particular treatment or procedure may involve risks to the subject (or to the embryo or fetus, if the subject is or may become pregnant) which are currently unforeseeable. Were the FDA to mandate the completion of animal reproduction studies prior to human testing, these provisions could be met. Instead, the 1993 guideline encourages sponsors to describe discoverable risks as unforeseeable.

36. For instance, an informed consent from a large New York City hospital of ACTG study #117 which compares ddI to AZT reads as follows:

This drug may cause problems to the fetus if you become pregnant or father a child. Women of childbearing age can only be admitted to the study if you are not breast feeding; if you are not pregnant (as determined by a prestudy blood test for pregnancy); if you have been surgically sterilized, or are using effective birth controls.

Another typical informed consent message is exemplified by the language contained in the informed consent form of ACTG #135 conducted in a large New York City hospital. The study tests five drugs in the treatment of Mycobacterium Avium Complex and anticipates the possibility of a woman becoming pregnant during the study. It does not, however, specify policies or procedures for dealing with the pregnant woman:

Pregnancy while you taking [*sic*] these drugs may expose your unborn child to significant hazards of deformity. If you are a woman, you are therefore strongly advised not to become pregnant while taking these drugs and, if you are sexually active, you must agree to use some form of barrier contraception (not the birth control pill) while you participate. If you do become pregnant while on this study, you must agree to immediately inform the Principal Investigator [name given], at [phone number given].

37. See *Mississippi University for Women v. Hogan,* 458 U.S. 718, 724 (1982). The FDA's role, through FDA 77–3040, of authorizing sex discrimination in drug testing constitutes state action sufficient to violate the equal protection clause of the federal Constitution. See, e.g., *West v. Atkins,* 487 U.S. 42, 56 (1988); *North Georgia Finishing, Inc. v. Di-Chem,* 419 U.S. 601 (1975).

38. See, e.g., *Frontiero v. Richardson,* 411 U.S. 677, 690 (1973).

39. See, e.g., *Planned Parenthood v. Casey,* 112 S. Ct. 2791 (1992).

40. *Id.*

41. The term "drug manufacturers" connotes investigators, sponsors, individuals, partnerships, corporations, associations, governmental agencies, scientific establishments, or organizational units thereof, or any other legal entity participating in the manufacture of drugs.

42. On July 22, 1993, the *Baltimore Sun* reported that the FDA acknowledged that drug companies may have liability concerns about the 1993 Guideline. Hoffman-LaRoche's Dr. Stots Reele stated, "It's not just a liability issue. There is a medical issue. We don't want to harm the fetus."

43. 21 U.S.C. 355.

44. See, e.g., 21 C.F.R. 314.50(d)(2)(iii).

45. See, e.g., *Chevron v. Natural Resources Defense Council,* 467 U.S. at 842–43 (if statute is silent, regulation must be based on a permissible construction of the statute); *American Trucking Ass'n v. United States,* 344 U.S. 298 (1953) (no requirement that authorizing statute specifically mention particular subject of regulation).

46. A 1992 report on the matter, mandated by Congress and conducted by the

General Accounting Office (GAO), found that 25 percent of drug companies deliberately do not recruit representative numbers of women as participants in any of their drug trials and more than 50 percent of drug companies claimed that they were unaware of the 1988 request by the federal government to recruit female drug trial participants.

47. In 1994, the author was appointed to the National Task Force on AIDS Drug Development. In January 1995, the Task Force unanimously recommended that the FDA publish the following regulations:

> *Recommendation 6a:* The Task Force recommends that the FDA amend existing regulations governing the Investigational New Drug (IND) and New Drug Application (NDA) process to require that a sponsor file gender accrual analysis in the annul IND report. In addition, for the NDA and the Product Licensing Application (PLA), the regulations will require sponsors to analyze clinical data by gender and assess potential differences between genders.
>
> *Recommendation 6c:* The Task Force recommends that the FDA amend the regulations defining circumstances under which it is appropriate to issue a clinical hold or terminate an IND to include instances where a trial sponsor imposes restrictions on the inclusion of women of childbearing potential in any phase of any clinical trial for life-threatening illnesses where there is no evidence of reproductive toxicities. The regulatory amendment should allow the FDA to employ these sanctions when there is evidence of reproductive toxicity but a less restrictive alternative than exclusion of women exists. If the FDA requests that women not be excluded and the exclusion continues, the FDA should first issue a clinical hold on the trial, and then, if the sponsor refuses to correct the exclusion of women, the FDA should force the sponsor to terminate the IND.
>
> *Recommendation 6e:* The Task Force recommends that the Public Health Service (PHS) develop a list of databanks, accessible to trial sponsors and the public, containing information on the known teratogenicity and mutagenicity of various drugs. [This recommendation was approved unanimously.]
>
> *Recommendation 6g:* The Task Force recommends that the Department of Health and Human Services (DHHS) amend its "Regulations Governing Human Subject Research" which limits research on fetuses and pregnant women. In particular, DHHS must eliminate the requirement that the father of the fetus must consent before a woman may participate in a clinical trial.

48. The language of 21 C.F.R. 312 and 314 should be interpreted to mandate the inclusion of results of by-gender analyses and animal reproduction studies. In 21 C.F.R. 312 subpart A "General Provisions" subheading "definitions and interpretations" of C.F.R. 312.3, preclinical testing should be included, and preclinical testing should be defined to include not only animal toxicology, as in how much of the drug is absorbed in the blood, how the substance is broken down chemically, the toxicity of the drug's metabolites, and the speed with which the drug is excreted from the body, but also by-gender analyses of all responses and results of the completed animal reproductive studies. The results of animal reproduction studies should also be included in subpart B "Investigational New Drug Application" under subheading "General Principles of the

IND" of 312.22(c) where it states that amendments should be supported by "additional information including the results of animal toxicology studies." The FDA could amend this to say, "including the results of animal reproduction studies." This would clarify extremely unclear language. Under 312.23(a)(5) "IND content and format" Section (5), the "Investigator's Brochure" should include a summary of the results of animal reproduction studies between subsections (ii) and (iii). The same information should be included in (8)(ii)(a) "nonclinical laboratory studies." In 314, governing New Drug Applications, 314.50(d)(2)(iii) "Content and Format of an Application-Nonclinical Pharmacology and Toxicology Section" states, "A section describing . . . studies, as appropriate, of the effects of the drug on reproduction and on the developing fetus." The regulations should make clear that "as appropriate" means "in all cases." Also, in 314.81(b)(2)(v) "other postmarketing reports—Annual Report—nonclinical laboratory studies," should include reproductive results as well as by-gender analyses.

49. Needless to say, drugs intended to treat persons with life threatening illnesses should be available to trial participants regardless of the mutagenic or teratogenic effects.

3

Caught in the Crossfire: Women and the Search for the Magic Bullet

Michelle Murrain

Michelle Murrain teaches biology and health issues at Hampshire College in the School of Natural Science. She is trained as a neurobiologist, and has been doing research on AIDS for several years, focusing primarily on women. Her recent work includes studies of opportunistic infections in women with AIDS and investigations of survival differences with AIDS in women and people of color. She also recently completed a study to look at how poverty might be related to HIV risk in Massachusetts. Michelle also has been active in community organizing around women-and-AIDS issues, and is presently cochair of the Western Massachusetts Women and AIDS Network, and she does training and workshops on these topics in the community.

Introduction

For quite a number of years, feminists have had an articulate voice in critiquing the method and application of scientific research. Especially eloquent has been the description of the ways in which science has studied the female body, and the problematic results of that study.[1] I have two goals in this essay. The first is to describe the situation regarding women and AIDS, and to describe a case study of research done on women that is deeply problematic, as well as the ways in which a combination of factors have come into play. The second is to use this example to encourage feminists and other scholars who study science to broaden their perspectives on the ways in which bias, not only by gender, but also bias in terms of "race," and political economy can influence and determine the path of scientific research.

Women and AIDS

It was quite some time before researchers admitted that women got AIDS, although there were AIDS cases in women from the beginning of the epidemic. When at last women were seen as potential people with AIDS, the first thought was how women could pass on the disease to others. This framing of women as "vectors" of HIV has been the dominant paradigm for research on women with AIDS, and although the amount of research on women and AIDS has increased greatly, this paradigm remains quite strong and continues to drive the majority of AIDS research done on women. It is important to note that the people that women might transmit the virus to (primarily their children) are considered "innocent victims."

At present, women are an increasing proportion of the new cases of AIDS in the United States (17 percent in 1994) and are at least half of cases worldwide. Thus, this research focus on women as vectors has broad impact on the lives and health of many women worldwide. Further, since clinical trials research in the United States (the primary research environment for testing of pharmacological treatments) on women has overfocused on decreasing vertical transmission of HIV (transmission from mother to infant), clinical information about the ways in which HIV and AIDS affects women differently and about potential differences in efficacy of drugs is not forthcoming as rapidly as is needed.

This is important and necessary research, because it is quite clear that women experience AIDS differently from men. Women get different sets of defined opportunistic infections,[2] and a host of gynecological infections[3] for which good treatment protocols need to be developed. However, to date there are no clinical trials that deal with these issues.

This is important to look at not only in terms of HIV, but in terms of the basic dearth of biomedical research on women. It has not been definitively found, for example that most pharmaceuticals work the same on women as they do on men, or that the side-effect profiles are similar. There is an inherent assumption that this is the case, but research on this issue is rarely carried out. Yet clearly this could potentially have serious impacts on women's health.

Who Are Women with AIDS?

It is important, before I continue, to make it clear what the population of women with AIDS is, and to suggest that the makeup of this population may have influenced the perceptions of and research around women and AIDS. Seventy-five percent of the women who have been diagnosed to date are women of color.[4] This proportion has remained relatively stable for most of the epidemic. Fifty-one percent are African American women, 22 percent Latinas (of various origins), and 1–2 percent Asian and Native American women. The majority of women with AIDS are poor, and many, but not most, are injection drug users. Many also have partners who are injection drug users.

In terms of risk, African American women are at sixteen times the risk of getting AIDS of White women, Latinas at eight times the risk, and Native American women twice the risk. Recent seroprevalence data suggests that this trend will continue. It is clear that people of color in general are at much higher risk for HIV infection, and poverty may be an important factor, beyond risk of injection drug use, in HIV risk.[5]

It is my argument that the makeup of the population of women with AIDS has affected the way in which the epidemic in women is framed. I have to wonder whether or not the racial and class characteristics of women with AIDS made it easier for the disease in women to be framed in the "vector" paradigm. Historically, poor people and people of color have often been perceived as the source of disease in our society.

AIDS Clinical Trials

As with basically all diseases that affect both men and women, the treatment of women with AIDS is based on the model of AIDS and HIV developed almost exclusively from research on men, even though, as I described above, it is known that women experience AIDS differently than men do. The lack of participation of women in AIDS clinical trials has been a particular bone of contention of women AIDS activists for quite some time. Until about 1992, the percentage of women involved in AIDS clinical trials was far less than their proportion of AIDS cases.[6] This disparity was not solely due to gender; people of color in general have had, and continue to have, problems accessing clinical trials.[7] This has a lot to do with overall access to health care facilities and the length of time that people of color survive with an AIDS diagnosis. Until recently, the majority of women of color were diagnosed at or very close to death. In the last few years, women have been able to participate in clinical trials at levels close to their representation of AIDS cases. However, a large proportion of that participation is in clinical trials that are not to their benefit, and not all of those clinical trials increase our understanding of how AIDS affects women, and how to treat women more specifically.

Only six clinical trials started so far as a part of the AIDS Clinical Trial Group (ACTG) focus entirely on women. There have been a number of smaller-scale trials of antifungal agents, most notably Fluconozole, for treatment of persistent vaginal yeast infections in HIV-positive women. The ACTG is the primary vehicle through which drugs gain approval as treatments. The first of these ACTG trials was a trial of the use of AZT in pregnant, asymptomatic, HIV-positive women to determine if AZT would decrease vertical transmission. This is the clinical trial I will look at in detail here. Another was a trial to determine whether the gp160 vaccine decreased vertical transmission in pregnant HIV-positive women. Two additional trials are similar to the AZT trial, determining whether using antivirals in women decreases vertical transmission. One of these focuses on women who are using methadone. Others are tests of AZT and specific immunoglobulins to see if those combinations reduce vertical transmission more than AZT alone. So, there have been few clinical trials to test treatments for known gynecological symptoms of AIDS and no clinical trials designed to determine if presently approved treatments (tested primarily on men) are as effective in women.

Thus, so far, the vast majority of the clinical trials that focus on women are (1) for pregnant and mostly asymptomatic women, and (2) not designed to help the women themselves, but to decrease vertical transmission. It is very important to put this in context: There is a range of rates at which HIV is transmitted from mother to infant. It has been seen to be as low as 10 percent and as high as 40 percent, but it appears that the standard estimate is 25 percent. Thus, all of these clinical trials are designed to reduce vertical transmission, even though basically three-quarters of infants will remain uninfected in any case, yet most if not all of the women will die of AIDS complications. This exemplifies the use of the "vector" paradigm in looking at women with AIDS. Further, the "success" of the first of these trials has spawned a whole set of legislative efforts to mandate testing in pregnant women, which has its own set of ethical and legal problems. In fact, mandatory testing will cause more problems than it solves, because women at risk will avoid testing by avoiding prenatal care, which will cause an increase in other problems, such as low birthweight, and may even cause an increase in transmission rates, since prenatal care is thought to be a factor in vertical transmission.

ACTG 076

ACTG 076 was a trial started in 1991 in a number of sites across the country, largely in urban areas in the Northeast, and again, the women in the trial were predominantly women of color. The results have recently been published.[8] Four hundred and seventy-seven women were recruited for this trial, of whom 391 were women of color (82 percent). These women had to be asymptomatic and in their second or third trimester of pregnancy. The trial was stopped in January 1994 because of the "early success" of the trial. This was a standard double-blind (meaning neither the patient, nor the person who gave the drug knew which group the patient was in), placebo-controlled trial. In the AZT arm, women were given AZT at 500 mg from either their fourteenth week (beginning of second trimester) or twenty-eighth week (beginning of third trimester). At the beginning of labor, they were given a dose of 2 mg per kg of body weight given intravenously for one hour, then 1 mg per kg of body weight during the rest of the birth process. The infant was given an AZT syrup for six weeks after birth. The rate of vertical transmission in the placebo arm was 25 percent. The rate in the AZT arm was 8 percent. This was hailed as a great success, got all sorts of press coverage as a "breakthrough," and was called one of the most important prevention successes to date. One can think of this somewhat differently, however. Without AZT, infants have a 75 percent or greater chance of being born uninfected, and AZT increases that to 92 percent. One could argue that this is a difference of 17 percent. But I guess that doesn't have the impact that saying vertical transmission is reduced by two-thirds, which is also true. Although it is true that reducing the number of infant infected by two-thirds is a laudable achievement, I'm still not quite convinced this is the breakthrough that everyone else seems to think. Transmission rates in Europe are significantly lower, sometimes as low as 13 percent.[9] The difference between 13 percent or 15 percent and 8 percent is not quite so dramatic. Serious consideration as to why rates are so low in Europe has not occurred, nor has research into how we could achieve those rates without pharmaceutical intervention. The ostensible purpose of this trial was to reduce vertical transmission, and thus decrease the number of infants who were getting AIDS and dying. This trial has a number of problematic aspects to it, which I will detail.

Reductionist Model

The first issue to deal with is the fact that this trial is based on a reductionist model of AIDS. The basic model of AIDS is this: HIV is the only causative factor. People get HIV through sex, sharing of intravenous drug works, or vertical transmission. HIV causes a progressive depletion of the immune system, which leads to AIDS. AZT specifically targets HIV, thus decreasing viral load, and decreasing vertical transmission. I think everyone at this point agrees that this model is too simplistic. This model does little to deal with the quite complex nature of the disease, or of vertical transmission. The reality of HIV and AIDS is much more complex than the standard model, and must involve some cofactors. Many basic scientists are engaged in this complexity to some degree, but this basic reductionist model still informs much of the epidemiological research and clinical trials at this point.

In looking at vertical transmission of AIDS, there are quite a few complex factors. It is not clear, for instance, how exactly the virus gets transmitted from women to their infants. It is thought that viral load is an important determining factor (thus treatment with AZT should help).[10] However, it has also been found that a variety of other factors may play quite important roles in vertical transmission.[11] There are a lot of complexities that are very slowly being looked at in terms of the determining factors of vertical transmission, and this trial really does nothing to increase that knowledge.

AZT Isn't for the Women, and It Isn't Fun

The AZT given to these women is not given to help them. It is not given to increase their T cells, or slow the progress of their disease, or increase their quality of life. These women are asymptomatic, and previous studies have suggested that AZT is not helpful in asymptomatic individuals. In fact, the dosage of AZT given to these women is larger than the dosage given to many people with full-blown AIDS. AZT is a toxic drug. AZT has been found to work in a very limited way for a limited time for a number of individuals with AIDS, although there is quite a bit of doubt that it is useful in the long run. It can have quite unfortunate and nasty side effects, which include peripheral neuropathy (damage to peripheral nerves, leading to sensory deficits in hands and feet), gastrointestinal problems, and severe anemia.

It is known that women will go through quite a lot to be mothers and will endure a lot for their children. Treating women who are asymptomatic with AZT to reduce vertical transmission asks these women to risk their own health and quality of life for the supposed "assurance" that their infant will be HIV negative. In fact, an infant has a 75 percent chance of being HIV-negative in any event. In addition, there are a variety of other methods which might reduce vertical transmission, such as counseling women at risk not to breast feed, counseling women who are further progressed in the disease not to continue the pregnancy, vaginal washing before birth, nutritional counseling, and others, all of which need intensive research. Now that AZT is the method of choice for reducing vertical transmission, research on these other methods and counseling for women about the kinds of things which could reduce the chances of an infant being infected will not be as aggressively pursued.

Another important point here. I've spoken to one woman, and heard about several HIV-positive women who, based on the hype around the results of this trial, now say that they want to get pregnant. This is something that they wouldn't have thought of before because of the possibility of passing HIV to their infant. In one woman's words: "I just wanted to feel like a normal woman again."

AZT Is Problematic for the Fetus as Well

Although my arguments are focused on women, on how the research has been biased, and on how the fallout from this clinical trial is problematic for women with HIV and AIDS, I think it is essential to outline a problem which in fact may end up to be quite important in terms of this trial and widespread subsequent treatment of women and fetuses with AZT.

As I mentioned above, AZT is a toxic drug. The way AZT works is to inhibit the action of a specific viral enzyme called reverse transcriptase. The drug has the effect of decreasing the replication of the virus by inhibiting this enzyme. AZT also has some nonspecific DNA inhibitory activity, which has the effect of slowing down the replication of all cells in the body. The cells most often affected by this are cells which rapidly reproduce, such as blood cells, which is why people on AZT treatment very often get anemia. In fact, AZT has been exploited recently for its so-called "cyto-static potency" (cyto = cell, static = stop) and was developed initially as an anticancer drug.

So, one might ask, what would such a drug do to a rapidly developing fetus, whose rate of cell replication is quite high, especially considering that the development of many aspects of the fetus is carefully timed? Very few researchers and people involved in AIDS treatment of pregnant women seem to be asking that very important question. In fact, it has become clear that this author is virtually the only scientist willing to publicly and vocally question this strategy for reducing vertical transmission. No physicians have, to my knowledge done the same, although there was a questioning editorial in the prestigious medical journal *Lancet* that has been all but ignored.[12]

The company which developed and now markets AZT (also called zidovudine; the brand name is Retrovir®) is Burrows Wellcome. In the merger mania of the nineties, Glaxo and Burrows Wellcome have merged to form Glaxo Wellcome. From information gathered from a Freedom of Information Act request from the FDA, it is clear that Burrows Wellcome did some very incomplete research to look at the teratogenic effects of AZT once it was determined that this drug might be tried as a method of reducing vertical transmission from mother to infant. They did a number of tests on rabbits and rats to determine the possible teratogenicity (the creation of birth defects of various types) of AZT. The tests are incomplete for a variety of reasons: testing only third trimester treatment of AZT (many mothers are given AZT at the second trimester), treatment protocols involving only one day of dosing with AZT, tests looking only at "skeletal abnormalities" (simply looking at gross morphology—whether there are the right numbers of fingers and toes, etc.), and very little histopathology (fine morphology—what the cells look like in various organs).

Interestingly enough, although I would argue that the testing is far too incomplete to suggest that AZT could be tried in pregnant humans safely, the little data that is there is suggestive of possible teratogenic effects. In fact, Burrows Wellcome's own pharmacologist says, "Under the conditions of these studies, AZT was embryotoxic and fetotoxic for rats at 150 and 450 mg/kg per day." This was the dosage given to the rats, and though quite high, again, Burrow's Wellcome's own pharmacologist says, "AZT serum levels in these animals are much higher than those attained in humans, but because of species differences in AZT toxicity, the high serum levels in the test animals does not mean that these studies overestimate the potential effects of AZT in humans." Further, independent testing of AZT given to pregnant rabbits suggested that there were problems with the viability of the offspring. Burrows Wellcome attempted to replicate that study, found some of the same effects, but at a lower (and not statistically significant) level, and stated that the differences in the results must have been due to "animal husbandry."

Of particular concern is nervous system development, which is quite dependent upon a very carefully orchestrated and timed set of developmental events. Decreasing the number of cells produced in the nervous system or the rate of that production may have severe effects on later cognitive development. In fact, other DNA synthesis inhibitors are known to have dramatic effects on the cellular architecture of the nervous system, which likely has severe behavioral effects. In fact, Burrows Wellcome's studies do suggest some behavioral effects in rats treated with AZT during development.

The Profit Motive

It is very important to look at the economic context of drug development in general and AIDS drug development in particular. The way in which the economic system drives scientific research and treatment has a clear influence on women. Drug development, especially of the most promising pharmaceutical therapies, is predominantly controlled by drug companies, whose primary purpose is to make a profit. Testing for specific treatments is only undertaken if a drug has profit potential. There are some exceptions to this, primarily in cases where the federal government subsidizes drug development for diseases with low prevalence. These are exceptions that I would argue prove the rule.

There are a number of drugs which are thought to show promise for AIDS, but because they are unpatentable, and therefore, unprofitable, they are not being very aggressively researched, and activists have had a very hard time getting any testing done. An example is the drug dinitrochlorobenzene (DNCB), which has been used by people with AIDS for years and which has shown some promise. Because it is a simple organic compound, and thus not patentable, no drug companies have been willing to sponsor clinical trials, and such sponsorship is critical in getting a trial started. AIDS has not been the only example of this. The ability (or lack thereof) of drug companies to make a profit has affected the development of birth control options for years. The profit motive has influenced a variety of other areas of women's health as well, such as the development of reproductive technologies.

In terms of AZT, the decrease in vertical transmission is now hailed as one of the best "successes" of AZT, and there are efforts underway to export this treatment to other countries. Of course, this provides a quite lucrative market for Burrows Wellcome, and clearly their interest in the potential use of their drug AZT for this purpose is the underlying factor for why such shoddy research was done to determine possible teratogenic effects. Again, this also continues the framing of women as "vectors" of HIV.

Conclusion

A reductionist paradigm for AIDS, a "vector" paradigm in looking at women with AIDS, the combination of race and gender bias, and a system driven by the profit motive combine together to form a particularly precarious situation for women who are HIV-positive and any children they might choose to bear. I think it incumbent on us as feminist critics of science that we begin, like our feminist counterparts in other fields, to closely examine not only gender bias in scientific research, but the intersection of race, political-economy, and gender issues in research that deals with women's bodies.

NOTES

1. Quite good work in this area has been done by M. Lowe and R. Hubbard, *Woman's Nature: Rationalizations of Inequality* (New York: Pergamon Press, 1983); Ruth Bleier, *Science and Gender: A Critique of Biology and Its Theories on Women* (New York:

Pergamon Press, 1984); and Emily Martin, *The Woman in the Body: A Cultural Analysis of Reproduction* (Boston: Beacon Press, 1987).

2. M. Murrain, "Different Rates of Opportunistic Infections in Women with AIDS," *Journal of Women's Health* 2 (1993): 243–50; and C.C.J. Carpenter, K.H. Mayer, A. Fisher, M.B. Desai, and L. Durand, "Natural History of Acquired Immunodeficiency Syndrome in Women in Rhode Island," *American Journal of Medicine* 86 (1989): 771–75.

3. R.P. Brettle and C.L.S. Leen, "The Natural History of HIV and AIDS in Women," *AIDS* 5 (1991): 1283–92.

4. Centers for Disease Control, HIV/AIDS Surveillance Report, 1994.

5. L.E. Krueger et al., "Poverty and HIV Seropositivity: The Poor are More Likely to be Infected," *AIDS* 4, no. 8 (1990): 811–14; and M. Murrain and T. Barker, "Poverty and HIV: The Unexplored Link" (manuscript in preparation).

6. Joyce Korvick, "Trends in Federally Sponsored Clinical Trials," in *Until the Cure,* ed. Ann Kurth (New Haven: Yale University Press, 1993), 94–103.

7. C. Hunter et al., "Selection Factors in Clinical Trials: Results from the Community Clinical Oncology Program Physicians Patient Log," *Cancer Treatment Reports* 71 (1987): 549–65.

8. E. Conner et al., "Reduction of Maternal-Infant Transmission of Human Immunodeficiency Virus Type 1 with Zidovudine Treatment," *New England Journal of Medicine* 331, no. 18 (1994): 1173–80.

9. A.E. Ades, M. L. Newell, C. S. Peckham, "Children Born to Women with HIV-1 Infection: Natural History and Risk of Transmission," *Lancet* 337 (1991): 253–60.

10. L. Boylan and Z. Stein, "The Epidemiology of HIV Infection in Children and Their Mothers—Vertical Transmission," *Epidemiologic Reviews* 13 (1991): 143–77.

11. Ibid.

12. "ZDV for Mother, Fetus and Child: Hope or Poison?" *Lancet* 344 (1994): 207–9.

4

Adolescent Underrepresentation in Clinical AIDS Research

Kate Barnhart

Kate Barnhart is a recent graduate of Hampshire College in Amherst, Massachusetts. She has served as Co-Coordinator of ACT UP/New York's Youth Education LifeLine committee for five years and has been arrested several times during protests at the New York City Board of Education. She is a founding member of New York City's Coalition of Peer Educators, and spends her summers training young felons to be HIV/AIDS peer educators. She sits on the Board of Directors of the National Child Rights Alliance, where she infuses AIDS activism into the youth liberation agenda and coordinates the annual Youth Summit conference. Her Division III research consists of interviewing HIV+ adolescents about their experiences with access to health care and clinical AIDS research.

What I don't find in my doctors is compassion, is understanding. I get this judgmental wall as I walk into the doctors' office, like: "Oh, here comes this fucked up kid that fucked up." I don't need that, especially if I'm going to try to sit in your office and get advice and if your advice is already coming from a jaded point of view or a biased point of view.   Ayisa Kennedy, 22 years old, HIV+

Despite rapidly rising HIV infection rates among adolescents, most resources are directed at primary prevention for uninfected youth rather than addressing the needs of those adolescents who are already infected with HIV. The number of young people who are currently infected is already alarmingly large, and more are infected every day. The World Health Organization estimates that half of the 14 million HIV-infected individuals in the world were infected while they were between the ages of fifteen and twenty-four.[1] In the U.S., about one-fifth of the 441,528 AIDS cases that had been reported to the CDC as of December 1994 were probably infected as adolescents.[2] Unfortunately, the commitment of resources to combating adolescent HIV infection lags way behind the infection rates. In May 1992 the U.S. House Select Committee on Children, Youth and Families estimated that less than 5 percent of the current federal AIDS budget funded research, programs, or services that benefited teens.[3] Primary prevention programs were included in this estimate, so the actual amount of money going to services for HIV-infected teens was just a fraction of that amount. As a result of this neglect, halfway through the second decade of this epidemic there is still very little known about HIV infection in adolescents. The limited information that does exist is based primarily on studies of hemophilic youth, who are not representative of most adolescents with HIV infection because they are primarily white males with access to health care.

This chapter will focus on one of the most invisible groups in the AIDS epidemic: HIV-infected adolescents. In this chapter, I will outline some of the gaps in knowledge about HIV infection in adolescence. These gaps include information about the epidemiology of HIV in adolescents, the natural history of HIV in adolescents, and correct drug dosage during puberty. I will then address some of the issues that contribute to the exclusion of adolescents from AIDS research, particularly issues around capacity to consent, access to care, and stereotypes of adolescents as noncompliant. In the final section, I will discuss how the historic exclusion of women from AIDS research combines with the exclusion of adolescents to create formidable barriers to understanding HIV infection in young women.

Essential to any discussion of adolescents is an agreement on what the term means. There is quite a bit of variation in how adolescence is defined from institution to institution. This creates problems because data collected by institutions that use different definitions of adolescence are not comparable. The American Academy of Pediatrics, the Centers for Disease Control and Prevention, and the World Health Organization consider adolescence to range from 13 to 21, 13 to 19, and 13 to 24, respectively. I have chosen to focus on young people between the ages of thirteen and eighteen in this article because this group has historically been the most neglected as a consequence of its falling above the pediatric cut off point at age thirteen and below the age of eighteen required for inclusion in adult research.

Another consideration that must be acknowledged in any discussion of adolescent HIV infection is that adolescents are not a homogeneous community; they are as diverse as the population of the world. In addition, there are subgroups of HIV-infected adolescents that each have their own needs and issues. These groups include adolescent hemophiliacs, chemical-dependent youth, ethnic and racial minority youth, sexual minority youth, homeless youth, sexually abused youth, and young women. A new distinct subgroup of HIV-infected adolescent long-term survivors of perinatal infection is beginning to be recognized. This group will require special attention as advances in clinical care enable more and more perinatally infected children to live into their teens and beyond. Issues this group may face include multisystem illness, growth failure, delayed puberty, and social isolation.[4] Undoubtedly, there will be major physical and psychosocial differences between young people who enter adolescence with HIV infection and those who acquire it during or after puberty.

Many of the gaps in knowledge about adolescent HIV infection are very similar to those that are just beginning to be addressed in women. Aspects of adolescent HIV infection about which little is known include epidemiology; natural history; pharmacokinetics and proper dosing schedules for anti-HIV and antiopportunistic infection medication for people in Tanner stages two, three, and four (during puberty); adolescent-normal lab values for markers of disease progression and toxicity; and rates of adverse reactions to commonly used prophylactic and antiviral medications. In addition, disease-stage classification systems, such as those promulgated by Walter Reed and the CDC, are not based on adolescent data and are therefore not necessarily as relevant for adolescents as they are for adults.

Epidemiology

The limited data available on the epidemiology of HIV infection among adolescents in the U.S. clearly indicate that both incidence and prevalence rates vary widely from community to community. In order to clarify the extent of the problem among adolescents, studies of both the incidence of HIV infection among adolescents and the prevalence of HIV in specific subgroups are needed. It is critical that this data be collected so that HIV services can be directed to areas in need.

Before further epidemiological research is undertaken, researchers should agree on a universal definition of adolescence so that data will be comparable from study to study.

Natural History

The natural history of HIV infection in adolescents is largely unknown, although some clinicians have suggested that it resembles the course of HIV infection in adults rather than children. Some studies of hemophilic youth have suggested that disease progression may be slower in people infected in adolescence.[5] In addition, developmental differences in the immune system at various stages of puberty may have an impact on both the natural history and infectivity of HIV.[6] Although it has been clear since the beginning of the epidemic that adolescents are a population at risk of HIV infection, the first natural history study of HIV infection in adolescence, ACTG 220, began enrolling in early 1993, twelve years into the epidemic. Since it was designed as a long-term, prospective study, ACTG 220 still has not produced any published data. Studies are needed to determine rates of opportunistic infections and cancers, as well as the role of cofactors in progression from HIV to AIDS in various populations of adolescents. Adolescent-specific values for markers of drug toxicity and HIV disease progression are largely unknown. For instance, CD4 cell counts are widely used to monitor HIV disease progression, but normal values during puberty have not been established.[7] Research is also needed to determine the impact of HIV infection on cognitive development in adolescents.

In addition to influencing the natural history of HIV infection, the physical and psychosocial changes which characterize adolescence may have an effect on the dosage, efficacy, and side effects of medications. The physical changes associated with puberty include several factors such as changes in body composition and organ function that may impact the optimum dose, drug half-life, and drug response of various prophylactic and antiviral medications. Organ function changes associated with puberty include changing activity of liver microsomal activities which could affect drug metabolism.[8] Uncertainty about dosing schedules for adolescents is not limited to HIV-related drugs. Michael Cohen, a professor and deputy chairman of the Department of Pediatrics at Albert Einstein College of Medicine and the Director of Adolescent Medicine at Montefiore Hospital, observes that "in spite of the several biologic factors just identified, the current approach to clinical drug dosage regimens in adolescent patients remains one of trial and error."[9]

Clinical Trials

Despite these major gaps in knowledge about adolescent HIV infection, the history of adolescent AIDS research has been one of neglect and exclusion. For the first eight years of the epidemic, young people between the ages of thirteen and eighteen were excluded from the clinical trials in which antiviral medications were developed because they were considered too old for pediatric trials and too young for adult trials. Although the trials were open to adolescents beginning in 1989, the few adolescents who enrolled were primarily hemophilic males. Underenrollment has continued to be a problem even with the establishment, in 1992, of seven clinical trial sites focussed on adolescents. As of September 1995, 95 of the 161 (59 percent) clinical trials listed in the AIDS Clinical Trials Information Service database were open to adolescents.[10] Although recently adolescents have been eligible to participate in more studies than they once were, many studies remain closed, and adolescents are not actively recruited even for those trials that are willing to include them. Adolescents are still not the focus of most studies, and even the few studies designed for adolescents tend to be underenrolled. The reasons for this, which will be discussed in greater detail, are a complex combination of physical needs and psychosocial issues. The physical needs include transportation and child care while the psychosocial issues include fears about confidentiality and deep suspicion of the medical establishment, especially in communities of color.

As of September 1, 1995, adolescents constituted only 1.4 percent of people enrolled in AIDS Clinical Group Trials.[11] The reasons for this are complex and involve societal attitudes about adolescents, legal issues around adolescents' capacity to consent, and adolescents' overall lack of access to health care.

Stereotypes of Adolescents

Stereotypes of adolescents play a major role in their exclusion from AIDS research. Researchers are often reluctant to design trials specifically for adolescents because of perceptions that adolescents are difficult to reach and frequently noncompliant with medical regimens. Similar stereotypes are also used to explain adolescent underenrollment in trials. Although adolescent psychology undoubtedly plays a role in trial enrollment, it is too frequently invoked while other issues, such as geographic accessibility, child care availability, and patient education are overlooked.

Compliance problems are one of the most common myths used to justify exclusion of adolescents from research. The societal construction of adolescence as a time of irresponsible, risk-taking behavior with little or no regard to consequences has caused adolescent noncompliance to be taken as a given although, as Michael Cohen points out, there is no data to suggest that adolescents are any less compliant with medication regimens than other populations:

> Until very recently most health professionals viewed the therapeutic drug taking behavior of adolescents as irresponsible or at best marginally appropriate for age. No data existed to support the contention that adolescents were any less compliant in their drug taking patterns than self-medicating adults or mothers asked to complete a specific treatment plan for their infants. . . . Anecdotal observations by clinicians who devote a significant amount of effort to the care of adolescents consider their abilities to receive drug information and drug taking instructions, accept and fill prescriptions, properly use medications at home, and return for periodic reassessment and prescription renewal to be no better or worse than those found in other age segments of the population.[12]

Compliance is a complex issue with a variety of contributing factors that remain largely unexplored. Although research into the determinants of compliance, especially among adolescents, is still in its infancy, several researchers have examined these issues. These include Iris Litt, Associate Professor of Pediatrics at Stanford University School of Medicine, and Walter Cuskey, Consulting Professor of Sociology at the same institution. Litt and Cuskey observe in their review of issues involved in medication compliance during adolescence that a great deal remains to be learned about compliance in general, and adolescent compliance specifically:

> The presumption of adolescent noncompliance has, until recently, precluded its thoughtful investigation. Are all adolescents noncompliant? Is noncompliance related to the characteristics of illness or features of the medical regimen? Does the adolescent's level of physical or psychosocial development influence compliance?[13]

Although there is still a lot to be learned about compliance, the history of community involvement in AIDS research suggests it is an issue that is very closely linked to access to care and trial design. People who view participation in a trial as their only option for primary care are likely to be less committed to following the trial protocol. Similarly, people participating in trials with a placebo control group may be tempted to determine whether they are receiving medication or placebo or to take steps to increase their chances of receiving active drug.

There are a variety of suggestions in the literature that might be adopted by investigators committed to adolescent AIDS research and concerned about compliance. Litt and Cuskey suggest that encouraging youth to be independent in terms of accessing health care may help improve compliance. They also note that satisfaction with both the care provided and the person providing the care were important determinants of compliance in their study.[14] Another recommendation for improving compliance comes from the Adolescent AIDS Program at Montefiore Medical Center, where they utilize a "one-stop shopping" approach that allows clients to receive multiple services at the same time in the same place.[15] This "one-stop shopping" program design model makes it possible for clients to receive medical services, counseling, and social services at one facility, eliminating the multiple conflicting appointments that are characteristic of AIDS services at many institutions. This is particularly important for clients with daytime obligations such as school, work, and child care. It eases the financial burden of paying for transportation to and from appointments, it allows clients to receive all their services in a setting they are familiar with, and it facilitates communication between professionals providing services to the same client.

Capacity to Consent

Another issue that contributes to researchers' reluctance to recruit adolescents actively is the legal confusion surrounding minors' capacity to consent. This issue is particularly important for HIV-related services, since the sensitive nature of many issues associated with HIV may make adolescents reluctant to disclose their HIV status to their parent(s). Laws regarding capacity to consent vary greatly from state to state and change frequently. Furthermore, in any given state there are three components of HIV care which may be addressed by separate laws: HIV testing and counseling, HIV treatment, and participation in research. Although, in some states, this separation means that there are statutes specifically authorizing minors to consent to HIV testing but not for treatment, the status of a minor with regard to HIV testing and/or treatment is often a precedent for whether minors will be able to consent to participate in research. One of the determining factors in whether an adolescent can consent to testing and treatment for HIV is that state's classification of HIV. All fifty states allow minors to consent to diagnosis and treatment of STDs without parental notification. Although this would seem to imply that minors can consent to HIV testing and treatment in every state, it is important to note that not all states classify HIV as an STD. In states that do not consider HIV an STD, minors may still have the capacity to consent to HIV testing because some states authorize minors to consent to diagnosis and treatment of communicable, contagious, or infectious diseases.[16] As of 1993, New York was one of sixteen states that had statutes specifically authorizing minors to consent to HIV testing.[17]

Factors that determine whether an adolescent will have the right to consent independently to participate in research in any given state may include the type of research, procedures, and risk involved, the maturity of the adolescent in question, and the adolescent's living situation. Most states allow providers to make decisions about an adolescent's capacity to consent on a case-by-case basis using a psychosocial determination of an adolescent's maturity. This puts providers on somewhat tenuous legal ground, because determining whether a minor is "mature" is a great deal more subjective than using chronological age. It does, however, increase minors' access to health care, especially since age of consent is essentially arbitrary. For instance, in one study, of sixty-seven pediatric hospitals in the U.S., only thirteen used chronological age as a yardstick for capacity to consent. The ages used by those thirteen ranged from five years to fifteen years, with seven years used by four hospitals and twelve years by three.[18]

A. S. Rogers, L. D'Angelo, and D. Futterman, respectively, from the Pediatric, Adolescent and Maternal AIDS Branch at the National Institute of Child Health and Human Development, cochair, and chair of the Adolescent Scientific Committee of the Pediatric AIDS Clinical Trials Group, have observed that the legal complexities around capacity to consent have a negative impact on the inclusion of adolescents in research:

> While many factors contribute to the underrepresentation of adolescents in community and clinical research proportional to their morbidity, one clear barrier results from the nebulous legal status of adolescents to consent to participate in research and the broad spectrum of interpretations of federal guidelines by local institutional review boards.[19]

Access to Care

Capacity to consent is just one of several issues that have made adolescents one of the populations in the U.S. with the least access to health care. Issues of payment for care, confidentiality, and disenfranchisement, as well as a lack of providers trained in adolescent medicine also contribute to the exclusion of adolescents from the health care system. Access-to-care issues are particularly significant for HIV-infected adolescents. Staff at the Adolescent AIDS Program of Montefiore Hospital estimate that only 5 percent of New York City's infected youth are in care.[20] The rest are either unaware of their HIV status or unable to access care. Young people with HIV not only face a variety of barriers when trying to access care, but interlinking ones as well: the issues of consent and confidentiality intersect with the problem of paying for care. For young people, issues of payment and disclosure are intricately linked because those adolescents who are covered by private health insurance are mainly covered as dependents under their parents' policies, making it difficult for them to receive services without their parents' knowledge and/or consent. New York State, for instance, has no independent Medicare program for youth under twenty-one who have not disclosed their HIV status to their parents.[21] In 1991, the Office of Technology Assessment found that one out of seven adolescents had no access to health insurance and one in three poor adolescents were not eligible for Medicaid.[22] In order to make health care accessible to young people, providers need to incorporate sliding fee scales and assistance with applying for benefits into health care delivery programs. This is especially important because adolescents are less likely to be familiar with the health care and related benefits systems than adults.[23]

Another barrier faced by young people seeking HIV care is the extreme lack of providers with knowledge of both adolescent medicine and HIV. Furthermore, groups of adolescents with special issues, such as sexual minority youth, face additional difficulty finding providers who are sensitive to their needs.

Young Women

Adolescents are not the only population who lack access to health care, nor are they the only group that has been systematically excluded from AIDS research. People of color, poor people, and women are just a few of the many communities whose marginalization has made them invisible to the people allocating resources for AIDS research and services. But these are not distinct groups: one person can be a member of multiple disenfranchised communities, compounding the difficulty in accessing care. An example of this is the intersection of age, gender, and ethnicity which renders young women one of the groups at the most risk of infection, as well as one of the most invisible groups in AIDS research. The long tradition of excluding women of reproductive age from clinical trials compounds the reluctance of researchers to recruit adolescents actively. This combination of factors leads to an extreme lack of information about the effects of HIV and medications on women's bodies in general, and young women's bodies in particular. To date, most of the limited information available about the course of HIV infection in adolescents is based on studies of hemophiliacs, who are overwhelmingly male because hemophilia is a sex-linked genetic disorder. The main types of trials young women are aggressively recruited for are those involving pregnancy. These trials focus not on the women, but on their infants, and therefore do not provide any useful data about HIV in adolescent women. The ignorance about HIV infection in adolescent women is especially appalling since, on average, young women are infected at earlier ages than men.[24] Young women are being infected at rates that, in some areas, equal or exceed those of their male counterparts. For instance, Job Corps data show higher rates of HIV infection among female sixteen- and seventeen-year-old applicants than among their male counterparts in the southeastern United States.[25] Young women of color, like their adult counterparts, have been disproportionately affected by the epidemic. Seventy percent of female adolescents with AIDS are racial or ethnic minority youth.[26] These young women bear the additional burden of institutionalized racism in both health care and AIDS research.

Conclusion

Despite the rapidly increasing number of adolescents infected with HIV, little is known about the clinical picture of HIV infection in this group. Areas in need of further research include the epidemiology of HIV in adolescents, the natural history of HIV in adolescents, "adolescent-normal" values for markers of toxicity and progression, and drug dosing schedules during puberty.

Stereotypes about teenagers that have historically contributed to their exclusion from research need to be overcome, as do access-to-care issues that prevent adolescents from participating in research. Issues of consent, disclosure, confidentiality, and payment need to be clearly addressed so that adolescents can both receive treatment for HIV infection and participate in research without parental consent or knowledge. Research on adolescent HIV infection needs to include adequate representation of all the populations of youth infected by HIV, particularly young women and racial, ethnic, and sexual minorities.

NOTES

1. M. Goldsmith, "'Invisible' Epidemic Now Becoming Visible as HIV/AIDS Pandemic Reaches Adolescents," *Journal of the American Medical Association* 270.1 (1993): 16–19; 18.

2. CDC AIDS Hotline, personal communication, Sept. 15, 1995. 3. House Select Committee on Children, Youth and Families, *A Decade of Denial: Teens and AIDS in America*, 1–394.

3. House Select Committee on Children, Youth and Families, *A Decade of Denial: Teens and AIDS in America*, 1–394.

4. D. Futterman and K. Hein, "Medical Management of Adolescents with HIV Infection," in *Pediatric AIDS: The Challenge of HIV Infection in Infants, Children and Adolescents*, eds. P. Pizzo and C.M. Wilfert (Baltimore: Williams and Wilkins, 1994), 757–72; 761.

5. J.M. Jason, J.S. Green, R.C. Holman et al., "HIV Infection in Hemophiliac Children," *Pediatrics* 82 (1988): 565–70; 569.

6. K. Hein, "Commentary on Adolescent Acquired Immune Deficiency Syndrome," *Journal of Pediatrics* 114.4 (1989): 144–49; 147.

7. D. Futterman and K. Hein, "Medical Care of HIV-Infected Adolescents," *AIDS Clinical Care* 4.12 (1992): 95–98; 98.

8. Hein 1989, 148.

9. M.I. Cohen, "Clinical Pharmacology and Adolescence," *Pediatric Clinics of North America* 27.1 (1980): 45–51; 48.

10. AIDS Clinical Trials Information Service, personal communication, Sept. 15, 1995.

11. AIDS Clinical Trials Information Service, personal communication, Sept. 19, 1995.

12. Cohen 1980, 49.

13. I. Litt and W. Cuskey, "Compliance with Medical Regimens during Adolescence," *Pediatric Clinics of North America* 27.1 (1980): 3–13; 3.

14. Litt and Cuskey 1980, 10.

15. R. Conviser, "Serving Young People at Risk for HIV Infection," in *Case Studies of Adolescent-Focused HIV Prevention and Service Delivery Programs* (Newark: National Pediatric HIV Resource Center, 1993), 59–66; 60.

16. A. English, "Expanding Access to HIV Services for Adolescents: Legal and Ethical Issues," in *Adolescents and AIDS: A Generation in Jeopardy,* ed. R. DiClemente (Knobbier Park, Calif.: Sage, 1992), 262–82.

17. T.A. DiLorenzo, D.M. Abramo, K. Hein, G.S. Clare, R. Dell, and N. Shaffer, "The Evaluation of Targeted Outreach in an Adolescent HIV/AIDS Program," *Journal of Adolescent Health* 13 (1993): 301–6; 302.

18. J.H. Pearn, "The Child and Clinical Research," *Lancet* (1984): 510.

19. A.S. Rogers, L. D'Angelo, and D. Futterman, "Guidelines for Adolescent Participation in Research: Current Realities and Possible Resolutions," *IRB: A Review of Human Subjects Research* 16.4 (1994): 1–6; 1.

20. Conviser 1993, 59.

21. Conviser 1993, 61.

22. DiLorenzo et al. 1993.

23. DiLorenzo et al. 1993, 302.

24. K. Hein, "Getting Real about HIV in Adolescents," *American Journal of Public Health* 83.4 (1993): 492–94; 492.

25. H. Kunins, K. Hein, D. Futterman, E. Tapley, and A. Elliott, "Guide to Adolescent HIV/AIDS Program Development, Module One: Epidemiology," *Journal of Adolescent Health* 14.5 (1993): 4S–15S; 8S.

26. House Select Committee on Children, Youth and Families, 1992.

5

Lesbians and the Medical Profession: HIV/AIDS and the Pursuit of Visibility

Nancy Goldstein

Nancy Goldstein, coeditor of this anthology, is an interdisciplinary scholar with a strong interest in the politics of biomedical research, public policy, and health care. She currently directs tutorials and senior theses for students in the Harvard University Women's Studies Program.

In the United States, both self-identified lesbians and women who have sex with women have traditionally been represented as no-risk or low-risk groups within standard AIDS medical discourse on those rare occasions when they have been acknowledged at all—and typically, little effort is made to distinguish between the two.[1] But this perfunctory clean bill of health reveals less about their actual at-risk status for HIV than it does about the traditional medical establishment's systemic failure to understand or address lesbian health issues in a thorough, informed manner. The myth of lesbian immunity from the AIDS epidemic was conceived, and continues to be disseminated, in an information vacuum that has no substantial basis in medical research at its core.[2] It has been constituted by a tendency on the part of medical researchers and clinicians alike to confuse sexual identity and behavior.[3] It has been authorized by the failure of the Centers for Disease Control and Prevention (CDC), which compile national surveillance data on persons infected with HIV, to include female-to-female transmission as a risk-exposure category in their AIDS case-reporting protocol, to define "lesbian" in a reasonable manner, or to collect data on what other smaller surveys show to be substantial numbers of HIV-infected women who have sex with women.

The myth of lesbian immunity has been sustained by misconceptions regarding lesbian identity and sexuality per se, and by the sheer lack of large-scale national research projects in the U.S. to gather information about women's health in general, let alone any project that focuses specifically on women's sexuality and drug-using histories.[4] (In the late eighties, one CDC physician remarked publicly that it was not necessary to study lesbians because "lesbians don't have much sex.")[5] The myth of lesbian immunity has been fostered by the inability or unwillingness of women who have sex with women to access health care, whether because of financial constraints, fears about disclosing same-sex sexual behavior to health care providers, a mistaken sense of invulnerability to diseases usually associated with reproduction and heterosexual sex, or some combination of all of these factors. It has been compounded by the failure of drug treatment programs and other AIDS education and outreach efforts to identify and target populations of women who have sex with women, whether in health care settings, community centers, prisons, homeless shelters, on college campuses, or through public transportation billboard campaigns.

The exclusion of women who have sex with women from most aspects of AIDS discourse, including research, education and prevention programs, publications and conferences is statistically sanctioned and perpetuated by the CDC's AIDS case-reporting protocol, which bars women who have sex with women entirely from its risk categories, employs hierarchical and mutually-exclusive categories for the attribution and distribution of cases, and makes no distinction between sexual behavior and identity. In 1991, Rebecca Cole and Sally Cooper were among the first critics to point out the intersection between the (then) CDC's methodology, its ideology, and the medical construction of the no-risk nonlesbian as a nonsubject:

> The CDC uses a hierarchy of exposure categories to determine HIV transmission date of AIDS cases in the U.S. If a woman has more than one possible exposure, she will be categorized by the highest risk only. . . . The CDC's hierarchy of exposure for women is as follows: 1. Intravenous drug use. 2. Recipient of blood products. 3. Heterosexual contact with an HIV-infected partner (or having specific risk for HIV). 4. No identified risk. . . . Female to female transmission is not classified as a possible exposure category in CDC surveillance data. Even though a case of female-to-female transmission was reported as early as 1984, such cases are counted in the "no identified risk" category. It is important to note that the percentage of "no identified risk" for women is *double* that of men. Clearly less is known about women's risk than about men's risk. (18)[6]

In the five years since Cole and Cooper published their article, "Lesbian Exclusion from HIV/AIDS Education: Ten Years of Low-Risk Identity and

High-Risk Behavior," the CDC has modified its "no identified risk" category, first to "other," and most recently to "other/risk not reported or identified." But what remains constant here is the disproportionate percentage of women in that category as compared to men and the ways in which the numbers keep growing: as of December 1994, 15 percent of women's cases were categorized this way, compared to 8 percent of men's cases; as of December 1995, the figures were 22 percent for women and 13 percent for men.[7]

The CDC's relegation of all cases with no possible risk factors other than female-to-female transmission to the very category of "other" serves as a paradigmatic gesture in a larger process of exiling women who have sex with women to the outback of AIDS discourse. But an equally important component of the CDC's structurally-predetermined erasure of women who have sex with women is their policy of consigning all cases with multiple risk factors to the single (allegedly) highest risk category. It insures that the statistics being compiled will confirm the medical community's earliest assumptions about risk factors, risk groups, and transmission routes. Rebecca Young, a Ph.D. candidate in sociomedical sciences at Columbia University, and her colleagues explain that "Cases with multiple risks are assigned to transmission categories based on epidemiological distribution of early AIDS cases in the U.S., with those *populations* in which the most AIDS cases were identified proxying for *transmission routes* that are then assumed to be most effective/risky."[8] The resulting reportage strategy is tautological, "preferentially assigning cases to categories deemed as 'more likely routes of transmission' (thereby inflating the number of cases in these categories), then asserting that these routes are more likely *because* of the greater number of cases in these categories." Ultimately, the CDC reportage strategy "actively seeks to *rule out* woman-to-woman transmission, while it seeks to *prove* transmission by routes that it has listed as more likely." In the July 1995 CDC report on women, children, and HIV/AIDS, the text confidently reports that while "An additional 19% were initially reported with no specific HIV exposure. . . . Historically, when these cases are investigated, it is found that most of these women—66%—have been exposed through heterosexual sex."[9] What it fails to describe is the mechanism whereby CDC methodology insures this conclusion.

The CDC's data-collection methodology fails to take into account the fact that self-definition depends upon a vast variety of factors—including ethnicity, sexual practices, class, and race—that may have little to do with their categories. Lesbian and gay health care activists have repeatedly tried to impress upon all health care researchers and providers the distinction— often the vast discordance—between sexual behavior and identity: women who identify as lesbians in terms of their community affiliation or the way in which they think of themselves (identity) may indeed have sex with men (behavior); women who identify as heterosexual in terms of their community affiliation or the way in which they think of themselves (identity) may indeed have sex with women (behavior). And many people choose not to identify in terms of their sexual practices or politics. Risa Denenberg, an FNP who works in the AIDS clinic at Bronx Lebanon Hospital, says most of her female clients who have sex with women "don't call themselves lesbians, but primarily identify themselves otherwise—as mother, intravenous drug user, woman in recovery, Puerto Rican, Black, butch, caretaker, or person with AIDS." Regardless of these complexities, the CDC's definition states that only women who report having sexual relations exclusively with female partners since 1977 can be considered lesbians.[10] When this arbitrary definition is combined with their policy of assigning cases to mutually-exclusive categories based on alleged risk, ontological absurdities ensue. As Patricia Stevens, RN, Ph.D., notes, "women with AIDS who have injected drugs at any time are recorded in the CDC's Injection Drug User category, whereas those who have not injected drugs but have had sex with men any time since 1977 are categorized in the heterosexual transmission category."[11]

Given these extensive barriers to lesbian documentation, it is no wonder that CDC-certified lesbians constitute a fraction of all reported cases of adult women with AIDS in the U.S. (0.8 percent as of 1989).[12] Nor is it surprising that lesbian health activists dispute this figure, arguing that it dramatically underrepresents the number of HIV-infected women who have had sex with women living in the states. Stevens observes that in the short term, the CDC's self-perpetuating logistical loop of denial and exclusion makes it "impossible to estimate lesbians' risks of exposure with any kind of accuracy." It also makes it more difficult for health providers to convince their female clients who have sex with women that they need to take precautions against contracting HIV. In 1994, when I spoke to Amelie Zurn, then head of Lesbian Health Care Services at Whitman Walker in Washington, D.C., she noted that, paradoxically, many of the same lesbians who usually shun the standard medical establishment still look to government-funded medical statistics and research to tell them what to do about practicing safer sex: "We question the health care community, but we'd still love to have them telling us what to do if they only had the "scientific" information to back up their claims. We keep begging the CDC for examples of female-female transmission so we can believe them." While Zurn disparaged the call for statistics as a prerequisite for beginning safer-sex education in the lesbian community—"After all, you can make them say anything you like"—she acknowledged that without statistics it's harder to sell safer sex to a community that perceives itself as immune. "People have a real hunger for statistical information. Women come to me and ask if the cases of female-female transmission that they've heard about are true. They're looking for a doctor to tell them whether or not to practice safer sex."[13] Above all, the CDC's failure to count lesbians accurately in its statistics has negative implications for the future of lesbian-inclusive research, treatment, prevention programs, and community education. In summary, as Stevens says, "Because CDC data about the number of AIDS cases determine funding [for these projects] this lack of data excludes lesbians from access to these resources and makes them essentially invisible in this epidemic."[14]

It is impossible to construct an HIV-infected person with a complex identity from within the confines of CDC-regulated AIDS discourse. The CDC subject is *either* a man who has sex with men *or* the recipient of blood products, *either* a heterosexual woman *or* an injection drug user—and never a woman who has sex with women. This normalizing regime purchases cultural comfort at the expense of accuracy: by creating easy-to-identify-and-discipline bodies and risk categories, the CDC's taxonomy constructs a more coherent, less uncontrollable epidemic, one that need not concern the average white putatively heterosexual person who does not inject drugs. If the CDC tracked the exposure risks of HIV-infected people using more behaviorally-focused, inclusive, and non-hierarchical methods, their findings might dispel the myth of "coherent" or "low-risk" social or sexual identity forever; and they might make available a more accurate picture of the virus's associated risk exposures, transmission routes, and epidemiology. Perhaps the rash of AIDS-related hate crimes which have risen steadily since the mid-eighties would decrease if people could no longer assume immunity based on identity or scapegoat "other" populations for bringing AIDS into "their" communities. But this cannot happen so long as the very research methodologies used to document HIV-infected people reify conventional assumptions and prejudices.

Although the CDC surveillance definitions play a significant role in obscuring the rate or cause of HIV infection among women who have sex with women, the construction of risk categories, and hence, responsibility for lesbian invisibility in the AIDS epidemic, also lies with other sectors of the scientific community.[15] (Another paradigmatic moment: while attempting to do a search on Med-line, the national data base for the National Libraries of Medicine [NLM], I find out that "lesbian" is not even listed in their subject headings.[16]) Among other barriers to research on women who engage in sexual behaviors with women, Nancy Warren lists "institutions that often refuse to sponsor such research, and journals that judge articles on the topic too controversial or insignificant to publish." The exclusion of lesbian and bisexual women from HIV/AIDS research, and from education and prevention programs, is particularly striking when compared to the extensive investigations of sexuality that have been undertaken in response to the epidemic's effect upon men:

> Questions that are routinely asked of men—including number and gender of sexual partners, exact sexual activities with partners, and discrepancies between sexual identity, orientation, and behavior—have not been asked of women. Motivated, no doubt, by the urgency of HIV transmission among men, HIV research has spearheaded groundbreaking studies on male sexual identity, orientation, and behavior. These important studies empirically document a significant minority of the general male population being studied, including: bisexual men; men who do not identify as gay or bisexual but who engage in sexual behaviors with other men to obtain money or crack; men who identify as gay but occasionally have sex with women. The results of such research have led to important HIV-related campaigns designed to target each of these specific male populations for education, prevention, and service delivery.[17]

In speaking of the differences in the treatment of men and women in the AIDS crisis by the American medical community, I think it is important to acknowledge that sexuality, not gender, most commonly distinguishes the population that accounts for almost 60 percent of all deaths from AIDS in this country.[18] It is not my intention, nor do I think that it is Warren's, to stir homophobic, addictophobic, or racist ire by implying that mostly white, mostly gay men are being provided with everything they need to address the AIDS crisis. But I *am* saying that women, particularly women who have sex with women, have been and continue to be miserably overlooked by government-funded medical researchers. And I think it is important not to evade the unpleasant fact that the sexism underlying the medical establishment's disregard for women is all too often echoed by male-dominated AIDS service agencies as well, including those in the gay male community. It is the policies of all of these institutions combined that continues to erase women from the health care system.[19]

Neglecting women in 1996 can only reap disastrous results. From 1985 to 1995 the percentage of AIDS cases in the United States documented among women rose from 7 percent to 19 percent.[20] The CDC reports that in 1995, "Among persons ages 25 to 44 years, HIV infection is now the leading cause of death in men and the third leading cause in women."[21] By 1993 it had already become the leading cause of death for black women in this age group (that same year it moved into fifth place for white women).[22] As early as 1990, AIDS had become the leading cause of death in New York City among Latinas ages 25–34.[23] By July of 1995, the CDC reported that "Although black and Hispanic women make up 21% of all U.S. women, more than three-fourths (77 percent) of AIDS cases reported among women in 1994 occurred among blacks and Hispanics . . . the AIDS rate for black and Hispanic U.S. women was approximately 16 and 7 times greater, respectively, than that for white U.S. women."[24] The combined factors of poverty and lack of access to health care, which often lead to late and/or incorrect diagnosis, contribute significantly to the fact that once diagnosed, "women become sicker faster and die sooner than men with AIDS."[25]

Speaking of the link between poverty, race, marginality, and HIV, Stevens notes that those women who are most excluded from access to health care services—economically-disadvantaged women, women of color, and women who have sex with women—are consequently those who are put at greatest risk for HIV precisely because they cannot access education, prevention, or treatment services:[26]

> In the US the most consistent pattern in the distribution of mortality and morbidity is their association with poverty. Death and disease rates vary inversely with social class. A disproportionate number of women and ethnic/ racial minority people live in low-income households. Their increased vulnerability to illness is significantly related to inequities in access to health care systems and differential quality of health care. . . . rates of death due to preventable and manageable conditions are 77% higher for African Ameri-

cans that for Euro-Americans and are associated with poor access to existing medical, public health, and preventative services.[27]

Miguelina Maldonado, the Executive Director of the Hispanic AIDS Forum, also examines the connection between poverty, race, and HIV. In "Latinas and HIV/AIDS: Implications for the 90s," she notes that "Strategies intended to stem the spread of HIV/AIDS among Latinas cannot be solely focused on promotion of safer sex and/or risk reduction related to IV drug injection. In addition, prevention approaches must address the economic, social, and environmental factors which impact on the very behaviors that are targeted for change." Maldonado reports that 50 percent of all Latina-headed households fall below the poverty level (61 percent in New York City) and that they represent 23 percent of all Latino homes. "Exacerbating the lack of access to quality health care is the fact that Latinos are the ethnic group least likely to have health insurance; approximately 33% lack private insurance or Medicare/Medicaid, as compared to 11% of the general U.S. population."[28]

Vallerie Wagner, cochair of the Black Gay and Lesbian Leadership Forum, only partially concurs with the image of the woman at risk for HIV as being "a low-income woman of color who may or may not be homeless or have children." She is wary about perpetuating stereotypes of risk based on race rather than behavior: "Women of color are most at risk because access to education and health care isn't available to these communities, and ignorance and fear go a long way in spreading the virus." Wagner felt that studies showing a higher prevalence of heterosexual sex among black lesbian and bisexual women, and a higher rate of IV drug use, were inaccurate representations of black culture, biased towards confirming racist stereotypes:

> I don't really know if IVDU is the number one lesbian risk for HIV. I think that there's a lot of pigeon-holing going on. Who is going into communities and asking these questions of lesbians of color, and what were they looking for and asking? If it's white straight men, the whole project is going to have a very racial slant. I want to know who's collecting the numbers before I listen to the statistics about who is at risk.[29]

All U.S. women, regardless of sexuality, race, class, or ethnicity, have been routinely excluded from clinical trials, allotted a marginal portion of the National Institutes of Health (NIH) budget, and underrepresented in articles and research. As Mary Beth Caschetta notes, an inventory conducted of the research activities supported by the NIH in 1987 "found that NIH spent approximately $778 million on women's health issues, approximately 13.5 percent of the budget; it was not until Spring of 1993 that the Food and Drug Administration (FDA) announced the lifting of a 16-year-old ban that prohibited women from participating in early experimental drug trials."[30] Caschetta observes that although the medical community has long regarded the normative human body as young, white, and male, its tendency to regard itself as objective has served as an iron-clad means of self-protection against the criticism of a host of other populations who are underrepresented in medical research. But the consequences of taking drugs that have been tested on this normative medical body have been disastrous for women, who are taking a range of medications, from aspirin to anti-depressant drugs, that have never been tested in female bodies.[31]

The CDC's failure to define AIDS in a manner that accounts for the specific symptoms that HIV disease manifests in female bodies is partly to blame for the pattern of late and/or incorrect diagnosis of HIV infection among women. Even though the CDC revised its definition of AIDS in January of 1993 (in response to years of organized protest, primarily from groups of female health activists that included many HIV-infected women), the new one is still inadequate to women's needs, since it includes only severe cervical cancer: "Cervical neoplasia, pelvic inflammatory disease, and chronic, severe vaginal candidiasis remain largely unexamined."[32] And even in a community where "The exclusion of females from medical research is so institutionalized that even female rats (except in reference to reproduction) are commonly excluded from early basic research on which many scientific decisions rest,"[33] women are shockingly underrepresented in AIDS research. At the time Caschetta published her article she noted that "Women's enrollment in trials nationwide has increased only slightly since 1990, when increased efforts to recruit women were said to have become a priority. The percentage of female enrollment from 1990 to 1992 increased from 6.5% to 7.8%." She comments, with more than a trace of irony, that these figures represent a dramatic improvement from earlier statistics.[34]

Warren notes that only a small percentage of medical research inquires after both its female participants' behavior and their identity. Those surveys that do are mostly small-scale and often go unpublished. Nonetheless, the statistics that are coming out of studies in New York City, San Francisco,

Seattle, and Sydney tell a complex story about the interplay between identity and behavior, and a troubling one as well. They find that "the number of HIV-infected women who engage in sexual behaviors with other women is higher than was originally presumed,"[35] that women who have sex with women practice far riskier sexual and drug-using behaviors than those who do not, and that their higher risk directly correlates to the lack of resources for education, treatment, and prevention available to them. As Warren reports, "Preliminary data from Bronx Lebanon Hospital in New York City found that over 30% of female HIV-symptomatic patients have had a female sexual partner. Similarly, preliminary data from Montefiore Medical Center at Rikers's Island Jail in New York City found that over 40% of HIV-infected inmates have engaged in sexual behaviors with other women at some point during their lives."[36] While Stevens sharply criticizes the absence of research or information on female-female sexual behavior, she also warns that "When we talk about lesbians and HIV, our focus cannot be exclusively on female-female transmission. Women who live as lesbians and call themselves lesbians are getting HIV a lot of different ways, including survival sex (sex with men for drugs or money), sex with men, and IV drug use. Lesbians are getting HIV the same way that all women are getting it."[37]

Early on, Denenberg noted both the link between IVDU and HIV infection in the lesbian community and the prevalence of women who have sex with women in the IVDU community. Further research has confirmed her conjectures,[38] but recent government-funded attempts to assess the health status and needs of the IVDU population barely acknowledges their existence:

> The National AIDS Demonstration Research (NADR) Project, established by the National Institute on Drug Abuse in 1987 and comprising 40 grants and contracts in 59 sites around the country, represents the largest research endeavor undertaken to date to assess sexual and drug-using behavior of IDUs and their sexual partners. . . . Only a handful of NIDA's 40 NADR programs explicitly sought out lesbian/bisexual IDUs and their sexual partners for inclusion in the research and education programs, and none received special funding for these efforts.[39]

Like the CDC, the NADR programs structurally impede the accumulation of data on women who have sex with women. Still, these women appear: Even in NADR programs that did not actively seek out lesbian/bisexual IVDUs, 9.5 percent of all female respondents reported at least one female sexual partner. As Young et al point out, this statistic represents a *minimum* estimate. Sites where the staff made an effort to identify and address lesbian IVDUs more than doubled that figure: 22.9 percent of their female IVDUs reported at least one female sexual partner.[40]

Despite the significant risk for HIV that IVDU poses to women who have sex with women, they are currently routinely excluded from drug and alcohol treatment program or misinformed and subjected to homophobia within them. Because research and outreach programs rarely target them, the vast majority of these women never make it to a drug treatment center at all. Those who do often encounter hostility from the staff and other clients alike. They face the strong possibility that their sexual orientation, rather than their drug use, will become the focus of their experience there. In our 1994 conversations about lesbian health care, Dr. Katherine O'Hanlan, the associate director of Gynecologic Cancer Services at the Stanford University Medical Center, noted of the high level of homophobia in this sector of the health care system that, "A questionnaire administered to 98 addiction center treatment providers revealed 26% scored in the homophobic or marginally homophobic range, a rate which may be an under-estimation because some providers refused to participate, stating that they believed that their personal attitudes toward homosexuality were not relevant to the quality of care they provided to gay and lesbian patients."[41] Routinely barred from access to unprejudiced counseling for their drug habits, or from information on how to practice safer behaviors around their sexual lives and their drug use, women who have sex with women are far likelier to practice far riskier sexual and drug-using behaviors than women who do not, and those riskier behaviors are translating into far higher rates of HIV infection. As Warren notes, "One small unpublished study of drug users entering treatment in Seattle found that women who had engaged in sexual behaviors with women were five times more likely to be seropositive (or 5,1, 95% CI: 1.8 to 14.7) than women who had only male sexual partners. Very similar findings were obtained from a New York City sample." And the list goes on.[42]

Equally dismal are the findings of a number of small research projects undertaken in the past decade that have focused, in whole or in part, on the sexual behaviors of self-identified lesbian and bisexual women. In contradiction to the CDC's narrow definition, these studies establish that most women who self-identify as lesbians have had or continue to have sex with men; more importantly, they confirm that many of these women are engaging in highly risky sexual behaviors during their cross-sex encounters. In a study of female sexual behavior conducted by the Kinsey Institute in 1987, 46 percent of self-identified lesbians had had sex with men since 1980. Nearly a third of the women knew that their partners were bisexual; still, although almost half of them reported penile-anal intercourse, only 8 percent of *all* of the women in the sample (including those who believed their male partners to be exclusively heterosexual) reported that they always used condoms. Of the self-identified lesbians who reported having sex with men since 1980, 88 percent had penile-vaginal intercourse, and less than 5 percent always used condoms.[43] In a more recent study of health behaviors among 483 lesbian and bisexual women conducted by the Prevention Services Branch of the San Francisco Department of Public Health AIDS office in October of 1993, 25 percent of self-identified lesbians and 84 percent of self-identified bisexual women had had sex with men in the past three years: 11 percent reported that their partners were gay or bisexual men, and 5 percent knew or believed that their male partner used injection drugs. But only half (47 percent) reported that they always use condoms, 37 percent said sometimes, 8 percent rarely, and 8 percent never. Similar findings appear in another report undertaken in the same year by a related branch of the San Francisco DPH and in a project undertaken by two private researchers in 1992.[44]

Because the U.S. government has never funded any research project on lesbian health, only two significant surveys exist. Both were initiated and funded by small organizations, and they are only large-scale surveys by the standards of small-scale research. Nonetheless their findings are significant, if only because they confirm an image of the lesbian community as underserved, underdocumented, and at greater risk than heterosexual women for a variety of health problems. As a commentary on the conditions under which lesbian health researchers work, it is worth noting that the largest grant given to the proposed National Lesbian Health Care Survey that Caitlin Ryan and Judith Bradford undertook in 1983 through the National Lesbian and Gay Health Foundation (NLGHF) was for $10,000 (from the Ms. Foundation for Women) and that although 1,925 questionnaires were returned by 1985, "lack of funding delayed analysis of the data until 1986."[45] AIDS-related homophobia also impeded Bradford and Ryan's efforts to complete their project:

It is perhaps a metaphor for the barriers in undertaking lesbian research to report the difficulties in inputting the survey data, once actual data were obtained. Four data keypunch firms were hired and with the exception of the last one, each reneged on their work, eventually refusing to complete the questionnaires and returning them to the Survey Research Lab, unentered. The last company stated that their keypunchers had walked off the job because they were afraid of getting AIDS from handling the questionnaires.

Ryan and Bradford's findings are corroborated by the Michigan Lesbian Health Survey, a comparable study undertaken in 1989 by the Michigan Organization for Human Rights (MOHR). Although the national survey drew respondents from all fifty states for a total of 1,925 respondents to the single-state study's 1,681, the parallels between the two studies suggest that the state of being a lesbian may be the primary factor in determining the kinds of health care that women who have sex with women seek out and receive: it includes lower incomes, greater stress, a disproportionate rate of uninsurance, higher rates of self-reported depression, obesity, and alcoholism,[46] impaired access to a variety of services, and a related history of less frequent health exams and later diagnoses.

There is a direct link between a lesbian's income, the type of insurance she has, and the health care she receives; the latter is often based on her ability to self-disclose. It is not only that a woman who has sex with women stands a better chance of getting the information she needs about self-care if her health care provider knows about her same-sex sexual behavior: her comfort level with her health care provider plays a substantial role in her decision to seek (or avoid) care at all. And that comfort level is only available at a certain income level. Despite the fact that both surveys' respondents were highly educated, incomes were disproportionately low. In the Michigan sample, the lesbian population's median income was $10,000 lower than the median income reported by all Michigan women to the U.S. Bureau of the Census in 1989. Heterosexist culture exacts heavy penalties from its unmarried women: the reduction in their income is reflected in their more limited access to basic health care:

> Lesbians are likely to have no health insurance for several reasons: lower incomes (reflecting women's lower earning power), inability to obtain "dependent" or "family" coverage on partner policies, and categorical restrictions on public health insurance programs like Medicaid. Without access to public programs or coverage on a partner's policy, most lesbians are a job loss away from being uninsured.[47]

Those lesbians who have access to standard insurance and the private fee-for-service sector are more likely to be able to find nonhomophobic health care providers, while women who are reliant upon HMO's and public sector services have little if any choice about whom they see. A significant number of the women in both studies (over half in the national survey) felt that they could not disclose their lesbianism to their providers and over 45 percent complained of their health care workers' heterosexist assumptions and rudeness. Women who cannot choose situations where they feel comfortable about disclosing their lesbianism to their health care providers will either not receive the care that they need when they do visit them or will avoid seeking health care entirely.[48]

The homophobia that pervades the contemporary medical community and the mistrust of the medical profession that pervades the contemporary homosexual community both represent a serious barrier to the frequency and quality of lesbian health care. The American Psychiatric Association (APA) may no longer officially pathologize homosexuality, but Stevens reminds us that "For most of the 20th century, lesbians and gay men suffered psychiatric confinement, electroshock treatment, genital mutilation, aversive therapy, psychosurgery, hormonal injection, psychoanalysis, and psychotropic chemotherapy aimed at 'curing' their homosexuality."[49] The legacy of the medical establishment's systematic persecution of lesbians and gays throughout the late nineteenth and twentieth centuries is still fresh in both parties' communal memory, and it continues to mark their interactions with one another:

> Significant numbers of physicians and nurses still consider lesbianism to be a pathological condition, make attributions of immorality, perversion, and danger to lesbian women, are uncomfortable providing care for lesbian clients, and regularly refuse service to women who are lesbian. . . . As a result of their negative experiences in health care encounters, many lesbians report hesitation in using health care systems and say they delay seeking needed treatment.[50]

Every study that gauges doctors and nurses' attitudes towards lesbians and gays in the past two decades reveals a high rate of homophobia among health service providers. A 1986 survey of M.D.'s attitudes towards lesbians and gays revealed that 23 percent were severely homophobic, 40 percent were uncomfortable treating lesbians and gays, 30 percent opposed admitting lesbians and gays to medical schools, and 40 percent would not refer clients to lesbian and gay colleagues.[51] Nurses were no less homophobic than doctors. A 1989 study of nursing educators' attitudes towards lesbians revealed that 52 percent considered lesbianism unnatural, 34 percent considered lesbians disgusting, 23 percent considered lesbianism immoral, 20 percent said that lesbians transmit AIDS, 19 percent thought lesbianism was illegal, 17 percent considered lesbianism a disease, 17 percent said that lesbians molest children, and 8 percent considered lesbians unfit as RNs.[52] In regard to their own behaviors, 54 percent of the bachelor of science in nursing (BSN) educators said that they never discussed lesbian issues in the classroom and 28 percent were uncomfortable teaching or providing care to lesbians.[53] Michele J. Eliason and Carla E. Randall observe, "The association of gay life-styles with AIDS may contribute to the high lesbian phobia scores identified in nurses": 28 percent of the sample considered lesbians to be a high-risk group for AIDS despite the fact that their classes had taught them that lesbians were a low-risk group.[54]

Not surprisingly, parallel studies also indicate that most lesbians and bisexual women feel uncomfortable disclosing sexuality-related information to their health care providers. Stevens and Hall report that 72 percent of the lesbians they interviewed reported "ostracism, invasive personal questioning, shock, embarrassment, unfriendliness, pity, condescension, and fear" after their identity was known: "Of the respondents, 36% described situations in which they had had to terminate the interaction or not return to that provider because of events following disclosure ... 84% described a general reluctance to receive health care."[55] Cochran and Mays' nationwide survey of self-identified black bisexual and lesbian women reports that of the women they interviewed, 67 percent of black lesbians and 18 percent of bisexuals had not disclosed their same-sex sexual behavior to their health care providers as opposed to 47 percent of white lesbians and 30 percent of bisexuals in an earlier study.[56] Bisexual women, who are at significantly higher risk for HIV if they are having unprotected heterosexual sex, "were significantly less likely than lesbians to have disclosed their same-sex sexual behavior to their physicians."[57]

Both the Michigan Lesbian Health Survey and the National Lesbian Health Care Survey report that lesbians visit health service providers less frequently because of a combination of poverty, fear of disclosure, and a false sense of immunity from health problems; the latter is partly due to the standard representation of women's health concerns as being reproductive or heterosexual in nature (not least by the fact that women's health clinics are often located in or near the OB/GYN sections of hospitals and health care centers). While nulliparity represents one of the best-known risk factors for breast cancer among women, lesbians' low health care visitation rate may contribute significantly to the fact that they appear to be at higher risk than heterosexual women for cervical, breast, endometrial, and ovarian cancers: over one-fourth of all lesbians over age forty in the Michigan survey had never had a mammogram, and 10 percent had either never had a pap smear or had one over ten years ago.[58] Susan Hester, the president of the Mary-Helen Mautner Project for Lesbians with Cancer, concurs, noting that:

> Lesbians don't go for primary care at the rate that heterosexual women do because they have lower motivation to do so. They aren't usually dealing with birth control and pregnancies. But this means that they aren't getting pap smears, pelvic exams, or breast health care. The profile of a woman at risk for breast cancer *is* the profile of a lesbian, particularly because we have a higher rate of nulliparity and less regular health care.[59]

Lesbian health activists agree that regardless of the actual risk behaviors a self-identified lesbian engages in, she needs to hear messages about how to decrease her risks through education and outreach within her own community; regardless of how a woman who has sex with women contracts HIV, her health care providers need to be able to respond in an appropriate and informed way to her sexual identity and/or behavior. Stevens notes that "We need to reach specific communities and speak about risk in a culturally competent manner. You have to reach lesbians as lesbians. Although we need to be talking about behavior once we have access to them, prevention is most effective if you target specific cultural groups and identities."[60] But few organizations exist that provide health services specifically targeted to the lesbian population: in fact, the misperception that lesbians' needs are being fulfilled either by the gay male or the women's community contributes to their continued marginalized status within the health care system despite the growth of alternative health centers.[61] Smaller still is the number of organizations that address the topic of lesbians and HIV, although those that do exist find that their services are in heavy demand.[62]

When I first spoke with lesbian health care activists in 1994, they pointed to three recent major triumphs as a sign that the U.S. medical community may be slowly beginning to come to terms with lesbians and their health needs. The first of these was the expansion of the federal funding for breast cancer research from $80 million in 1990 to $400 million in 1993, a victory won primarily due to the efforts of the National Breast Cancer Coalition, which includes the Mautner Project for Lesbians with Cancer on its board. The second and third victories concerned the inclusion of questions about women's sexual behaviors and/or orientation on major research projects including the $625 million Women's Health Initiative (WHI) and the Harvard Nurse's Study (HNS), a triumph that a number of organizations and individual activists rallied to achieve.

Paula Ettelbrick, then Director of Health Policy for the National Center for Lesbian Rights (NCLR), characterized the WHI as "a large-scale ten-year study of the causes of disease and frailty in postmenopausal women" and the HNS as "a long-term study of more than 100,000 female nurses that obtains general health information in all areas of women's health." The first is set to enroll approximately 160,000 women to study "the effect of low-fat diets, estrogen replacement therapies, and calcium supplements in preventing diseases." In the NCLR memorandums on the WHI letter-writing campaign that went out to members in 1993, a sanguine Ettelbrick described the WHI as "*the* study on women's health care for decades to come," predicting that it was "bound to be the most statistically valid profile of women's health ever—the study from which all future policy will emanate, not to mention money for future research."[63] But not everyone shares her optimism. A number of epidemiologists remain concerned that the WHI will not be as informative as the lesbian health community once projected it would be.

Moreover, the questions on the WHI are not precisely what lesbian health activists had hoped for, and they may not produce as accurate a profile of the lesbian community as they might have. While question number 22 of the Harvard Nurse's health study now reads, "Whether or not you are currently sexually active, what is your sexual orientation or identity?", the WHI survey asks its participants two questions related to sexual *behavior*. The first inquires, "Regardless of whether you are currently sexually active, which response *best describes* who you have had sex with over your adult lifetime?" The second question asks for the same information, but for sex partners participants have had after the age of forty-five. Women can respond "have never had sex," "sex with women," "sex with men," "sex with both men and women," or "prefer not to answer."

When I spoke with Marj Plumb in 1994, she called the NIH decision not to include an orientation question "short-sighted," noting that "while behavior questions are important in terms of assessing and addressing risk, identity questions are important for health education and outreach." By her account, the National Gay and Lesbian Task Force (NGLTF), where she had just left her post as Health Policy Director, also fought to have the question expanded because it did not establish a time frame: "In fact," said Plumb, "the limited response options construct a subject who is necessarily bisexual if she has indeed partnered with women, when in fact the subject may have been exclusively heterosexual first, then homosexual, or vice versa—not bisexual at all in the sense of having sex with both men and women during the same period of one's life." [64]

Whether or not any of these putative breakthroughs in lesbian health care will produce a more accurate picture of women who have sex with women and their health care risks and needs remains to be seen. The same goes for whether these studies will have any bearing on the medical profession's willingness to address issues related to lesbians and HIV: the government's willingness to fund such research is entirely unknown. Despite the NIH's professed commitment to seek out lesbians to include in the WHI actively, there is no real system in place to monitor their actions. At least one request for a site in San Francisco, one of the major centers for lesbian life in the U.S., was rejected in the spring of 1994.

The activists and health care providers with whom I spoke in 1994 agreed unanimously that the WHI and HNS decisions were positive ones, but their responses ranged from cynical to guardedly hopeful when I asked them what kinds of changes they thought these decisions would bring to the picture of American health care for lesbians or the future of research on lesbians and HIV. After all, the Harvard Nurses' Study is precisely that, a study conducted on 100,000 members of a profession that is simultaneously populated by a considerable percentage of lesbians and statistically verifiable as negative in its attitudes towards homosexuals.[65] And the WHI questions will be asked of a generation of women, many of whom, arguably, grew up before the lesbian/gay liberation movement in a time when it may have been quite dangerous to disclose one's sexual identity or behavior. Rebecca Young, Nancy Warren, and Risa Denenberg all commented that the ability to conduct a client intake is an art, one that the average medical professional involved in research is not likely to have. Noted Young, "The amount of interviewer training required to ask sex questions well and to get accurate information is something that the government is just not going to invest in. And people are not going to disclose if they don't feel safe." Going beyond the intricacies of science and medicine, those allegedly neutral disciplines, she foregrounds the political issues that rule the intersection of any meeting between women who have sex with women and members of the dominant health care culture when she says that she strongly believes "that the biggest thing we could do to improve our collection of data on lesbian health is civil rights work. Without full civil rights protection we're never going to get representative sampling."[66] Like Young, Amelie Zurn considers the whole issue of lesbian health care and HIV part of a larger discussion about the values of the American health care system and the quality of lesbian existence. Summing up the transition that she believes must happen before HIV can be adequately addressed, she sighs, "We live in a country that values death care; much of the health care in this country is devoted to decreasing morbidity, not increasing the quality of life. And we can't make a dent in homophobia until we care about death and life."[67]

NOTES

1. The original version of this article was made possible by a grant from the Brandeis University Sachar Fund. I would still like to extend my sincere thanks to the members of the grant committee for supporting my work. It is dedicated with respect and gratitude to the activists, health care providers, and researchers whose work makes lesbian health care reform possible. I would especially like to thank those who took the time to speak with me, send me material, provide references, and familiarize me with the maze of issues and disciplines that converge on the topic of lesbian health care, both in 1994 and in 1996. Special thanks to Patricia Case, Io Cyrus, Risa Denenberg, Gale Dutcher, Paula Ettelbrick, Jenifer Firestone, Susan Hester, Amber Hollibaugh, Melissa Jones, Jean McGuire, Marian Millbauer, Kate O'Hanlan, Marj Plumb, Jim Shortridge, Patricia E. Stevens, Janice Swiatek, Vallerie Wagner, Alice Weiss, Ellie Weiss, Rebecca Young, Nancy Warren, Anne White-Olsen, Sally Zierler, and Amelie Zurn. Any inaccuracies that still exist in this piece do so despite their patient attempts to eradicate them.

I use the terms "lesbian" and "women who have sex with women" throughout this article with as much accuracy as the limitations of space and language will allow to distinguish between women who self-identify as lesbians and women who self-identify in terms that prioritize other aspects of their lives but whose sexual behaviors include sex with women. Usually I use the latter term when I am trying to refer to the whole broad spectrum of women who have sex with women, including self-identified lesbians; at other times I use "lesbian" for the sake of sound and coherence (as in "myth of lesbian immunity" and "lesbian health care").

2. In fact, no significant study of any aspect of lesbian health has been undertaken by U.S. government-funded researchers since the American Psychiatric Association's

official pathologization of lesbians and gay men ended in 1973 with the removal of homosexuality from its list of disorders (the DSM III).

3. For the purposes of this article, I will be using the sexual identity definition provided by the SIECUS organization (Sex Information and Education Council of the U.S.) in their comprehensive sexuality education fact sheet. "Sexual identity is an inner-sense of oneself as a sexual being, including how one identifies in terms of gender and sexual orientation."

4. The 1994 SIECUS sexuality and orientation fact sheet notes that "there are no current U.S. population research studies on sexual behavior, identity or orientation." In 1996, this is still the case. In July 1995 Kennedy et al. noted that

> Only one prospective study involving WSW and HIV has been reported (Raiteri R, Fora R, Sinicco A: No HIV-1 transmission through lesbian sex. *Lancet* 1994;344:270). Researchers in Italy followed 18 lesbian HIV-1 discordant couples in steady relationships (seronegative partners had monogamous relationships of at least three months with seropositive partners). None of the seronegative partners had seroconverted six months after study enrollment. The validity of this study has been questioned, however, because of the small number of subjects and short follow-up time. One researcher suggested that if the risk of transmission for each couple was 5%, there was a 40% probability no seroconversions would occur over the study period; thus, the reported finding of no seroconversions could result from chance alone (Reynolds G: HIV and lesbian sex. *Lancet* 1994: 344;544). (Quotation from Meaghan B. Kennedy, Margaret I. Scarlett, Ann C. Duerr, and Susan Y. Chu, "Assessing HIV Risk among Women Who Have Sex with Women: Scientific and Communication Issues," *Journal of the American Medical Women's Association* 50, nos. 3 and 4 [May/August 1995]: 103–7; 103.)

5. This incident is reported by Patricia E. Stevens. See "Lesbians and HIV: Clinical, Research, and Policy Issues," *American Journal of Orthopsychiatry* 63, no. 2 (April 1993): 291. It reappears in Laura Ramos's article in this volume.

6. Rebecca Cole and Sally Cooper, "Lesbian Exclusion from HIV/AIDS Education: Ten Years of Low-Risk Identity and High-Risk Behavior," *SIECUS Report* 19:2 (December 1990/January 1991): 18.

7. Centers for Disease Control and Prevention. *HIV/AIDS Surveillance Report* 7, no. 2 (1995): 1–39; 11.

8. Rebecca M. Young, Gloria Weissman, and Judith B. Cohen, "Assessing Risk in the Absence of Information: HIV Risk Among Women Injection-Drug Users Who Have Sex with Women," *AIDS & Public Policy Journal* 7, no. 3 (Fall 1992): 178.

9. CDC National AIDS Clearinghouse, "Women, Children, and HIV/AIDS" (July 1995): 1.

10. Susan Chu et al., "Epidemiology of Reported Cases of AIDS in Lesbians, U.S. 1980–1989," *American Journal of Public Health* 80 (1990): 1380–81. Thanks to Sally Zierler for pointing out the asymmetry "whereby men who report any sex, ever, with a man since 1978[?] are classified as 'gay/bi.'" (Personal communication, May 1996.)

11. Stevens, "Lesbians and HIV," 290.

12. Chu et al., 1381.

13. Personal communication, March 25, 1994.

14. Stevens, "Lesbians and HIV," 290. As the CDC itself states, "Surveillance is essential to know where HIV infection is decreasing, stabilizing, and increasing so that programs can be directed where they are most needed." (CDC National AIDS Clearinghouse, "Women, Children, and HIV/AIDS": 2.)

15. For further reading, see Charles E. Rosenberg, "Disease and Social Order in America: Perceptions and Expectations" in *AIDS: The Burdens of History,* ed. Elizabeth Fee and Daniel Fox (Berkeley and Los Angeles: University of California Press, 1988), 12–32.

16. When I first researched this article in the spring of 1994, the new 1994 update listed "see homosexuality" under "lesbian" even in the annotated alphabetical list of medical subject headings. In 1995 the subject heading changed, but only to "Homosexuality, female."

17. Nancy Warren, "Out of the Question: Obstacles to Research on HIV and Women Who Engage in Sexual Behaviors with Women," *SIECUS Report* 22, no. 1 (October/November 1993): 14.

18. Statistics provided by Centers for Disease Control, US AIDS cases through December 1994, HIV/AIDS surveillance, 1994. I would like to thank Paul Morrison for his observation about sexuality rather than gender being the determinant of difference in American AIDS discourse. The 1995 report states that "Although the incidence of estimated AIDS—OIs (opportunistic illnesses) is increasing most rapidly among persons infected heterosexually, men who have sex with men continue to represent the largest number and proportion of persons estimated to have AIDS—OIs. . . . Among men reported with AIDS in 1995, male-to-male sexual contact again accounted for the largest proportion of cases (51%), followed by injecting drug use (24%)." (Centers for Disease Control and Prevention, *HIV/AIDS Surveillance Report* 7, no. 2 [1995]: 6).

19. In Rebecca Cole's 1991 overview of lesbian projects and organizations in the United States, she notes that while "Homophobia in society at large as well as within specific health areas was the biggest impetus to begin a lesbian specific or lesbian sensitive project. . . . Sexism in all of society, including the gay community, was also reported by a majority of project coordinators as a reason for initiating a lesbian project." See "Lesbian Projects and Organizations in the United States: An Overview (Astraea National Lesbian Action Foundation: New York, 1991): 1.

20. Centers for Disease Control and Prevention. *HIV/AIDS Surveillance Report* 7, no. 2 (1995): 6.

21. Centers for Disease Control and Prevention. *HIV/AIDS Surveillance Report* 7, no. 2 (1995): 6.

22. CDC National AIDS Clearinghouse, "Facts about Women and HIV/AIDS" (December 1994; revised February 13, 1995): 1.

23. Miguelina Maldonado, "Latinas and HIV/AIDS: Implications for the 90s," *SIECUS Report* 19, no. 2 (December 1990/January 1991): 11.

24. CDC National AIDS Clearinghouse, "Facts about Women and HIV/AIDS," 1–2. The year-end 1995 report notes that in 1995,

blacks and Hispanics represented the majority of cases among men (54%) and women (76%). The reported AIDS incidence rate per 100,000 among blacks (92.6) was 6 times higher than that among whites (15.4) and 2 times higher than that among Hispanics (46.2). Rates were lowest among American Indians/Alaska Natives (12.3) and Asians/Pacific Islanders (6.2). *However HIV/AIDS surveillance data collected from medical records do not include measures of socioeconomic status such as education and income that may more accurately predict risk of HIV than demographic factors such as race/ethnicity."* (Centers for Disease Control and Prevention, *HIV/ AIDS Surveillance Report* 7, no. 2 [1995]: 6, emphasis mine.)

25. Eunice Diaz, "Public Policy, Women, and HIV Disease," *SIECUS Report* 19, no. 2 (December 1990/January 1991): 4.

26. Patricia E. Stevens, "Marginalized Women's Access to Health Care: A Feminist Narrative Analysis," *Advanced Nursing Science* 16, no. 2 (1993): 39–56; 40.

27. Patricia E. Stevens, "Who Gets Care? Access to Health Care as an Arena for Nursing Action," *Scholarly Inquiry for Nursing Practice* 6, no. 3 (1992): 185–200; 193.

28. Maldonado, 12.

29. Personal communication, May 27, 1994.

30. Mary Beth Caschetta, "The Identity Politics of Biomedical Research: Clinical Trials, Medical Knowledge, and the Female Body," *SIECUS Report* 19, no. 2 (November/December 1993): 1. The entire passage that follows is indebted to Caschetta's article.

31. Caschetta reminds us that female bodies are,

regardless of essentialist vs. constructionist debates, different in some undeniable aspects from men's bodies. For instance, women have smaller body mass, more fat, different hemoglobin levels, and varying hormonal levels due to their menstrual cycles. The original researchers of anti-depressant medication did not anticipate these differences; in fact, they did not even ask the question (3).

32. Caschetta, 3.

33. Caschetta, 3.

34. Caschetta, 3. As of 1995, women account for only 5,091 of the 37,146 adult participants in the AIDS Clinical Trial Group (ACTG) Study Entries, or 14 percent (Centers for Disease Control, Demographic Summary of ACTG Study Entries from Beginning to 2/23/96).

35. Warren, 13.

36. Warren, 13.

37. Personal communication, May 1, 1994.

38. Samuel Friedman, who ran an NADR program in New York City, corroborates Denenberg's unpublished findings from the early nineties, reporting that "drug injection is the major risk factor for HIV infection among women who have sex with women."

In a May 1993 article, Rich et al. report that of the "Four prior cases in which transmission of HIV virus was presumed to have occurred via female-to-female sexual contact . . . female homosexual activity was listed as the sole risk behavior for acquisition of HIV infection in only two cases," and that of the 164 women with AIDS who qualify as lesbians according to the CDC's definition, "152 (93%) were IV drug users and the remaining 12 (7%) had received blood transfusions before March 1985." See Josiah D. Rich, Arlene Buck, Ruth E. Tuomala, and Powel H. Kazanjian, "Transmission of Human Immunodeficiency Virus Infection Presumed to Have Occurred via Female Homosexual Contact," *Clinical Infectious Disease* 17 (December 1993): 1004. The four prior cases are documented in the following articles: M. T. Sabatini, K. Patel, and R. Hirshman, "Kaposi's Sarcoma and T-Cell Lymphoma in an Immunodeficient Woman: A Case Report," *AIDS Research* 1 (1984): 135–37; M. Marmor et al., "Possible Female-to-Female Transmission of Human Immunodeficiency Virus" [letter], *Annals of Internal Medicine* 105 (1986): 969; O. T. Monzon and J. M. Capellan, "Female-to-Female Transmission of HIV" [letter], *Lancet* 2 (1987): 40–41; S. Perry, L. Jacobsberg, and K. Fogel, "Orogenital Transmission of Human Immunodeficiency Virus (HIV)" [letter], *Annals of Internal Medicine* 111 (1989): 951–52.

39. Young et al., 179.

40. Young et al., 180.

41. Personal communication, May 14, 1994.

42. Warren notes further that

> Some published studies reporting HIV-related risk from intravenous drug use, or from exchanging sex for drugs, reveal high numbers of women who are or were once sexually involved with other women. . . . A 1993 study examining the risk of sexual transmission of HIV among injection drug users reported that 19% of 72 women had a female partner within five years of the interviews. A recent Australian study on sexually transmitted diseases (STDs) found that 32% of 325 female intravenous drug users were either bisexual or lesbian. Another study of drug-using women in California found that 21% of 711 women interviewed regarded themselves as bisexual, and 3% identified as exclusively lesbian. (Warren, 13)

43. Young et al., 177.

44. *A Study of Health Behaviors among Lesbian and Bisexual Women:* A Community-Based Women's Health Survey conducted by the San Francisco Department of Public Health AIDS Office, Prevention Services Branch, October 1993: 27, 24, 32. Other significant recent studies include the following: *HIV Seroprevalence and Risk Behaviors Among Lesbians and Bisexual Women:* The 1993 San Francisco/Berkeley Women's Study conducted by the San Francisco Department of Public Health AIDS Office, Surveillance Branch, October 19, 1993; Gretchen B. Van Boemel and Elaine Vaughan, "Risk Behaviors Associated with HIV Transmission in the Lesbian Community," paper presented at the 98th Annual Convention of American Psychiatric Association, Boston, August 13, 1990. Analysis of these findings attribute the increased risk for women who have sex with women to the dearth of education, outreach, and health care available to

them; in turn, this lack of lesbian-related services is the direct result of the CDC's AIDS case-reporting protocol, which indicates no need for them.

45. Caitlin Ryan and Judith Bradford, "The National Lesbian Health Care Survey: An Overview," 1988; 33.

46. "Self-reported" is the operative term here. Lesbians may or may not actually consume more alcohol or have more food issues than heterosexual women. Dr. Katherine O'Hanlan reminded me that the early samples reporting a higher rate of alcoholism among lesbians and gay men have been criticized for their opportunistic selective sampling techniques, i.e., their tendency to do surveys of bar patrons, who have been shown to be more likely to abuse drugs or alcohol, regardless of sexual identity or behavior. As for the later samples, which continue to show a higher rate of alcoholism, drug abuse, and food issues among lesbians, their statistics may indicate a greater incidence of these issues in the lesbian community, heightened self-awareness leading to higher self-reportage, or the peculiarities of selective sampling yet again.

47. Michigan Organization for Human Rights special report, August 1991. In Stevens's 1993 sample, 36 percent of her lesbian participants did not have health coverage, and of those who did, copayment and prepayment policies often prevented them from seeking care. See Stevens, "Marginalized Women's Access to Health Care," 45.

48. This entire paragraph is indebted to Patricia E. Stevens, "Who Gets Care? Access to Health Care as an Arena for Nursing Action," *Scholarly Inquiry for Nursing Practice* 6, no. 3 (1992): 185–200.

49. Patricia E. Stevens and Joanne M. Hall, "A Critical Historical Analysis of the Medical Construction of Lesbianism," *International Journal of Health Services* 21, no. 2 (1991): 291–307; 298.

50. Stevens and Hall, "A Critical Historical Analysis," 291.

51. Patricia E. Stevens, "Lesbian Health Care Research: A Review of the Literature from 1970 to 1990," *Health Care for Women International* 13 (1992): 91–120.

52. Ironically, lesbians comprise the largest minority in nursing, 7 percent. See Michele J. Eliason and Carla E. Randall, "Lesbian Phobia in Nursing Students," *Western Journal of Nursing Research* 13, no. 3 (1991): 363–74; 363.

53. Stevens, "Lesbian Health Care Research," 95. Of the 1,009 M.D.'s surveyed in the first study, 93 percent were male. The nursing study consisted of 100 nurses teaching in bachelor's of science in nursing programs.

54. Eliason and Randall, 371–72. Of course, neither one of those beliefs is acceptable, but I cite this statistic as part of a larger point about the impact of homophobia on a putatively scientific, rational population.

55. Patricia E. Stevens and Joanne M. Hall, "Stigma, Health Beliefs and Experiences with Health Care in Lesbian Women," *IMAGE: Journal of Nursing Scholarship* 20, no. 2 (Summer 1988): 69–73; 72–73.

56. Susan D. Cochran and Vickie M. Mays, "Disclosure of Sexual Preference to Physicians by Black Lesbian and Bisexual Women," *Western Journal of Medicine* 149, no. 5 (Nov. 1988): 616–19; 618.

57. Cochran and Mays, 617.

58. As far back as 1981, Patricia Robertson and Julius Schachter reported similar

findings to those made by the two lesbian health surveys of the late eighties and early nineties regarding episodic health care among lesbians. They noted that among the women who had sex with women in their survey, "the average time interval from the last Papanicolau smear was 21 months as compared with the eight months for the general population of women using the same clinic" and speculated that the high-normal range of cervical dysplasia among the lesbians in their sample (2.7%) might reflect that lower health care provider visitation rate. See Patricia Robertson and Julius Schachter, "Failure to Identify Venereal Disease in a Lesbian Population," *Sexually Transmitted Diseases* 8, no. 2 (1981): 16–17; 17.

59. Personal communication, May 26, 1994.

60. Personal communication, March 25, 1994.

61. Coles, *Lesbian Projects*, 2–3; 7. As she notes,

In 1989, only 4.3 percent of government, foundation, and private funding dollars went to women's organizations. That same year, only 0.26 percent of foundation dollars went to gay and lesbian organizations, and there is no way of knowing how much of this tiny percentage went to lesbian projects. According to those interviewed, funders are either not interested in the reasons why lesbians do not seek services, or they believe lesbians are always welcome and comfortable at either gay or women's organizations. . . . All those interviewed spoke of the tremendous difficulty of confronting sexism within gay male organizations and homophobia within women's organizations.

62. *LAP Notes*, the newsletter of the New York City Lesbian AIDS Project (LAP), one of only three organizations worldwide committed entirely to serving the lesbian community in regard to HIV/AIDS issues, reports that "for the year ending June 31, 1995, LAP [had] answered 4200 individual requests for information and assistance; given presentations about Lesbian AIDS issues to over 240 groups, reading an additional 3600 people; and distributed over 51,000 LAP information packets, fliers, bibliographies, newsletters, resource guides, HIV prevention brochures and other written information." *LAP Notes* 3 (summer 1995): 23. For more information, see Nancy Goldstein's interview with Amber Hollibaugh, the Coordinator of LAP, *Deneuve* 4 (July/August 1994): 4.

63. Paula Ettelbrick, NCLR memorandums on the Women's Health Initiative letter-writing campaign, August 16, 1993, and on the Harvard Nurse's Study letter-writing campaign, December 1, 1993.

64. Personal communication, May 3, 1994.

65. See documentation regarding homophobia among health care providers earlier in this article.

66. Rebecca Young, personal communication, May 1, 1994.

67. Personal communication, March 25, 1994.

Part II

Institutional(ized) Myopia

6

Seeing AIDS: Race, Gender, and Representation

Evelynn M. Hammonds

Evelynn M. Hammonds is Assistant Professor of the History of Science in the Program in Science, Technology, and Society at MIT. Her research is in the history of science and medicine in the United States, specifically the history of disease, and topics on race and gender in science and medicine. Currently, she is completing a manuscript on the history of the control of diphtheria in the United States. Her new work is a historical study of conceptions of race in biology, medicine, and anthropology in the United States since the nineteenth century.

If one speaks about women and AIDS, one is speaking about African-American women.[1]

One of the more moving moments for me at the NGO Forum on Women, held in Beijing, occurred in a workshop on women and AIDS.[2] The panelists were all HIV positive. One of them, a young woman from South Africa, recounted her experiences living with AIDS in that country. She told us how she had been tested for the disease without her permission; she was given no counseling or support when she was told of her positive status. At the university she attended, she was not allowed to take a chemistry lab because instructors feared she would contaminate other students if there was an accident in the laboratory. Despite her anger and despair she volunteered to be a part of an AIDS prevention campaign. She agreed to this because she "wanted to put a face on AIDS, an African woman's face." It was her fervent hope that her face and her story would help other African and South African women recognize that they too were at risk for AIDS.

In December 1994, *Essence,* the leading national magazine for African-American women featured a beautiful young woman on its cover.[3] Without the accompanying text, the cover looked similar to every other issue of the magazine with its endless images of young, stylish, impeccably groomed, upwardly mobile black women. The text however, disrupted the image of youthful innocence and beauty. It read, "Facing AIDS: "I'm young, I'm educated, I'm drug-free, and I'm dying of AIDS." The accompanying story was a first-person account of this young woman's life with AIDS. I'm told that AIDS hotlines around the country reported increases in calls from African-American women after the appearance of the *Essence* story. Many of the callers remarked that they had not known they were at risk for HIV until they read the *Essence* article.[4]

Both these anecdotes indicate that despite the increasing rates of HIV infection among women of color, specifically among African-Americans and Hispanics/Latinas in the United States, and despite the widespread knowledge about how HIV is transmitted, women of color do not see their "faces" in representations of AIDS. As Sander Gilman has argued, the act of "seeing disease" is socially coded in many complicated ways. Images of disease tell us a great deal about the social construction of disease categories *and* they tell us about the internalization of such constructions in individuals from groups who are labeled as being at risk.[5] Thus, for African-American women, AIDS reflects a crisis of representation. The first African-American woman with AIDS was reported in 1982, and since that time African-American women have accounted for three-fourths of the females and two thirds of the children with HIV/AIDS.[6] Currently, African-American women account for 57 percent of the AIDS cases among women: this is sixteen times higher than the rate for white women.[7]

While these data show the increasing risk of HIV for African-American women, the representations of women with AIDS do not highlight this risk. In this essay I want to examine how the risk of AIDS to women is defined specifically with regard to African-American women. How is race depicted and/or elided in representations and narratives of women and AIDS? As many scholars have noted, representations of AIDS serve to draw the boundaries of risk and construct identities for whom the epidemic is meaningful; however, the complexities of the representations of African-American women and AIDS have not been taken up by cultural studies scholars writing about AIDS.

While scholars initially focused on the invisibility of women in the representations of AIDS in the early days of the epidemic, it is now recognized that there are many women depicted in AIDS narratives. As

Paula Treichler has noted, there are several identities and narratives readily available for women in relation to AIDS: "loving helpmeet/swinging single, Madonna/whore, good mother/bad mother and so on."[8] Alexandra Juhasz identifies six types of women in AIDS narratives: "middle-class, single yuppie; unmarried procreating low-income woman of color; the teenager forced to say no; the procreating white wife; the promiscuous prostitute (the African/Haitian woman gets tossed into this category as well, because of her assumed promiscuity); and the unseen and therefore unsexed lesbian."[9] Each of these categories carve up "woman" into "a series of women-who-do-not-count-as-women," which produces in turn "women" who are deserving of protection and empathy and another group of "women" rendered outside of the boundaries of protection, but whose behaviors must be policed and controlled.[10] African-American women in these narratives fall within the categories of women who are not deserving of protection or consideration without respect to their class or educational background. Most importantly, however, this is not a new categorization of African-American women. The task of the critic is to show how, and to what effect, such constructions arise historically, how they persist, how they are perceived by African-American women, and how they are used by the media and the medical/public health establishment in representations of the risk for AIDS.

Media constructions of women with AIDS use race to "shore up racist ideas that African-American women's sexuality is categorically different than 'white' heterosexuality."[11] In so doing African-American women are not rendered invisible in AIDS narratives in any simple way; rather, they are simultaneously made invisible *and* exposed. As I have argued elsewhere, early media representations of persons with AIDS greatly contributed to the invisibility of African-American women. On the one hand, when the threat of AIDS to women is discussed, no mention is made of African-American women. When they do appear, they are relegated to the drug abuser category, or partners of drug abusers or the supremely negative category of bad mother. These women's lives are described as "unruly," "chaotic," and "despairing." Secondly, they are rendered invisible because of the tendency of the media to make symbols out of AIDS victims in order to represent to the public a particular aspect of the epidemic. African-American women do not fit into the categories of: innocent child; victimized patient of irresponsible health care workers; creative artist; or African-American male super-athlete.[12]

In addition, African-American women with AIDS have eloquently spoken about their invisibility in the AIDS epidemic. Margaret Rivera's testimony is illustrative of this point: "Nobody is ever in to see me or to hear my complaints. They're never there when I try to make an appointment to get anything done. Nobody cares. I continue to get sick over and over again and nobody listens to what I have to say. I don't think that's fair because I feel I deserve better, because not only am I a woman, I am also a human being, and its hard enough for me to deal with the issue of having AIDS, dying a day at a time and to have to live under the circumstances that I am under." [13] Though Rivera's testimony poignantly and vividly speaks to the material effects of her invisibility in the AIDS epidemic, African-American women are not simply rendered invisible: they are simultaneously profoundly exposed.

Many newspaper articles that address women and AIDS typically do not carry headlines that signal that the articles are about women of color, nor do the headlines emphasize that women of color are at greater risk for AIDS. The text usually begins by reporting statistics which confirm that indeed the *only* women who should be concerned about AIDS are women of color. This disjuncture between a headline that calls attention to "women" followed by text which focuses on women of color in effect simultaneously erases and stigmatizes women of color. In fact, white women have begun to respond to this representation by emphasizing their risk for AIDS. A white woman from Long Island wrote, "I want to tell my story and I want people to see me so that they realize that AIDS has a face, a middle class white face." [14] In the same article another white woman remarked, "I'm not an i.v. drug user or a poor woman. I'm not a self-destructive woman. AIDS happens to normal middle class professional single women who date. It happens to nice Jewish girls like me." [15] This struggle for the "face" of AIDS indicates that the dependence on stereotypes in the representation of women and AIDS has become a barrier to all women in assessing their risk from AIDS. All women then engage in distancing themselves from the stereotypes in AIDS narratives. The representation of the woman at risk for HIV/AIDS as a woman of color either produces classist, racist, and addictaphobic declarations of difference from white women or exposes these as necessary if not fundamental aspects of white middle-class female culture.

Everyone who confronts AIDS narratives and representations experiences a desire for some boundary, some demarcation between themselves and the chaos and stigma that the disease represents. The declarations of some white women suggest that the white woman with AIDS *must* be innocent. AIDS happens to these women: it is an accident—an unfortunate bad choice and an ultimately undeserved fate. Here race—that is, whiteness—joined by educational and class privilege, is the sign of this innocence and the most significant boundary between these women and the stigma associated with HIV/AIDS. This is the obverse of how race is deployed as a risk factor for women of color. Furthermore, white women can read AIDS prevention messages in a way that invokes race to preserve this boundary. Meghan Daum does this when she argues that since she is a middle-class, white woman graduate of an elite college who doesn't sleep with bisexual or i.v. drug-using men; and since "less than three-fourths of one percent of white non-Hispanic men with HIV infection contracted the virus through heterosexual sex with a non-iv drug using woman," she is not at risk.[16] More disturbingly she writes, "until more people appear on television, look into the camera and tell me that they contracted HIV through heterosexual sex with someone who had no risk factors, I will continue to disregard the message."[17] Such declarations by white women are certainly racist by default if not by intent.[18]

For African-American women, race is used in a way that overdetermines their risk for HIV/AIDS. As African-American women are, on the one hand, rendered invisible in certain aspects of AIDS narratives, they are also made explicitly visible because they are considered the only women at risk. Yet they are visible in journalistic narratives in ways that sustain their invisibility. In many newspaper articles the women of color with AIDS rarely have names; the authors usually assert that the women want it this way because they fear exposure and censure from family, community, or employers. These nameless women are typically described by age, race, maternal status, and drug use history, but only rarely by first name and last initial. Very intimate details of their lives are revealed including their lack of economic resources; their fears of dying; their inability to care for their children; their mistrust and dependence on unreliable male partners; their sense of despair about the future.[19] Their powerlessness is graphically exposed in these narratives, but they have no "face," no fully articulated identity that culturally signifies African-Americans or Latinas as "women."

The experts that figure in such articles lament the fact that African-American women do not accept the fact that they are at risk for AIDS. African-American women's so-called denial of risk is cast by the experts as unreasonable and irresponsible given the scientific evidence which points to their greater risk. Thus the experts argue that the behavior of women of color suggests an inability to simply "face the facts."[20] The portrait of the woman with AIDS is explicitly one who is African-American or Latina, poor, an i.v. drug user, single mother, partner of drug abuser, living a chaotic life in some urban center usually in the northeastern United States, who refuses to accept her risk for HIV infection. This refusal is read not as a refusal of the stigmatized stereotypes embedded in these narratives, but rather as a rejection of medical and scientific authority.

Implicitly these narratives also articulate that such women pose a threat to the larger public and thus do not deserve the protection of their rights but rather must be controlled by the state. African-American women thus see in such narratives a profoundly negative representation of themselves, one that is based on familiar and frightening stereotypes as well as the attendant specter of an insensitive and intrusive medical/public health establishment. The narratives of women and AIDS are just one more example of the joining of race and gender into a narrative which ultimately erases/exposes and pathologizes African-American women. Both newspaper accounts and the article in *Essence* magazine speak to the dual narratives of African-American women long given currency in American culture—the "black lady" and the "welfare mother." As literary critic Wahneema Lubiano has argued,

> Categories like "black woman," "black women," or particular subsets of those categories, like "welfare mother/queen," are not simply social taxonomies, they are also recognized in the national public as stories that describe the world in particular and politically loaded ways—and that is exactly why they are constructed, reconstructed, manipulated, and contested.[21]

Within AIDS narratives, the irresponsible African-American mother/welfare queen and the African-American lady are two figures which exist side by side as narratives which are powerful because they are guaranteed to divert attention away from the historical and contemporary neglectful treatment of all African-American women within the health care system. To paraphrase Lubiano, it is difficult to conceive of a "normal," unproblematic space in our historical moment for black women outside of the demonic-narrative economy of the welfare queen or the betrayal-narrative economy of the black-lady overachiever (as represented by the *Essence* woman). The disproportionate and increasing presence of AIDS in African-

American communities signals that the black-lady overachiever is always precariously placed to fall to the level of the welfare-queen as the differences between and among African-American women is collapsed within AIDS narratives. In addition, critics must recognize that neither the "African-American welfare queen" nor the "African-American lady" are accurate representations of real African-American women.

> With the representation of AIDS, as with other images of disease, it is the historically determined variations that mark the function and place of the sufferer in relation to the society in which he or she dwells. From such images we can begin to understand how such models of disease evoke the most deep-seated sense of the self's fragility. Those suffering the very disease about which such fantasies are spun are themselves not immune; they respond to the isolation and stigmatization that is the social boundary of their disease not part of the disease itself.[22]

How do African-American women evaluate their risk within AIDS narratives? There is clearly much social science research that needs to be done examining how cultural constructions of African-American women with AIDS affect perceptions of risk and, of course, risk reduction behavior; however, some preliminary conclusions can be drawn. First, many social scientists have documented that risk from AIDS is constructed against the backdrop of other risks—"the benefits of heterosexual interaction and possible pregnancy and childbearing outweigh risks of disease, when not risking this could lead to more immediate consequences such as verbal and physical abuse, the loss of a partner, or childlessness,"[23] and the loss of economic support and community. Anthropologist E. J. Sobo argues that community-level HIV/AIDS risk denial among African-Americans is part of a self-protective strategy adopted in the face of racist finger-pointing and blame-laying; therefore, risk denial is essential for maintaining group pride. For African-American women, she argues, individual risk denial is constructed in relation to "idealized cultural constructions of gender and heterosexual relationships, which are used in rhetoric that supports claims of social position and bolsters self-esteem."[24]

Sobo's analysis focuses on the narratives that poor inner-city African-American women construct about risks. She identifies two important ones. The first, she calls the "wisdom narrative" where African-American women try to maintain their ability to identify "clean" (i.e. disease free) and upstanding male partners. The second is the "monogamy narrative" in which African-American women describe an idealized, monogamous, heterosexual union which they use to deny the infidelity of their partners and promote their own self-esteem.[25] These narratives indicate that risk for HIV/AIDS for African-American women is constructed within the context of African-American culture. Rather than risk denial, these poor African-American women are trying to construct an image of themselves in relation to their male partners that allows them some agency and self-esteem while locating themselves within the dominant category of woman. To use Gloria Anzaldua's term, they are "making face," constructing identities.[26]

But Sobo's analysis does not include the perceptions of middle-class African-American women. Another narrative evident in the account of Rae Lewis-Thornton in *Essence* is the "redemption narrative." Lewis-Thornton begins by distancing herself from the prevailing view of women (African-American women) with AIDS, "I am the quintessential Buppie: I'm young—32. Well educated. Professional. Attractive. Smart. I've been drug- and alcohol-free all my life. I'm a Christian. I've never been promiscuous. Never had a one-night stand. And I am dying of AIDS."[27] By her list of negatives, she foregrounds the prevailing view of African-American women with AIDS as uncontrolled, drug abusing, uneducated, and poor. She is a victim of AIDS because she "had one partner too many," and she continues, "I'm here to tell you that one is all it takes." In this instance a Black professional woman's declarations distancing herself from the stigma of AIDS speaks to the aspect of AIDS narratives that suggest that race is an inherent risk factor for AIDS. The goal for Lewis-Thornton is to overturn the negative stigma associated with AIDS by acknowledging her mistake through an appeal to religion for forgiveness and redemption. "Surrendering myself to God is the smartest decision I have made in this odyssey. As I let go of the old person, God created a new one. This new Rae has a purpose." The stigma associated with AIDS is removed in this account; equally importantly, through this process of redemption she also finds a new partner: "God, sent me a man grounded in Christianity and bursting with compassion, love—and fun."[28] At the end of the article Lewis-Thornton's image as an upstanding African-American woman deserving of compassion is preserved. The image of the African-American woman that *Essence* magazine sells—educated, upwardly mobile, committed to community uplift, religious, drug-free, monogamous and heterosexual—that was threatened by the association with AIDS is preserved through the narrative of redemption, thus allowing *Essence* readers to embrace an African-American woman with AIDS. The message in this article is again not a simple denial of risk but rather a revaluation of risk and the stigma associated with infection with HIV in light of specific African-American cultural values.

By accepting uncritically the notion that African-American women engage in risk denial, with its connotations of failure and irresponsibility, Sobo and other researchers cannot see the complicated negotiations that African-American women must go through to acknowledge their risk while denying their own demonization and that of their partners in dominant representations of AIDS. The discourse of race in the United States has constructed African-American women as "all-that-is-not-white," inherently different from white women. In order to articulate their risk from AIDS, African-American women have developed complex narratives to claim a place within the category of protected women including, but not exclusively, by appealing to their similarity with the idealized image of white women and normative heterosexuality rather than to their presumed inherent difference from these. The "face" of AIDS that African-American women want to see is one that does not allow a demonized image of themselves to stand as a norm for all African-American women, especially with respect to an issue tied to both sexuality and disease.[29]

The irony of this move on the part of African-American women is that the decision to claim a similarity with white women in order to enter the category of protected women makes it more difficult to acknowledge that no "women" are protected in this epidemic. The refusal of racial stereotypes does not remove the problems associated with gender and sexuality with respect to AIDS. Moreover, through this move African-American women lose one of the critical insights that their situation brings to bear on this epidemic: that heterosexual relationships have to be reconstructed in the age of AIDS in order for women to reduce their risk.

Cultural critics writing about women and AIDS have noted the ways in which African-American women and other women of color have been stigmatized in this epidemic. Few, however, recognize that what is happening on the level of representation mirrors what is occurring at the level of research and prevention. African-American women continue to provide disturbing reports of the moral scrutiny they face regarding their reproductive choices when they seek health care services for HIV, and they undergo significantly more forced sterilizations because of their HIV status or drug use.[30] The task for critics is to relentlessly emphasize that the representations of the demonization of African-American women are necessary for the preservation of the notion of the purity of (some) white women. African-American women as figured in AIDS narratives consistently become the site where whites' fears of disease are banished. The tragedy is that what is obscured by situating African-American women as "other" is the fact that the AIDS epidemic is becoming the great leveller of women. "Fear of becoming infected and an inability to ensure that they remain uninfected are common to virtually all heterosexually active women, irrespective of their race, their education, their social class, their lifestyles, their marital status, their legal rights, or any other socioeconomic variable."[31]

While health care workers and cultural critics have argued that AIDS prevention messages must grow out of and reflect the diverse realities of women's lives, the question remains how to do this. Is it possible to produce representations of African-American women's lives without confronting the problems in the representations, both visually and in narratives, of the binary of white women as "women" versus African-American women as "women-who-do-not-count as women"? At the core of this representational problem is the problem of race. Health care workers, policy analysts and scholars all acknowledge that race has been used in problematic and materially damaging ways in the AIDS epidemic. Most analysts have been clear that in large part race has been used to separate women or treated as a barrier or indeed as a risk factor itself.[32] In addition, many national commission reports make clear that there is no biological link between race and AIDS. This explication, however, is insufficient for dislodging the links between race and AIDS that sensationalized media reports note and prevention material represent. In particular, neutral-sounding disclaimers denying a biological link between race and AIDS do not address the pervasive view that race is a biological fact rather than a social myth.[33] This remains a key problematic in representations of AIDS because there is no adequate explanation available as to *why* African-American women are at greater risk from AIDS nor as to why it is spreading faster in communities of color.

This is not just a problem for AIDS prevention: it is the familiar one that feminists have been engaged with over the last ten years in confronting the problem of race and gender and the attendant disappearance of the black woman in feminist theory. Feminist theorists are still struggling with how to think about race and gender relationally. This is the perspective that is lost when race and gender are discussed separately or within a binary oppositional construct.[34] Though there is still much theoretical work to do: representations of women and AIDS need to incorporate feminist theory in order to depict the relationship between race and gender, and to disrupt stereotypes of both, if they are to be effective and meaningful for all women.

A first step would be to acknowledge that our understanding of race in the U.S. is profoundly dependent upon the visual. One of the most provocative examples of a representation of women and AIDS that embodies the complex history of representations of African-American women and also speaks to all women is provided by artist Lorna Simpson (Figure 1). Simpson's photograph for the Art Against AIDS Project depicts the torso of a dark-skinned woman dressed in a white sheath. Her arms are crossed just below barely discernible breasts. The figure seems to be vulnerable in the way she holds herself and yet also determined. There is no face. The body speaks the text written upon it:

> *a lie is not a shelter*
> *discrimination*
> *is not protection*
> *isolation is not a remedy*
> *a promise is not a prophylactic*

Simpson's photograph is a critique of the prevailing representations of Black women's bodies, and of women and AIDS. The photograph is both specific and universal: the body of a dark-skinned woman—she could be African-American or Latina—dressed in a sheath that is similar to the gown any woman would wear in a medical setting. It is the text that disrupts dominant representations of women's risk for AIDS. Rather than speaking *for* women of color with AIDS, the photograph speaks *to* the questions AIDS prevention raises for any woman: the potential infidelity of partners; the discrimination that women encounter in the health care system; the silence that accompanies the fear of loss of community and family; and the too often futile hope that "love" can protect women from AIDS. And finally the figure's embrace of herself can be read as a call for self-empowerment. Simpson's photograph evokes race and disrupts racial stereotyping at the same time; it speaks to Black women, not for them; it speaks to all women from the perspective of a Black woman and thus highlights both the subjective and the universal. The viewer cannot inscribe upon this woman of color the familiar litany of stereotypes first, because Simpson refuses to "expose" the Black female body, and her refusal to show a face "mirrors the refusal of the world to know these black women."[35] In addition, as Saidiya Hartman has noted, "Simpson's self-imposed limits—her choice

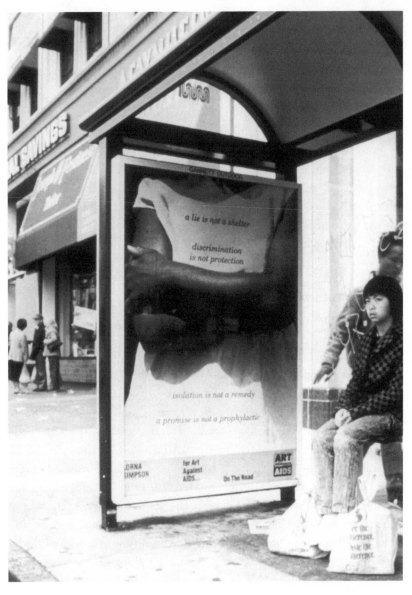

6.1. "Art Against Aids" illuminated bus shelter by Lorna Simpson, San Francisco, CA, 1989, by kind permission of Lorna Simpson, Sean Kelly, NY.

not to show faces—articulate the limits of dominant representations of black women, which have shown everything only to de-face black women as subjects."[36] Finally, Simpson's Black female body cannot be seen in familiar racialized terms because it speaks against such a reading, and thus it counters a reading of race in the body, as biology. Simpson successfully and powerfully disrupts the negative representations of African-American women by her skillful insistence that representations must be challenged by articulation. Her example is one we should all follow if we want to produce effective and empowering identities that all women can claim in the midst of this epidemic.

NOTES

1. National Commission on AIDS, "The Challenge of HIV/AIDS in Communities of Color," Washington, D.C., December, 1992, p. 34.

2. The NGO Forum in Beijing (August 30–September 8, 1995) was part of the Fourth World Conference on Women of the United Nations.

3. Rae Lewis-Thornton, "Facing AIDS," *Essence,* December 1994, p. 63.

4. Personal communication from case workers at AIDS projects in New Jersey and Georgia.

5. Sander Gilman, *Disease and Representation: Images of Illness from Madness to AIDS* (Ithaca, N.Y.: Cornell University Press, 1988), 4.

6. National Commission on AIDS, 5.

7. Centers for Disease Control, *Morbidity and Mortality Weekly Report* 44, no. 5 (February 10, 1995): 82.

8. Paula A. Treichler, "Beyond Cosmo: AIDS, Identity and Inscriptions of Gender," in "Imaging Technologies, Inscribing Science" *Camera Obscura,* no. 28 (June 1992): 1–2.

9. Alexandra Juhasz, "The Contained Threat: Women in Mainstream AIDS Documentary," *Journal of Sex Research* 29, no. 1 (February 1990): 25–46.

10. Cindy Patton, *Last Served? Gendering the HIV Pandemic* (London: Taylor and Francis, 1994), 1–2.

11. Ibid., 11.

12. See my essay, "Missing Persons: African-American Women, AIDS and the History of Disease," *Radical America* 24, no. 2 (April-June 1990): 7–24.

13. Testimony of Margaret Rivera, report of the public hearing, "AIDS: Its Impact on Women, Children and Families," June 12, 1987 (New York State Division on Women, 1987): 21.

14. Cheryl P. Weinstock, "For Women, Growing Risks from AIDS," *New York Times,* October 21, 1990, sec. 12: 1, 19.

15. Ibid.

16. Meghan Daum, "Safe-Sex Lies," *New York Times Magazine,* January 21, 1996, 32–33.

17. Ibid.

18. Thanks to Nancy Goldstein for her insightful comments on this point.

19. See "A Woman with AIDS Asks: Who Will Care for Her Children?" *New York Times,* April 20, 1991, B2.

20. "AIDS in Women Rising, but Many Ignore the Threat," *New York Times,* December 28, 1990, B1.

21. Wahneema Lubiano, "Black Ladies, Welfare Queens, and State Minstrels: Ideological War by Narrative Means," in *Race-ing Justice, En-gendering Power,* ed. Toni Morrison (New York: Pantheon, 1992), 330–31.

22. Gilman, 272.

23. E. J. Sobo, "Inner-City Women and AIDS: The Psycho-social Benefits of Unsafe Sex," *Culture, Medicine and Psychiatry* 17 (1993: 455–85.

24. Ibid., 463.

25. Ibid., 469.

26. See Gloria Anzaldua's Introduction to *Making Face, Making Soul: Creative and critical Perspectives by Women of Color,* ed. Gloria Anzaldua (San Francisco: Aunt Lute, 1990), xv.

27. Lewis-Thornton, 63.

28. Ibid., 130.

29. See discussions by Black feminist critics Deborah McDowell, Hazel Carby, and Patricia Hill Collins among many others on the complexities of the representation of African-American women's sexuality.

30. National Commission on AIDS, 36.

31. Elizabeth Reid, "Population and Development Issues: The Linkages to HIV and Women," in *Defining the Women and AIDS Agenda* (Arlington, Va.: AIDSCAP Women's Initiative, 1995), 27.

32. Center for Women Policy Studies, "National HIV Prevention Policy Agenda for Women" (Washington, D.C.: Center for Women and Policy Studies, 1995), draft, 2.

33. For an excellent discussion of race and class and epidemiology see Nancy Krieger, Byllye Avery et al., "Racism, Sexism and Social Class: Implications for Studies of Health, Disease, and Well-being," *American Journal of Preventive Medicine* 9, 6 Suppl. (November—December 1993): 82–122.

34. For a recent discussion by a feminist theorist on the notion of racialized sexuality see Judith Butler, *Bodies That Matter: On the Discursive Limits of "Sex"* (New York: Routledge, 1993), especially chapter six.

35. Lorna Simpson, quoted in Saidiya V. Hartman, "Excisions of the Flesh," in B. Wright and S. Hartman, *Lorna Simpson: For the Sake of the Viewer* (Chicago: Museum of Contemporary Art, 1992), 61.

36. Ibid.

7

"*Sí, tenemos sexo con mujeres, pero no somos marimachas.*" (Sure, we have sex with women, but we're not lesbians.): Sexual Diversity in the Los Angeles *Latina* Community—Ethnographic Findings, 1987–95

Laura J. Ramos

Laura J. Ramos is a specialist in the field of sexually transmitted disease (STD) and HIV/AIDS prevention. She focused on utilizing ethnographic methods in order to discover and understand *Latinas*' and WSW's sexual and other risks for STDs/HIV. She's been an AIDS activist since 1986 and would love to see HIV and other STDs eradicated from the planet.

Psssst! Hey *ése!* Hey you over there! I know this is supposed to be an academic book, you know, for those professors and doctors, but what I got to say, can't be said that way, you know? I got to tell it from here, from L.A. man, not from the ivory tower. I jes' want to invite you into my world for a moment. Come listen to me and my friends, we'll tell you some things sure. Mind your manners though, boys and girls, 'cause it can be dangerous down here. Yeah, I know, you think we all talk like this in the *barrio*. Just like in those gang movies and shit. Let's get real.

Actually, here in Los Angeles, most of us *Latinas* can talk like that if we want to, if we need to, but most of us don't use it all the time. Sometimes we talk that way just to aggravate other folks or sometimes just to feel at home with someone. Lots of us don't have a Spanish accent, except when speaking Spanish, of course! But you'd be amazed at the percentage of the time *Latinos* are portrayed as being heavily accented, slang-mouthed, ignorant immigrants in the major media. Ruins our image, you know? I would like to extend you all a *bienvenidos* (a big welcome) to Los Angeles. *Nuestra casa es su casa.* Our home is yours too for the moment. Sit down and make yourself comfortable. I want to introduce you to *mi familia.* No, I don't mean all my brothers and sisters, I mean my extended *Latina* lesbian family here in L.A. No, not all of us call ourselves lesbians, but that's getting ahead of myself, let's begin at the beginning.

We're inviting you into our home so that you can begin to see the AIDS and Sexually Transmitted Disease (STD) epidemics from our point of view. Most of us don't have a lot of access to education, medical care, and preventive health messages. We've got to get the information about how these diseases are affecting our community from our friends, neighbors, and the other women like us who are afraid to ask questions. Yeah, it helps that we've got some women who've gone on for that fancy education and many other lesbians who've been working against AIDS since the beginning, but it's pretty confusing down here. We're trying to cope the best ways we know how, but the "powers that be" (the CDC, doctors, researchers, etc.) don't really study us much at all. Yet we're told that "Lesbians don't get AIDS," "Lesbians don't get STDs," "Lesbians don't have much sex," etc.[1] Heck, at the beginning of the epidemic when our gay brothers were feeling cursed and condemned by the fearmongers, we were touted as "God's chosen people" because we weren't supposed to be at risk. *¡Ay! Hermanos y hermanas,* my brothers and sisters, I just have to ask: If we're not supposed to be at risk, how come so many of us have HIV and STDs?

I want you to meet some of my *lesbianas Latinas* and *Latinas*-who-have-sex-with-women (*LSW*) sisters who have or are at varying risk for HIV or STDs. Then I want to discuss some of the bases for the debates about how HIV or STDs can be passed from one woman to another during sex. Mind you, I've met or ethno-graphically observed hundreds of *Latina LSW* in Los Angeles[2] alone, but I only have space to introduce you to a few of us. All of the names are changed to protect the privacy of these *Latinas.* For this book chapter, I'd like you to meet Esmerelda, Olga, Hortensia, Fabiola, Guadalupe, Cristina, Ana, Yolanda, and Gloria. Each history represents a few of the ways that *LSW* are at risk for HIV and STDs.

Esmerelda

Esmerelda is a 34-year-old *Dominicana* who was diagnosed with HIV ten years ago. She's had many struggles, the worst of which is trying to get the

Latina lesbian and the general lesbian community to believe that she, as an HIV + lesbian, exists. In exasperation one day she said,

> Why can't they see me? They got to know I'm out here. I keep talking 'til I'm blue in the face and I still feel invisible. Hell, I can't stand to cry and every time I go out telling my story I cry. Why can't they even see my tears?

Esmerelda thinks she got HIV from using drugs, but she's not sure because she also had a lot of unprotected sex.

> They say I got it from sharing needles back before I stopped using drugs. But I don't know, I did a lot of things I'm not proud of. I had a lot of unprotected sex—with men and with women. Yeah, I fucked around a lot. But *coño,* everybody did. It was a way to belong, especially when we were high and stuff. Sometimes it was a way to cop some stuff or to make your high better. Especially when we did uppers, that made me do all kinds of crazy shit. One time I was out with some guys and we were doing coke and some other shit. Then we all started having sex. Yeah, I had sex with all of them. And we did everything, you know, from the front, up the ass, you name it we did it. One of the guys took some of the coke and put it on my cunt and then licked it off. Didn't do that much though, 'cause you don't get much of a high that way and the stuff costs too much to waste.

On another occasion, Esmerelda talks about her experiences with women:

> Some girlfriends and I would go out drinking and doping. Sometimes we'd make out together. But I never really discovered my love for women until after I got sober. Yeah, but just as I was falling for my first woman, I got my HIV diagnosis. It almost sent me back to using—you never know, it still could. It's a fight, a fight every day to survive—if it ain't HIV, it's my addictions. Then I thought, oh my God, I can't ever have sex again! I could give this thing to somebody. Damn it, I was just beginning to live, and now I'm going to die!

Many years later, she finally got involved with another *Latina* lesbian (Olga).

> I just couldn't believe it when she said she liked me too! When we decided to go steady, I must have told the whole world! They all told me, 'You Go Girl!' But it wasn't that easy for Olga, her friends couldn't understand why she'd go out with an HIV + woman. They told her she was crazy and should know better. We were just trying to be happy together. It was good to feel wanted, loved. But this safer sex thing was not easy. See I thought I'd never have sex again, so I never paid any attention to how women have safe sex. I didn't know what to do, she had to explain everything to me. I just wanted to dive in with my whole heart. It was hard to not to go for it all! But I

knew I didn't want to ever put her at risk for HIV, so I really tried to behave myself.

Olga

Olga, a 30-year-old *Cubana,* was Esmerelda's lover for two years. The stress of dealing with HIV was complicated by the fact that she also has an incurable STD, human papilloma virus (HPV), which had given her cervical cancer. She said,

> In many ways it was the easiest safer sex discussion I ever had with a new lover. Everyone else had all kinds of reasons why lesbians didn't have to practice safer sex. Esmerelda just said "of course!", but she didn't know how. The main problem between us was that she only knew about her HIV and wouldn't believe that I could possibly have anything that risky to give her. I mean, a lot of women with HIV are dying from cervical cancer 'cause their bodies can't fight off the HPV, and she's telling me she doesn't care. Right in the middle of sex, she'd ask me if she could go down on me! I mean, damn it, it's hard enough to negotiate about safer sex when I'm not doin' it, but it was an emotional nightmare to have to tell her not to right then. I mean my entire body is praying that I can have the feel of her mouth, hands, cunt directly on my skin, inside of me, you know? And I got to tell her no? It was just too much. It was one of the reasons we had to break up, I couldn't take the stress of taking on so much of the responsibility, you know?

Olga and Esmerelda always practiced safer sex even though they were tempted not to at times. Neither one could bear the thought of giving their disease to the other. They explained that,

> We always used gloves to touch each other's cants, with lots of water-based lube so we didn't get irritated by the rubber. We tried to be creative, like putting a large bowl of warm water by the bed so that it was easy to rinse the powder off of the gloves. It was also useful to have at least two wastebaskets lined with plastic bags within throwing distance of the bed. That way we didn't have to worry about spreading stuff through latex we'd used when cleaning up later. Especially since Esmerelda often had yeast infections too. We didn't use dental dams, 'cause we didn't do oral sex. Given the two STDs and the yeast, we thought it was too risky. Some other dykes would have, but every woman or couple has to make these decisions by what they know and how they feel. We tried not to do anything that would make one or both of us feel scared. Scared of getting something or giving something. But it was pretty rewarding. Oh yeah, when we used toys—you know, dildos or vibrators and stuff—we always covered 'em with condoms too.

How did Olga get the HPV?

Well, they don't really know for sure. When I was diagnosed with the cervical cancer, I'd been out as a dyke for eight years already. They say that the HPV can be latent for a long time or it can hit you right away. If it hits you right away it can take as little as eighteen months to develop cancer. By that time I'd already had three lovers and certainly I'd done stuff with them which I think could have spread HPV. See it's really contagious—it's easy to get, not like HIV which is hard. All you got to do is touch the skin which is infected. In my case I'd never have known I had anything, 'cause it never made any warts or anything. I never had any symptoms. I just went in for my pap smear and BAM, I had cancer! I could have caught it from a woman 'cause my first woman lover gave me a "trich" infection, so she could have had HPV too. And I had clit-to-clit contact with all my girlfriends up till the time I really realized that dykes could get STDs too. But by the time I really caught on, it was already too late for me. I wish I could go back in time and just wash it all off. So I could feel clean again, you know?

This couple represents the many *LSW* and their lovers who face the uncertainty and dangers of one or more STDs/HIV in their love relationship. Their relationship occurred in the early 1990's when more information and debate was taking place regarding woman-to-woman transmission of HIV/STDs. They were much better informed on safer sex practices than the vast majority of the *LSW* communities. Although the next participant history happened in the late 1980s, Hortensia and her lover represent the situation which still exists for most WSW worldwide—a basic lack of definitive information regarding female-to-female sexual risks and the dreadful uncertainty we live with on a daily basis.

Hortensia

Hortensia was a *Chicana* lesbian who hung out with a group of *lesbianas* in the late 1980's. She was a sweet butch, with a great sense of humor. Sometimes she'd talk about her White lover, who couldn't hang out with this group most of the time 'cause it was for *Latinas* only. I met Hortensia in April one year, saw her a few times, and then in August she vanished. Rumor had it that she was very sick. Then in March the next year, I got a phone call saying that they'd found out that Hortensia was in an AIDS hospice and they were suggesting everyone send cards or letters of support. She was so upset about what was happening to her body that she really didn't want any visitors. I tried calling the hospice, but Hortensia died the day before my call.

A few weeks later, I had a talk with Maggie, Hortensia's lover. Maggie was understandably grief-stricken, but she was also very concerned about her own health. She didn't know what to believe about HIV. She didn't know if she'd done anything to get it from Hortensia. Not that they did that much after she'd been diagnosed, but before that, well . . .

> They told me at the hospice that I'd be fine. Lesbians couldn't pass it to one another. Now I'm not so sure. They seemed to wave away my concerns without another thought. But were they really listening? They never asked me what we did together. If they didn't know that, then how could they be so sure. I know it's terrible to say, but I don't want to die like Hortensia did. She was such a sweet, warm woman. She taught me so much and gave me so much in this life. I can't believe she's gone.

So Maggie and I talked about her risks. Certainly, for most of their time together they practiced low-risk behaviors, especially since Hortensia was mostly a "stone butch" (she would please Maggie and be pleased by that sexual release herself as well), so that Maggie never went down on her, or "kissed clits," or came into contact directly with her genitals or blood. After that, Maggie felt somewhat relieved, but she wasn't sure if she should get tested for HIV. I encouraged her to go get tested if it would help ease her mind, but suggested that she shouldn't get the test if she couldn't face receiving a positive result. I never found out if she got tested or not, as we lost contact with each other after a memorial service was held for Hortensia. Even though the memorial service was announced to our crowd, almost none of the other *lesbianas Latinas* showed up. They couldn't deal with the thought that one of us could have fallen to AIDS. To this day they don't talk about what happened to Hortensia. Even though they knew that what had happened to her could have happened to any of us—she got HIV from a blood transfusion during an operation.

Fabiola

Fabiola is a fortyish *El Salvadoreña* who had recently immigrated to the United States. She is a very proper and respected member of the *Latina* lesbian community. She came to the United States after breaking up with her lover of nineteen years. This woman had helped raise Fabiola's children and then left her to be with a man. Fabiola found that she had fallen in love with this woman while she was still married to her children's father. After a time, she moved herself and the children into a house which she shared with her lover, Lourdes. In this relationship, Fabiola very much identified as the butch or "*marimacha*," while Lourdes played the role of the "feminine" woman. I don't say "fem" or "femme" as those are terms usually reserved for women who identify as lesbian. Lourdes did not identify as lesbian, she felt that she had a "special relationship" with Fabiola. She did believe that Fabiola was a lesbian, because Fabiola was "*marimacha*"; she wore pants or suits and not "women's clothing." Fabiola took on the role of breadwinner and supported the family the best she could.

At first she told me that she and Lourdes exclusively practiced "*sexo de vagina a vagina*." When asked why, Fabiola responded, "*No pude darle más de eso.*" To give her partner anything less would have been an insult, just as it was the "ultimate behavior between men and women." Later she admitted to "going down on her partner," especially when she had her period. She said, "*Me gusta ver el sangrado*" (I liked to see her blood). However, if her partner's period was particularly heavy, she stated, "*Cuando hay mucha sangre se para de tener relaciones hasta al tiempo que el sangre disminuye*" (they waited until the blood diminished). She didn't like for her lover to do anything except touch her "*vagina.*" She felt that the point of any other sexual activity was to culminate in "*sexo de vagina a vagina.*"

Eventually Fabiola disclosed that while she'd previously stated that she'd not had sex with a man in the past ten years, that perhaps she did have, just twice. I asked her to explain.

> *Cuando vine a los Estados Unidos, yo no tenía mucho dinero. Necesitaba algún dinero para crear un negocio. Conocía un hombre bien honorable a quien me ofreció algún dinero para mi negocio a cambio de tener sexo con él.* (When I came to the U.S., I didn't have much money. I needed some money to start a business. I knew a respectable man who offered me money in exchange for having sex with me.)

She explained that she'd known that this man was interested in her for some time and that she thought it was a reasonable exchange. She said proudly that he'd received his "money's worth" from her end of the bargain. She made sure to add that she'd only done it for the money and that she still was and always would be a lesbian.

Guadalupe

Another *LSW* who'd had sex with a man, was a young Mexicana named Guadalupe. Guadalupe, her baby daughter, her sister Amelia and Amelia's lover Veronica all lived in the same house. Of these three women, only Amelia, who was "*marimacha*" identified as "*Lesbiana*." Veronica felt that she was only in this relationship, because she'd fallen in love with Amelia; she was one of the few *LSW* who thought of herself as "*bisexual*." Guadalupe really didn't believe in these labels, all she knew was that she was attracted to and wanted to be with women. She wasn't "masculine" or "*marimacha*" like her sister, so she didn't identify as "*Lesbiana*." Guadalupe was twenty-three and at the age which she thought she should be having children, so she decided to get pregnant. In this densely populated *Latino barrio* on the east side of L.A. was a man from Guatemala whose goal in life seemed to be focused on having sex with as many women in the neighborhood as he could. Guadalupe "let herself be alone with him one day." She "let him take her" and in five minutes (she explained that he just pulled her skirt up and underwear down, having sex standing up against the wall in an empty apartment), she not only got pregnant, she got gonorrhea. She got the infection treated and now has a healthy, beautiful baby girl.

None of the AIDS literature addresses WSW, particularly women of color, who have sex with men to get pregnant. That literature has focused on the risk from transmission via artificial insemination.[3] However, women of color, particularly lesbians, have little or no access to formal insemination clinics. We need to look at all the reasons WSW are having sex with men and stop treating all occurrences of vaginal-penile intercourse the same. Often *LSW* choose to have sex with bisexual or gay *Latino* men in order to get pregnant, because they know that these men will not harass them about their stigmatized lifestyle or because they wish to share parenting roles with these men. This increases the chance that they may be infected with HIV.

Cristina

Cristina is a 23-year-old *Chicana* who is attending graduate school. She's very active in politics, the queer community, women's sports, and participates in a wide variety of activities in the lesbian bar, club, and sex-club scene. She knew a lot of lesbians and bisexual women who were part of their school's sports teams. As with other college teams, wild parties followed games, often involving drinking, drugs, and sex.

At one point, Cristina went into a "slut phase" where she "fucked everyone I could. You name it I did it." During this time she decided to stretch the limits of convention as far as she could. She discovered the lesbian sex club and leather or S&M club scenes. At the lesbian sex clubs or parties, she could also find women who would participate in S&M fantasies and scenes. At the leather or S&M clubs or parties, she could find bisexual or lesbian women to "play with." During this time, she began coming to me with questions about how to have safer sex in the context of S&M play. It was her admission to the S&M sexual community which gave her incentive to practice safer sex. She also admired the S&M cultural practice of gaining explicit consent for sexual activities from one's partners, negotiating what you wanted before having sex.[4] Yet while she described the S&M community as being "real up on safer sex practices," she also described some possibly unsafe S&M practices which could spread not only HIV but other diseases as well (e.g., hepatitis B), or cause serious injury to those participating in the behavior. One example was,

> I went into the XX club last Sunday. It was awesome. There were people everywhere engaged in sexual activity or watching and getting off on what other people were doing. In the middle of the club was a stage where one man was wearing chains, he had numerous piercings, and of course leather harnesses. Right on stage a woman came up to him and pierced his nipple. Blood squirted everywhere and he really got off on what she'd done.

While this history may seem unusual to some, during the course of my ethnographic study the leather and S&M communities were expanding by leaps and bounds into the WSW and *Latina* communities of Los Angeles. Particularly the younger generation, 15–25, of WSW have experimented with or added S&M practices to their sexual repertoires, or joined the S&M or leather community.

Another risk for this group is the vast increase in "piercings" for either adornment or for S&M practices. Women are having their genital lips and clitoris, nipples, noses, navels, etc., pierced. Disease and injury risks are threefold: (1) from sharing piercing equipment; (2) from damage caused to the genitals or other areas by having piercings poorly placed (e.g., nerve damage) or poorly cared for (infection); (3) pulling, tugging, or otherwise rubbing on the piercing and its jewelry can cause tears which makes it easier to catch various STDs.

This age group is also more likely to identify as "queer." "Queers" tend to take a more "in your face" attitude towards expressing their gay, bisexual, lesbian, transgendered, and/or transsexual lifestyles. A relatively new phenomenon, has been that of "queer sex" where lesbian or bisexual young women will have sex with their gay or bisexual "brothers." It's not seen the same as "straight sex" and often occurs without using any safer sex precautions.

Ana

Ana is a 45-year-old *Mexicana* who is currently married to a man. She does what she can to be a good mother to her two children and a good wife to her husband. However, at the same time that she's keeping up this long-term relationship, she's got a lover, Carmen, of ten years who she's also married to. Carmen, a *Chicana,* just found out about Ana's other family. She's shocked and heartbroken that she could have been so deceived by Ana. And now Carmen is worried that she'd been exposed to HIV/STDs because of Ana's relations with her husband.

Such a double life is common among men in *México,* but thought to be rare for women. However, many women who are married to men may carry on affairs with other married women behind their husbands' backs, never identifying as lesbians nor thinking about leaving their marriages and families. Sometimes these arrangements are condoned by husbands who spend a great deal of time away from home (e.g., migrant workers) as they believe this means that their wife will not stray with other men. These *LSW* are a very hidden population.

Yolanda

Yolanda is a *Latina* of mixed heritage who just turned thirty and who believes in nonmonogamous relationships. Of all the members of the community whom I've introduced you to today, she's the most active in the political lesbian community. She's keen on discussing everything from radical lesbian separatist feminism to antipornography campaigns to the antipatriarchal structure of nonmonogamy. As such she believes in using consciousness-raising groups, food co-ops, going to political rallies, and generally supporting women's rights. She strongly believes that women are better than men. She tends toward androgynous styles of dress, "women's music," and the norms of the overt U.S. White lesbian feminist culture. She conducts her love relationships as nonmonogamous arrangements.

She's had the following types of nonmonogamous relationships:

1. "Primary lovership": A romantic and sexual relationship where the two women are primary to each other's lives. They may have secondary sexual relationships on the side. Please note that in the lesbian community, the term "lover" most often indicates a woman committed relationship similar to that of the straight communities' use of the term "wife," so this arrangement is similar to an "open marriage."

2. "Primary sexual partner": A relationship where they commit to being each other's main sexual partner, but are not committed romantically the same way that lovers are. They can have other sexual and/or romantic interests. Often this arrangement is made after the women have been screened for HIV/STDs, so that they will agree to have unsafe sex with each other, but use safer sex with the other sexual partners.

3. "Sweet friends": These are women who begin as friends and then arrive at a rewarding emotional and casual sexual relationship. They do not expect this to lead to a committed union, rather it is a gift they give each other at the time. Some other WSW would label these arrangements as "fuck buddies," but in Yolanda's definition, "sweet friends" have more of a friendship relationship than that typically attributed to "fuck buddies."

4. "Affairs": Women who she would have sex with due to a mutual attraction, but which would not be expected to lead to friendship or ongoing sexual relationships.

It is important to include women like Yolanda as many WSW, including *LSW,* who are very active in the Lesbian Feminist and Separatist communities have created similar nonmonogamous relationship structures, based on the political ideology that monogamy is a patriarchal structure used by men to control women. Many of these women still believe that HIV/STDs cannot be spread through sex between women and do not practice safer sex. Obviously, having unprotected sex with many partners can lead to a culture where STDs may be rapidly spread.

Gloria

The last woman I'd like to introduce you to is Gloria, a delightful 50-year-old *Mexicana*. By day you'd never know that she was anything more than a stereotypical, middle-aged, soft-spoken *Latina* who works as a janitor at an educational institution in L.A. After an interview, she insisted that we make arrangements to meet at a club over in West Hollywood. This place, she assured us, would be full of *"lesbianas Latinas y mujeres bisexual."* At the club we found Gloria transformed into one of the most dapper, distinguished looking butches you'd ever find. She wore a white suit coat, black pants, white shirt, and tie. Her hair was stylishly slicked back and she acted like she owned the place. In fact, many of the young women (in their twenties and thirties) were trying to get her attention. She introduced us to women throughout the evening. She also introduced us to her *novia* (girlfriend). Gloria's rules of "monogamy" dictated that she only have one *novia* at a time. Her *novia* could see only her, never straying, flirting, or playing around with anyone else. However, Gloria was "entitled to" have "flings." "Flings" were women that she usually only saw once or twice. Gloria had mixed feelings about her risks for HIV/STDs. On the one hand, she felt, like many other *Latinas,* that you can get it from being around people with AIDS by breathing the same air. She'd already known eight people who'd died from AIDS. One who was an *LSW* who'd had sex with a *Latino* bisexual man. On the other hand, she felt that she was safe, because two women couldn't give HIV or STDs to one another. Also she said, she always had her girlfriends "checked out," which meant she made sure they went in and had a physical and a blood test. She believed that if they had a blood test, then she'd know if they had HIV or not. She didn't know that one needed to have a special blood test to check for HIV nor did she feel that her "flings" had to be checked out. She didn't have a lot of sex with them, so what did a little "fooling around" matter? She never practiced safer sex.

    Instead of focusing on determining the cultural norms for sexual behavior within the various *lesbianas Latinas* communities, my ethnographic research attempted to describe the range of sexual and other risk behaviors expressed throughout Los Angeles. Too often, researchers will decide before going out into a community what the norms are and limit their investigation of the variety of sexual practices within a community to the study of those "normative" behaviors. By using ethnographic methods to go out into the neighborhoods, churches, bars, clubs, homes, beaches, etc., of *LSW* throughout Los Angeles County, I found a broad range of sexual behaviors which had never before been written about nor studied. At most, these behaviors had been documented in lesbian and *LSW* fiction, poetry, songs, and other forms of cultural expression. Even though I introduced you to quite a few of my "sisters," I jes' want to let you know that there are many more who did not get introduced today—the *cholas* (some *LSW* are involved in gangs), the homeless, those in prison, the prostitutes and pimps, the clergy, the *curanderas,* the politicians, the rich and elite. We don't all jes' have risk from sex with women, we can get it through sharing needles and other things that pierce the skin or through sex with men or transfusions, or in any other way that any other person might get it. But I had to emphasize our risks about sex between women, 'cause no matter how an *LSW* gets HIV or STDs, once she has it, she could give it to another woman 'cause what we all got in common is sexy, sensuous sex between women. So that's what we got to find out about. Studying the diversity of sexual behavior, cultural interpretations of sexual orientation and sexuality, and perceptions of HIV/STDs and prevention methods provides valuable data which may transform the scientific debate regarding woman-to-woman transmission from one envisioned in the laboratory to one which accounts for risks faced by WSW and *LSW* in real life.

Woman-to-Woman Transmission—Biomedical Theory vs. Ethnographic Findings

In 1986, I went to meetings on AIDS at the American Public Health Association conference and almost no one talked about women at all. So I asked one of the presenters, "How come you have all these statistics on the risk of HIV for men by various sexual behaviors, but not for women?" He told me to go talk to Dr. Peter Drotman of the Centers for Disease Control (CDC), who was waiting for the next session to begin. So, being an enthusiastic graduate student, I went up to him, introduced myself and asked, "Why do we have epidemiological information on the variation in sexual risk of HIV for men but not for women?" And he told me, now you've got to picture him putting his right index finger in and out of a circle made by his left index finger and thumb at the same time as he says, "Well, lesbians don't have much sex." From that moment on, I decided that in no way should such an important epidemiological question be answered by such ignorance. So I decided to become not only an AIDS researcher, but a sex researcher as well.

Mind you, I had to do a lot of reading and learning about a bunch of stuff they don't teach you generally in high school, college, graduate school, medical school. . . . In fact, this stuff about the intimate details of women's sex lives is more accessible in cheap women's magazines, on talk shows, at the movies, etc. Professionals and research types tend to treat those studying sex like some kinds of sleazes. Or they want to study sexual behavior from a distance. Like using telephone surveys where some person you never heard from before calls you up and within twenty minutes you're supposed to tell them all the nasty things you've done. . . . *Híjole, mami,* most of the time you can't even understand their questions. And if we don't even talk about sex with the ones we're doing it with, how're we supposed to talk to these people on the phone? Especially, since they want to find out if you're selling yourself on the street, dealing drugs, or fucking lots of guys, but they never bother to ask you about your sweet girlfriend. Even if you thought, OK, so maybe they really want to know. It might be important. Hey, maybe they might even be able to answer some questions you got, you know? So you try to get the interviewer to pay attention and tell them they're asking the wrong questions. "If you really want to know about me, I got this girlfriend and we . . ." They don't want to listen to you. They don't have no answers for your questions neither. What's the use?

Or they do all these studies on White, middle-class, educated folks and then tell the rest of us, we're all like them. How the hell do they know? When did they come down here and see for themselves? When did they let us tell them our ways of doing things? When did they stay for a while and donate some time to getting to know us and maybe answer some of our questions first? Did they ever listen to how we talk about things? Can they even understand Spanish or street Spanish? Do they know that *Chicanos, Mexicanos,* and *Puertorriqueños,* etc., we all got different ways of saying these important things? Or did they learn their Spanish in some book based on that stuff we don't understand from Spain? Or even their English. Some of it sounds like they've been on drugs reading the encyclopedia or something so they forgot how to talk to folks entirely. Some things you can't learn from a book, in an ivory tower, from your e-mail newsgroup, nor from your phone-fax-modem-removed from reality office. Some things are better learned through ethnography, by getting off that campus and into the homes, streets, bars, churches, clinics, and beaches of the friendly folks you want to find out about. The best thing about good ethnographers is that they listen to you. In fact, they listen to you so well, that you're talking for hours and hours about your whole life, before you even knew you wanted to. Then you introduce them to your whole neighborhood.

I discovered anthropology and ethnography in graduate school. I decided that since no one had ever written about the actual diversity in sexual behavior for different groups of *Latinas,* that it would be the most appropriate methodology to use for my master's thesis and dissertation research. So I've spent the last eight years going off campus and into the neighborhoods, cities, homes, schools, beaches, bars, churches, clubs, support groups, etc., of the *Latina* lesbian, bisexual and *LSW* communities of Los Angeles County. I've been from the San Fernando Valley to Pomona to the shores of Santa Monica and Long Beach. No we're not all in East L.A., we're everywhere. Don't you know that L.A. is between 40–50 percent *Latino?*

What was really amazing about analyzing the background literature for this research was that men and women were studied very differently.[5] Men were investigated with the premise that the totality of their sexual expression made a difference in their exposure to STDs, but women were not. Men were rarely if ever studied in relation to their reproductive and contraceptive practices. Women, on the other hand, were studied primarily in relation to their reproductive and contraceptive practices. The range of their actual sexual behaviors was never investigated at all, even though researchers implied time and again that the reproductively related sexual behaviors with men included the entire range of behaviors important to the study of the family, sex roles, family planning, and sexually transmitted disease control. An exception to this pattern seemed to be the study of prostitution.[6] Here women were still not studied for the meanings they gave to their sexual behavior nor for fertility-related events, but in relation to the assumption that they certainly were disease transmitting creatures who were putting men at risk. The study of prostitutes (female and male) has also been limited as no one asks if women were ever paying clients. Without the concept that women were actually at risk for contracting HIV/STDs or that they were actually full-fledged sexual beings themselves, the sexual behavior reality and diversity of risk could never be described nor even conceived of by theorists, researchers, or HIV/STD prevention specialists.

Not even when one reads the literature on *Latino* culture could one find studies investigating women's actual sexual behavior.[7] The literature is full of papers and books on investigations of *Latina's* sex-role behaviors and saturated with stereotypical modeling of *machismo* and *marianismo* behaviors. It seems like everything about sex and women was defined by her relationship with a man. It appeared to me that the cultural norms had permeated academia as well as popular culture.

A few people in the academic literature who wrote about women's sexual behavior and sexuality differently were those actually studying lesbians or bisexual women. However, no studies at that time had been done with lesbians of color, most were done with White, middle-class, educated, self-identified lesbians who either had access to health care or who happened to go to college or women's festivals.[8] Remarkably, the majority of the academic literature on lesbians did not address sexual behavior directly either. Sex roles, identity, politics, general lesbian health, homophobia and other forms of oppression were examined, but not sexual behavior. So even lesbians weren't written about as sexual beings. With the notable exceptions of Pat Califia and Joann Loulan, who write about lesbian sex and sexuality, but not *Latinas* nor women of color.[9]

In fact, when sex between women is mentioned as a way to transmit STDs or HIV, most researchers and health care providers glaze over and ask, "What do two women DO anyway?" It's as if their imaginations have shriveled up and died. As if the very idea of having sex without a penis being inserted into a vagina is impossible.[10] The other major myth, if people can imagine it in the first place, is that lesbian sex must be dry— why else do they believe that fluids can't be passed from one woman to another? Even lesbian researchers have had difficulties with this notion.[11] Since 1986 various organizations have attempted to come up with "safer sex guidelines" for lesbians. Most of the time the riskiest behavior on the list is oral-genital sex (that means "eating out," "going down on a woman," or putting your mouth on her pussy). Except that oral-genital sex ain't the riskiest thing two women can do together. It's like somewhere under the guise of being PC or egalitarian or something they forgot that two women can, as they say in the street, "fuck each other." By that I don't mean the use of dildos for vaginal or anal penetration, which also happens (and if these sex toys are shared may pass STDs or HIV from one woman to the other), but actual genital-to-genital contact between women. That's often referred to as "rubbing," "tribadism," "humping," "kissing clits," etc.

Now I'm not sure why, even in the lesbian community, genital-to-genital contact is not asked about. It's been left off of all of the major research projects studying WSW[12] and any review articles on the topic of woman-to-woman HIV transmission by the folks at the CDC.[13] For those who don't know, HIV and STDs may be present in women's vaginas, their mucous membranes, cervical and vaginal secretions (sexy juices), their menstrual blood, and in any lesions (sores, warts, etc.) that are caused by STDs.[14] No one has checked into female ejaculate (this is the fluid which squirts out from the urethra when some women orgasm—no it's not pee.)[15] There have been articles in the medical literature which have shown that certain STDs (chlamydia and trichomonas) can live for years in the paraurethral ducts or glands which are on both sides of the urethra.[16] But no one knows if HIV can live there as well, nor if it could be transmitted through contact with the female ejaculate.

Now when I say that genital-to-genital contact is the riskiest behavior two women can share, I say that for some very specific reasons:

1. There can be a LOT of fluid, particularly if you've got a woman who multiply orgasms and ejaculates (we call that "soakin' the sheets" or "making lesbian lakes").

2. The fluid cannot be contained the same way as a man's ejaculate as there's no place to hang on a condom. Dental dams and saran wrap placed over the vulva (over your *"parte íntima de la mujer"* or *"panocha"*) cannot contain the fluid. They may redirect some of the fluid. Even latex panties or Saran Wrap worn as a sort of loose shorts[17] doesn't work as the fluid runs out over the edges of the panty or down the legs of the shorts.

3. Many organisms which are present in or on one woman's vagina or vulva have direct access to the nice, soft, wet, and warm mucous membranes of the other women's vagina or vulva. Many of these organisms (Human papilloma virus, gonorrhea, syphilis, candida (yeast), etc.) do not need tears or abrasions in tissue in order to transmit from one person to another. In fact, HIV also does not need to be passed through a tear in order to infect a mucous membrane.[18] Finally, many of these other STDs, both ulcerative (like herpes which causes sores) and nonulcerative (like trichomonas which doesn't cause sores) STDs increase the possibility that HIV will be transmitted from one woman to the other.[19]

4. Most women with HIV, whether they know they're infected or not, have much higher rates of vaginal candidiasis (vaginal yeast infections).[20]

Candida albicans has been shown to be one of the organisms which may help HIV transmit from one person to another. So even if the woman without HIV has the yeast infection, the presence of this infection is may increase the likelihood that HIV will be transmitted during this behavior.

5. In addition to the possible presence of female ejaculate, the mucous membranes are being rubbed together against the pressure of muscles and bone causing a great deal of friction which may increase the likelihood of microscopic tearing and abrasion (which is probably pretty high for this activity as mucous membranes are much more fragile and sensitive than regular skin).

6. There may be the presence of multiple infectious fluids at one time (menstrual blood, blood from tears, urine, female ejaculate, vaginal and cervical secretions, and even fluid from feces or the anal canal [which may be more infectious for diseases like hepatitis A and B]). So genital-to-genital contact between women involves more compounding of risks on a microscopic and biologic scale than penile-vaginal or penile-anal penetration for women.

Whoa, radical idea or what?! Now I can hear people out there screaming that I'm some kind of lunatic and a sex-negative lesbian alarmist, but hold on there. Let's look at the theory which says that sex between men and women is more risky for the woman than for the man.[21] It has been stated that there is a higher risk of sexual transmission of HIV from a man's penis to a woman's vagina, or even riskier to her anus. The reasons given are as follows:

1. A man's penis has skin rather than mucous membrane so it makes it more difficult for the HIV to penetrate.

2. Even a man who is uncircumcised is thought to have less of a risk than the woman, but more of a risk than a man with a circumcised penis as it is thought that the skin on the head of his penis would be more sensitive and fragile. The prepuce or foreskin is thought also to harbor harmful bacteria and aid in transmission that way.[22] Even so, his risk is thought to be less than a woman's fragile vaginal membrane.

3. A vaginal membrane is thought to be tougher than an anal membrane (because the anus is supposedly "not made for that kind of activity" and more prone to tearing).

4. A man leaves a large amount of possibly infectious fluid inside the woman's vagina, right there on her mucous membrane.

5. The sperm may act as agents of transmission as they have been found to carry HIV. Therefore if the sperm penetrate the cervical canal and enter the uterus, they may bring HIV into a more protected environment where transmission may be more likely to occur. In addition, sperm have been known to penetrate through the mucous membranes of the vagina, and therefore may assist HIV in finding the blood system.[23]

6. The latest debate is around women's localized vaginal immune response to HIV. Some women in Africa were found to be HIV + vaginally but not in their blood. So some researchers thought that perhaps these women were not "really infected" or possibly not infectious. Other researchers believe that since HIV attacks certain immune system cells in order to establish infection, this makes women even more vulnerable to infection as those cells are right there for the HIV to attack. And some immune system's cells' purpose is to absorb harmful germs, so that would make women more vulnerable than we thought.[24]

7. It is thought that some STDs (candida, herpes simplex, etc.) are more easily transmitted from women to men.

Therefore, when one compares the reasons that women are thought to be more susceptible to HIV transmission from men, then one can take that reasoning one more step. Genital-to-genital contact between women has none of the protection in it which reduces men's risk during sexual intercourse with women. In fact, both women have fragile mucous membranes in contact with possibly multiply infectious agents, sores, fluids, blood, etc. During this type of contact the membranes probably sustain a fair amount of microscopic tearing which increases the likelihood that the fluids and germs could enter the blood stream directly. The fluids also have ample opportunity to get inside the women's vaginas, urethras, and (less likely) their anal openings. Due to the reasoning used to establish estimates of risk of sexual transmission between men and women, I believe that direct genital contact between women may be even riskier than women receiving penetrative vaginal or anal intercourse with men.

You know about this transmission risk thing, a lot of people are really confused about it. Women are trying all kinds of things to reduce their risk, but we haven't really got the data we should have to really give anybody a good idea of what they should do. After all, some of these mathematicians and epidemiologist model-developer types seem to believe that most people participate in only one sexual activity at a time or during any one session of sex play. I mean how accurate can an estimate be for transmission of HIV (or any other STD) via one kiss, etc.? Who kisses only once? How long a kiss are they estimating? We've got a long way to go before we really understand sexual behavior and these quantitative types are already trying to put numbers on risk. We need to be more realistic about risk.

Oh yeah, I almost forgot, oral-genital sex with a woman is probably riskier than going down on a man (particularly if the woman doesn't swallow the semen) for all the same reasons as previously stated (you know, the mucous membrane-to-mucous membrane argument). Although there might be some small reduction of risk due to saliva's inactivation of HIV, that's probably offset by the fact that other STDs increase the likelihood that HIV will be transmitted (including yeast which may also be present in the mouth or vagina—especially for HIV+ people). No one's really doing much investigation of this type of transmission yet, even though it is the most talked-about risk behavior in the WSW community. For those of you who read Kennedy et al.'s 1995 article in JAMWA reviewing these very issues, please don't be confused. Somehow these authors from the CDC felt that oral-genital sex was riskiest to the woman receiving the oral sex. However, the risk is not primarily from the mouth to the vulva, but from the vulva to the mouth. Although if an HIV+ woman had herpes sores, HPV lesions, or candida in her mouth, then the odds of HIV being transmitted from mouth to vulva might be very real. The problem is that most of the transmission research has been done with the idea that HIV is this little isolated organism, rather than the notion that HIV actually lives in crowded germ city.

Another thing I've learned from the field is that when two women are engaged in oral-genital sex, especially activities like "69" (both women going down on each other at the same time), the fluids don't just come in contact with the anogenital and oral mucous membranes. The fluids go everywhere! In your mouth, up your nose, in your eyes, everywhere. There have been cases that I've heard about from researchers and clinicians in the field[25] where women have contracted chlamydia trachomatis in the eye. If the women also use drugs (like sniffing cocaine), have bad allergies, or have medical problems where these other mucous membranes are made even more fragile, then HIV may be transmitted through these membranes without even having to worry about the mitigating factor of saliva.

People really need to think about this stuff more clearly. After all we aren't having sex in laboratories, we're doing dirty, wild, crazy, beautiful love-making down here in L.A. And it's not as if there were not reported cases of the transmission of HIV and other STDs from nonpenile penetrative behavior reported in the literature[26] nor seen in clinician's practices,[27] it's just that these reports are never taken on as a conceptual whole— examined all at the same time. Instead these reports are dismissed out of hand by clinicians and researchers as a nonissue the vast majority of the time. What we'd like to see researchers and clinicians do is to make more use of methods like ethnography and leave the sterile laboratories, clinics, and academic institutions and come down to our neighborhood. Bring your mobile clinics and good listening skills; work with us to find out what's really going on, going down, right here in our bodies, minds, and souls about these important things like love, sex, and STDs/HIV. Respect us and treat us as partners, after all we're the experts on what we do in bed, in the streets, and what it all means to us. We're the most invested in this. We're afraid, but we don't know what to do to protect ourselves. We're getting sick and ain't no one noticing. We're dying and no one cares. Except us. Come join us in our fight to live sexy and healthy lives.

NOTES

I would like to acknowledge the many women who opened their hearts and their lives to contribute to this research, I couldn't have done any of this without them. I am particularly indebted to WSW and *LSW* with STDs/HIV and their lovers who brought me their fears and hopes and put themselves on the line to participate in this work. They hope that this work will create change in how they and all WSW are treated by clinicians, scientists, and researchers. I would also like to acknowledge the following funding sources who also made this work possible: The University of California, Universitywide AIDS Research Program, AIDS Behavioral Traineeship; The Bixby Fellowship; Affirmative Action Research Assistant/Mentorship; UCLA Institute of American Cultures; Charles F. Scott Fellowship; the UCLA School of Public Health; and the Lambda Alumni Association of UCLA. Finally, I would never have made it through this chapter without the support and encouragement of my friends and colleagues: Pat, Sabrina, Patricia, Sandy, my son John, and particularly Liza Rankow and Carole Browner.

1. Peter Drotman, Centers for Disease Control, personal communication, October 1986. And see citations from Chu et al. 1994, 1990; Chu, Hammett, and Buehler 1992; and Kennedy et al. 1995.
2. Latinas and AIDS Research Project (LARP), UCLA School of Public Health, 1987–present. See Ramos 1995; and Ramos, Fischbach, and Samaniego 1993. I would

like to note that the LARP project provided free individual and small group HIV/STD prevention workshops for women throughout Los Angeles County during this study in order to provide a needed service to the individuals and the communities participating in this research.

3. See Chiasson et al. 1990, 3:69–72; and Eskenazi et al. 1989, 2:187–93.

4. For more details read Califia's *The Lesbian S/M Safety Manual* (Boston: Lace Publications, 1988).

5. See Wasserheit et al. 1991 and Voeller et al. 1990 for thorough background on these issues.

6. See Alexander 1987, 248–63; and Bezemer 1992, 31–36.

7. See Singer et al. 1990 for a good literature review on this topic.

8. In 1987 few studies had been done on lesbian and bisexual women's health, let alone on sexual behavior, STDs, or HIV: Bell and Weinberg 1978; Hill 1987; Johnson et al. 1981; Johnson and Palermo 1984; Johnson et al. 1987; McCall 1981; Parker 1982; Robertson and Schachter 1981; Smith et al. 1985. Since then, a number of studies have been conducted, which primarily used convenience samples of lesbian and bisexual identified women who attended women's festivals, certain health clinics, and/or predominantly educated, White middle-class women. A few such studies are mentioned in the bibliography: Case et al. 1989; Conway and Humphries 1994; Edwards and Thin 1990; Einhorn and Polgar 1994; Eskenazi et al. 1989; Garcia et al. 1993; Hunter et al. 1992; Hunter, Rosario, and Rotheram-Borus et al. 1993; Jones et al. 1993; Lemp et al. 1993; Magura et al. 1992; Mills et al. 1993; Raiteri et al. 1994; Reardon et al. 1992; Sasse et al. 1992; Warren et al. 1993; Weiss et al. 1993; and Weissman and Young 1993.

9. See Califia 1988, 1979; Loulan and Thomas 1990; Loulan and Nelson 1987; and Loulan 1984. Some of the previously mentioned studies have included questions regarding lesbian and bisexual women's sexual practices and STD/HIV risks, but this was secondary to examining the women's sexual health concerns rather than the primary focus of the research.

10. For explicit details see Caster 1993; Sisley and Harris 1986; as well as Califia 1988, 1979.

11. In personal communications with several lesbian AIDS activists and researchers over the years (1986–present), many held very narrow definitions of what activities defined "lesbian sex," therefore limiting their abilities to imagine how transmission could occur from one woman to another.

12. On one of the San Francisco studies (Garcia 1993), I was informed that a group of twelve lesbians met to determine what sexual behaviors to ask about in the study. Not one mentioned genital-to-genital contact, and I believe this to be the result of long-term prevention messages which indicate that "rubbing" or "tribadism" is "safer sex." See also Lemp et al. 1993 and Mills et al. 1993.

13. See Kennedy et al. 1995; Chu et al. 1994, 1990; Chu, Hammett, and Buehler 1992; Petersen et al. 1992; and Drotman and Mays 1988.

14. See Belec et al. 1989, 385–91; CDC 1993; Clemetson et al. 1993, 2860–64; Holmberg et al. 1989, 116–25; and Zorr et al. 1994, 852.

15. See Heath 1984, 194–215; Huffman 1948, 86–101; Sevely and Bennett 1978, 1–20; Zaviacic et al. 1989, 564–66; and Zaviacic and Whipple 1993, 148–51.

16. See Pec et al. 1991, 430.

17. *Don't try this with tight Saran Wrap—you can hurt yourself when you try to move.*

18. Fultz et al. 1986, 896–900; and Plummer et al. 1991, 35–45.

19. See Hook et al. 1992, 251–55; Laga et al. 1993, 95–102; LaGuardia et al. 1994, 553–62; and Wasserheit 1991, 47–72.

20. See Baker 1995, 935–38.

21. See Padian, Shiboski, and Jewell 1991, 1664–67; Padian et al. 1987, 788–90; Plummer et al. 1995, 35–45.

22. See Plummer et al. 1995, 35–45.

23. See Anderson et al. 1990, 311–33.

24. See Forrest 1991, 835–36; and Lu et al. 1991, 323–24.

25. Personal communications: Case 1995, Carroll 1994, Denenberg 1994.

26. See Conway and Humphries 1994; Edwards and Thin 1990; Gill, Loveday, and Gilson 1992; Marmor et al. 1986; Monzon and Capellan 1987; Oates 1979; Pancini et al. 1992; Perry, Jacobsberg, and Fogel 1989; Rich et al. 1993; Sabatini et al. 1984; Sivakumar et al. 1989; Spencer 1993; Spitzer and Weiner 1989; Walters and Rector 1986.

27. Personal communications with the following clinicians between 1987 and 1995: Robertson; Gage; Denenberg; Carroll; and one who reported a hepatitis A sexually transmitted outbreak among lesbians at a college in the northeastern U.S. in the early 1990s.

REFERENCES

Alexander P. "Prostitutes Are Being Scapegoated for Heterosexual AIDS." In *Sex Work: Writings by Women in the Sex Industry*, ed. F Delacoste and P Alexander. Pittsburgh: Cleis Press, 1987.

Anderson DJ et al. "Immunology of the Male Reproductive Tract: Implications for the Sexual Transmission of Human Immunodeficiency Virus." In *AIDS and Sex,* eds. B Voeller et al. Oxford: Oxford University Press, 1990.

Belec L et al. "Antibodies to Human Immunodeficiency Virus in Vaginal Secretions of Heterosexual Women." *Journal of Infectious Diseases* 160.3 (1989): 385–91.

Bell AP and Weinberg MS. *Homosexualities: A Study of Diversity among Men and Women.* New York: Simon and Schuster, 1978.

Bezemer W. "Women and HIV." *Journal of Psychology and Human Sexuality* 5.1/2 (1992): 31–36.

Bybee D. *Michigan Lesbian Health Survey: Results Relevant to AIDS.* March 1990, unpublished.

Califia P. *Sapphistry: The Book of Lesbian Sexuality.* Tallahassee, Fla.: Naiad Press, 1993.

———. *The Lesbian S/M Safety Manual.* Boston: Lace Publications/Alyson Publications, 1988.

————. "Lesbian Sexuality." *Journal of Homosexuality* 4.3 (1979): 255–67.

Case P et al. "The Social Context of AIDS Risk Behavior among Intravenous Drug Using Lesbians in San Francisco. *Fourth International AIDS Conference.* Abstract no. 8023. 1989.

Caster W. *The Lesbian Sex Book.* Boston: Alyson Publications, 1993.

Centers for Disease Control and Prevention. "1993 Sexually Transmitted Diseases and Treatment Guidelines." *Morbidity and Mortality Weekly Report* 42 (1993): 19.

Chiasson MA et al. "Human Immunodeficiency Virus Transmission through Artificial Insemination." *Journal of Acquired Immune Deficiency Syndromes* 3 (1990): 69–72.

Chu SY et al. "Female-to-Female Sexual Contact and HIV Transmission" (letter). *Journal of the American Medical Association* 272.6 (1994): 433.

————. "Epidemiology of Reported Cases of AIDS in Lesbians, United States 1980–89. *American Journal of Public Health* 80.11 (1990): 1380–81.

Chu SY, Hammett TA, and Buehler JW. "Update: Epidemiology of Reported Cases of AIDS in Women Who Report Sex Only with Other Women, United States 1980–1991." *AIDS* 6.5 (1992): 518–19.

Clemetson DBA et al. "Detection of HIV DNA in Cervical and Vaginal Secretions: Prevalence and Correlates among Women in Nairobi, Kenya." *Journal of the American Medical Association* 269.22 (1993): 2860–64.

Cole R and Cooper S. "Lesbian Exclusion from HIV/AIDS Education: Ten Years of Low Risk Identity and High Risk Behavior." *SIECUS Report,* December 1990/January 1991, 18–23.

Conway M and Humphries E. "Bernard Clinic Meeting Need in Lesbian Sexual Health Care." *Nursing Times* 90.32 (1994): 40–41.

Drotman DP and Mays MA. "AIDS and Lesbians: IV-Drug Use Is the Risk." *Fourth International AIDS Conference.* Abstract no. 8022. 1988.

Edwards A and Thin RN. "Sexually Transmitted Diseases in Lesbians." *International Journal of Sexually Transmitted Diseases AIDS* 1 (1990): 178–81.

Einhorn L and Polgar M. "HIV Risk Behavior among Lesbians and Bisexual Women." *AIDS Prevention Education* 6 (1994): 514–23.

Eskenazi B et al. "HIV Serology in Artificially Inseminated Lesbians." *Journal of Acquired Immune Deficiency Syndromes* 2 (1989): 187–93.

Forrest BD. "Women, HIV, and Mucosal Immunity." *Lancet* 337 (1991): 835–36.

Fultz B et al. "Vaginal Transmission of HIV to a Chimpanzee." *Journal of Infectious Diseases* 54 (1986): 896–900.

Garcia D et al. "Lesbian and Bisexual Women: Indications of High-Risk Behaviors with Men." *Ninth International AIDS Conference and Fourth STD World Congress.* Abstract Book, vol. 1, no. WS-C07-6, p. 88. Berlin, 1988.

Gill SK, Loveday C, and Gilson RJ. "Transmission of HIV-1 Infection by Oroanal Intercourse." *Genitourinary Medicine* 68.4 (1992): 254–57.

Heath D. "An Investigation into the Origins of a Copious Vaginal Discharge during Intercourse: 'Enough to Wet the Bed'—That 'Is Not Urine.'" *Journal of Sex Research* 20.2 (1984): 194–215.

Hill I. *The Bisexual Spouse: Difference Dimensions in Human Sexuality.* McLean, Va.: Barlina Books, 1987.

Holmberg SD et al. "Biologic Factors in the Sexual Transmission of Human Immuno-deficiency Virus." *Journal of Infectious Diseases* 160.1 (1989): 116–25.

Hook EW et al. "Herpes Simplex Virus Infection as a Risk Factor for Human Immu-nodeficiency Virus Infection in Heterosexuals." *Journal of Infectious Diseases* 165 (1992): 251–53.

Huffman JW. "The Detailed Anatomy of the Paraurethral Ducts in the Adult Human Female." *American Journal of Obstetrics and Gynecology* 55.1 (1948): 86–101.

Hunter J et al. "Sexual and Substance Abuse Acts That Place Lesbians at Risk for HIV." *Eighth International AIDS Conference.* Abstract no. PoD 5208. Amsterdam, 1992.

Hunter J, Rosario M, and Rotheram-Borus MJ. "Sexual and Substance Abuse Acts That Place Adolescent Lesbians at Risk for HIV." *Ninth International AIDS Conference and Fourth STD World Congress.* Abstract no. PO-DO2-3432. Berlin, 1993.

Johnson SR et al. "Comparison of Gynecological Health Care Problems between Lesbians and Bisexual Women: A Survey of 2,345 Women." *Journal of Reproductive Medicine* 32.11 (1987): 805–11.

———. "Factors Influencing Lesbian Gynecologic Care: A Preliminary Study." *American Journal of Obstetrics and Gynecology* 140.1 (1981): 20–28.

Johnson SR and Palermo JL. "Gynecologic Care for the Lesbian." *Clinical Obstetrics and Gynecology* 27.3 (1984).

Jones M et al. "Prevalence of HIV-1 among Lesbians and Bisexual Women in San Francisco (SF) and Berkeley, CA: The Women's Seroprevalence Survey." Session 3251, *APHA Abstract,* October 1993.

Kennedy MB et al. "Assessing HIV Risk among Women Who Have Sex with Women: Scientific and Communication Issues." *Journal of the American Medical Women's Association* 50.3/4 (1995): 103–7.

Laga M et al. "Non-Ulcerative Sexually Transmitted Diseases as Risk Factors for HIV-1 Transmission in Women: Results from a Cohort Study." *AIDS* 7.1 (1993): 95–102.

LaGuardia KD et al. "Genital Ulcer Diseases in Women Infected with Human Immu-nodeficiency Virus." *American Journal of Obstetrics and Gynecology* 172.2, pt. 1 (1994): 553–62.

Lemp G et al. *HIV Seroprevalence and Risk Behaviors among Lesbians and Bisexual Women: The 1993 San Francisco/Berkeley Women's Survey, October 1993.* Surveillance Branch, AIDS Office, San Francisco Department of Public Health.

Loulan J. *Lesbian Sex.* San Francisco: Spinsters/Aunt Lute, 1984.

Loulan J and Nelson MB. *Lesbian Passion: Loving Ourselves and Each Other.* San Francisco: Spinters/Aunt Lute, 1987.

Loulan J and Thomas S. *The Lesbian Erotic Dance: Butch, Femme, Androgyny, and Other Rhythms.* San Francisco: Spinsters Book Co., 1990.

Lu NS et al. "Enhanced Local Immunity in Vaginal Secretions of HIV Infected Women." *Lancet* 338 (1991): 323–24.

Magura S et al. "Women Usually Take Care of Their Girlfriends: Bisexuality and HIV

Risk among Female Intravenous Drug Users." *Journal of Drug Issues* 22 (1992): 179–90.

Marmor M et al. "Possible Female to Female Transmission of Human Immunodeficiency Virus" (letter). *Annals of Internal Medicine* 105 (1986): 969.

McCall MC. *Health Needs Assessment of a Lesbian Population.* Unpublished master's thesis, Emory University School of Nursing, 1981.

McCombs SB et al. "Epidemiology of HIV-1 Infection in Bisexual Women." *Journal of Acquired Immune Deficiency Syndromes* 5.8 (1992): 850–52.

Mills S et al. *Health Behaviors among Lesbian and Bisexual Women: A Community-Based Women's Health Survey.* San Francisco Department of Public Health, AIDS Office, Prevention Branch. October 1993.

Monzon OT and Capellan JM. "Female-to-Female Transmission of HIV." *Lancet* 2 (1987): 40–41.

Oates JK. "Recurrent Vaginitis and Oral Sex" (letter). *Lancet,* April 7, 1979, 785.

Padian NS et al. "Male-to-Female Transmission of Human Immunodeficiency Virus." *Journal of the American Medical Association* 258.6 (1987): 788–90.

Padian NS, Shiboski SC, and Jewell NP. "Female-to-Male Transmission of Human Immunodeficiency Virus." *Journal of the American Medical Association* 266 (1991): 1664–67.

Pancini PB et al. "Oral Condyloma Lesions in Patients with Extensive Genital Human Papillomavirus Infection." *American Journal of Obstetrics and Gynecology* 167 (1992): 451–58.

Parker GL. *Sexually Transmitted Diseases among a Lesbian Population.* Unpublished master's thesis, Emory University School of Nursing, 1982.

Pec J et al. "Female Paraurethral Ducts and Glands as the Sites of Agents of Sexually Transmitted Diseases" (letter). *Journal of Genitourinary Medicine* 67.5 (1991): 430.

Perry S, Jacobsberg L, and Fogel K. "Orogenital Transmission of Human Immunodeficiency Virus (HIV)." *Annals of Internal Medicine* 111.11 (1989): 951–52.

Petersen LR et al. "No Evidence for Female to Female HIV Transmission among 960,000 Female Blood Donors." *Journal of Acquired Immune Deficiency Syndromes* 5 (1992): 853–55.

Plummer FA et al. "Factors Affecting Female to Male Transmission of HIV-1: Implications of Transmission Dynamics for Prevention." In *AIDS and Women's Reproductive Health,* ed. Chen et al. New York: Plenum Press, 1991.

Raitieri R et al. "Lesbian Sex and HIV-1." *International AIDS Conference.* Abstract #PC0103. August 7–12, 1994.

———. "Seroprevalence, Risk Factors and Attitude to HIV-1 in a Representative Sample of Lesbians in Turin." *Genitourinary Medicine* 70.3 (1994): 200–205.

Ramos LJ. "Are Latina Lesbian and Bisexual Women at Risk for HIV/STDs? A Review of Ethnographic Findings, the LARP Project, Los Angeles County 1987–1994." In *Universitywide AIDS Research Program Conference Abstract.* University of California, San Francisco, 1995.

Ramos LJ, Fischbach LA, and Samaniego LM. "The Latinas and AIDS Research Project: Exploring the Differences in AIDS Sexual Knowledge, Beliefs and Behaviors for Mexican, Mexican American, and White Women of Different Sexual Orientations and Sexual Behavior Groups in Los Angeles County 1987–1992." *Ninth International Conference on AIDS and Fourth STD World Congress.* Abstract Book, vol. I, no. WS-D18–6, p. 121. Berlin, 1993.

Reardon J et al. "HIV-1 Infection among Female Injection Drug Users (ID) in the San Francisco Bay Area, California, 1989–1991: Increased Seroprevalence Rates for ID Who Are Lesbian/Bisexual, Racial/Ethnic Minorities or Cocaine Injectors." California HIV Seroprevalence Studies Coordinating Group. *Eighth International AIDS Conference.* Amsterdam, 1992.

Reinisch JM, Sanders SA, and Ziemba-Davis M. "Self-Labeled Sexual Orientation, Sexual Behavior, and Knowledge about AIDS: Implications for Biomedical Research and Education Programs." In *Proceedings of NIMH/NIDA Workshop on Women and AIDS: Promoting Healthy Behaviors,* eds. SJ Blumenthal, A Eichler, and G Weissman. Washington, D.C.: American Psychiatric Press, 1990.

Reynolds G. "HIV and Lesbian Sex." *Lancet* 344 (1994): 544–45.

Rich JD et al. "Transmission of Human Immunodeficiency Virus Infection Presumed to Have Occurred via Female Homosexual Contact." *Clinical Infectious Diseases* 17 (1993): 1003–5.

Robertson P and Schachter J. "Failure to Identify Venereal Disease in a Lesbian Population." *Journal of Sexually Transmitted Diseases* 8.2 (1981): 75–76.

Ross M et al. "Sexually Transmissible Diseases in Injecting Drug Users." *Journal of Genitourinary Medicine* 67 (1991): 32–36.

Sabatini MT et al. "Kaposi's Sarcoma and T-cell Lymphoma in an Immunodeficient Woman: A Case Report." *AIDS Research* 1 (1984): 135–37.

Sanders SA, Reinisch JM, and Ziemba-Davis M. "Self-Labeled Sexual Orientation of Sexual Behavior among Women." Presented at the Fifth International Conference on Aids. Montreal, June 1989.

Sasse H et al. "Potential Routes of HIV Transmission among Women Engaging in Female-to-Female Sexual Practices." *Eighth International AIDS Conference.* Abstract no. PoD 5209, p. D421. Amsterdam, 1992.

Sevely JL and Bennett JW. "Concerning Female Ejaculation and the Female Prostate." *Journal of Sex Research* 14.1 (1978): 1–78.

Singer M et al. "SIDA: The Economic, Social and Cultural Context of AIDS among Latinos." *Medical Anthropology Quarterly* 4.1 (1990): 72–114.

Sisley EL and Harris B. *The Joy of Lesbian Sex.* New York: Pocket Books, 1986.

Sivakumar K et al. "Trichomonas Vaginalis Infection in a Lesbian" (letter). *Genitourinary Medicine* 65 (1989): 399–400.

Smith EM et al. "Health Care Attitudes and Experiences during Gynecological Care among Lesbians and Bisexuals." *American Journal of Public Health* 75.9 (1985): 1085–87.

Spencer B. "Orogenital Sex and Risk of Transmission of HIV." *Lancet* 341 (1993): 441.

Spitzer PG and Weiner NJ. "Transmission of HIV Infection from a Woman to a Man by Oral Sex." *New England Journal of Medicine* 320 (1989): 251.

Stevens PE. "Lesbians and HIV: Clinical, Research, and Policy Issues." *American Journal of Orthopsychiatry* 63.2 (1993): 289–94.

Voeller B et al. (eds.). *AIDS and Sex: An Integrated Biomedical and Biobehavioral Approach.* Oxford: Oxford University Press, 1990.

Walters MH and Rector WG. "Sexual Transmission of Hepatitis A in Lesbians." *Journal of the American Medical Association* 256.5 (1986): 594.

Warren N. "Out of the Question: Obstacles to Research on HIV Women Who Engage in Sexual Behaviors with Women." *SIECUS Report,* October/November 1993, 13–15.

Warren N et al. "Women Who Have Sex with Women among an HIV Infected Incarcerated Population." *APHA Abstract,* October 1993.

Wasserheit JN. "Epidemiological Synergy: Interrelationship between HIV Infection and Other Sexually Transmitted Diseases." In *AIDS and Women's Reproductive Health,* ed. Chen et al. New York: Plenum Press, 1991.

Wasserheit JN et al. *Research Issues in Human Behavior and Sexually Transmitted Diseases in the AIDS Era.* Washington, D.C.: American Society for Microbiology, 1991.

Weiss SH et al. "Risk of HIV and Other Sexually Transmitted Diseases (STD) among Bisexual and Heterosexual Women." *Ninth International AIDS Conference and Fourth STD World Congress.* Abstract Book, vol. 1, no. WS-D04–4:107. Berlin, 1993.

Weissman G and Young RM. "HIV among Lesbian and Bisexual Injection Users." Session 3251, *APHA Abstract,* October 1993.

Young RM, Weissman G, and Cohen JB. "Assessing Risk in the Absence of Information: HIV Risk among Women Injection-Drug Users Who Have Sex with Women." *AIDS and Public Policy Journal* 7.3 (1992): 175–83.

Zaviacic M et al. "Enzyme Histochemical Profile of the Adult Human Female Prostate (Paraurethral Glands)." *Histochemical Journal* 17 (1985): 564–66.

Zaviacic M and Whipple B. "Update on the Female Prostate and the Phenomenon of Female Ejaculation." *Journal of Sex Research* 30.2 (1993): 148–51.

Zorr B et al. "HIV-1 Detection in Endocervical Swabs and Mode of HIV-1 Infection." *Lancet* 8901 (1994): 852.

8

Midlife and Older Women and HIV/ AIDS: My (Grand)mother Wouldn't Do That

Diana Laskin Siegal and Christie Burke

Diana Laskin Siegal and *Christie Burke* are coauthor and contributing author of *The New Ourselves, Growing Older: Women Aging with Knowledge and Power.* Ms. Siegal is currently with the Elder Health Programs, Division of Family and Community Health and Ms. Burke with the Division of Sexually Transmitted Diseases Prevention in the Massachusetts Department of Public Health.

Recently available data suggest that reported cases probably underrepresent the actual numbers of women over forty-five who have HIV disease. Most health care providers, even those who have experience diagnosing and treating HIV/AIDS, may not consider HIV testing when treating older women.[1] Even when HIV disease is identified in the older adult, this is less likely to happen in a timely fashion.

> I did not fit the stereotype of someone who is HIV+ so I had to go from doctor to doctor before I was even tested. This happened even though I had many of the symptoms of HIV. I don't really trust doctors anymore.
>
> A 48-year-old HIV+ woman infected by her husband

Retrospective chart audits of older adults diagnosed with HIV infection demonstrated that clinicians may not consider the possibility of HIV infection until late in the course of infection despite a high prevalence of prior sexually transmitted disease among the patients being evaluated. In one study of twenty-four older patients presenting with signs and symptoms of HIV infection, testing was often delayed, in some cases as long as ten months. Eleven patients were worked up for other malignancies first and three were diagnosed with organic brain syndrome.[2]

One reason for this lack of awareness by health care providers is the generally ageist attitude of providers, especially their assumption that older adults and the elderly are disengaged from sexual activities. Health care providers rarely ask appropriate questions of older people, especially women. This is because older women's sexuality is so discounted and invisible. It's hard enough for health care providers to deal with their parents' sexuality (and by extension the sexuality of patients the same ages as their parents) let alone deal with the sexuality of their grandparents. While jokes are made about "dirty old men" (namely any old man interested in sex), the common assumption in society and among most health care providers is that there aren't any "dirty old women."

> They never even asked me about my sexual behavior.
>> The same 48-year-old HIV + woman

In contrast to the stereotype, what little research has been done shows that older adults are sexually active.[3] However, older women, particularly those who may have internalized society's view that sexuality is unacceptable in women, especially in older women, may have difficulty in asking questions and getting the information they need from their medical providers—even more so if their providers are also uncomfortable with the subject. For women of color, issues of actual or perceived racism,[4] as well as belonging to cultures that may stress the virtues of sexual innocence,[5] may make sexual communication even more difficult. In addition, ageism combined with homophobia within the health care system makes it difficult for older women who have sex with women to assess their risk and receive adequate information.[6]

The assumption that older adults and the elderly are not sexual has another serious implication for the prevalence of HIV in that group. Prior to 1985, when a large number of older adults (who are the greatest consumers of blood products) became infected with HIV through blood transfusions and went on to develop AIDS, providers and policy makers assumed that this infection, not being of a sexual nature, would not spread. This myth that older adults infected through transfusion would not go on to infect others sexually has been one basis for the lack of education of the older adult population regarding the risks from this phase of the epidemic. Since so many cases of HIV among older adults are not identified, we do not know how many partners of those who were infected by transfusion are unaware of their exposure and may continue to transmit the virus.

Where women have been the subject of study, the focus has been on women of childbearing age. This is usually defined as fifteen to forty-four years of age, even though women have always become pregnant and given birth past the age of forty-five right up to menopause (which still occurs on average a few months past the age of fifty). Underreporting of AIDS in women certainly occurred before the recently changed case definition.

Underreporting may also result from underdiagnosis in the older adult and elderly population as a whole. Several recent studies of elderly patients have confirmed high rates of undiagnosed HIV disease. One retrospective study published in 1995 of elderly hospital patients in a high-risk community revealed that 8.9 percent of the women ages 60–79 who had died within the year of the study were actually HIV-positive, even though before the study none of these patients was identified as HIV-positive.[7] Another study of women in an emergency room setting in New York City showed that none of the HIV infections in women over forty-five retrospectively identified had been previously identified.[8]

Manifestations of HIV Disease in Older Women

Basic biomedical information on older women and HIV/AIDS is still lacking. There are articles that indicate that disease progression from HIV to AIDS is faster in the older adult population.[9] However, it is difficult to interpret this phenomena, especially since study cohorts identified have not included samples of older women. Faster disease progression among women as a whole has been due partly to delayed diagnosis. Since diagnosis is also delayed in older women, rapid disease progression could be caused by either a delay in case identification, immune suppression as a function of age, or perhaps a combination of the two. This is an area where research is needed.

Little is known about the particular opportunistic infections that are most likely to affect older women. Some people thought to have Alzheimer's disease have been found to be suffering from AIDS dementia. In some older women, the aging process may reduce the production of antibodies and decrease the effectiveness of the blood-brain barrier, possibly making them more susceptible to infection as well as AIDS-related dementia.[10]

HIV-infected older individuals appear to have an overall lower quality of life than younger persons with the same CD4 T-cell count[11] and the normal CD4 count may differ between older and younger people.[12] CD4 tracking as a tool for measuring disease progression and for making medication decisions may need to be more carefully evaluated when used for the care of older women.

One unique and relatively unexplored area of HIV disease in older women is the interrelationship of HIV disease and menopause. Little research exists on how HIV affects the timing or experiences of menopause nor how menopause affects the manifestation or progression of HIV disease. There is some evidence that hormone replacement therapy may contribute to HIV risk through the immunodepressive effects of estrogen and progesterone.[13]

> When I have night sweats, I don't know whether it's menopause or HIV. . . .
> The doctor doesn't know what is what either.
>   A 51-year-old HIV+ woman also infected by her husband

Another area of particular concern to older adults with HIV infection is the effectiveness and correct dosages of medications. The side effects and effectiveness of HIV antiviral drugs are not well known among the older adult and elderly population. As individuals age, the possibility of adverse drug reactions and the need to carefully monitor drug dosages increases. Testing of the safety and efficacy of drugs in women, especially in older women, is generally inadequate.[14]

AIDS clinical trials are set up to test drugs for preventing or treating HIV-related diseases. There are no clinical trials exclusively on women except for gynecological conditions and none on older women. There is no requirement for testing on older women.[15] More research is needed in this area. For those women who are also menopausal, the medication issues are very complex and relatively unknown. And, in addition, little is known about other drug interactions for those older women who may be more likely to be on medication for other conditions.

HIV/AIDS Risk for Older Women

In spite of all the awareness campaigns, many older women are still oblivious to the dangers of HIV transmission. What little research has been done shows that the sexuality of older people is often not in the context of a safe or monogamous relationship.[16]

When asked, "What are you doing to protect yourself when sleeping with a male partner?" many postmenopausal, heterosexual women will interpret the question as they always did—namely that "to protect yourself" means birth control. They will respond, "Oh, I don't need to worry about that, I'm past menopause." An awareness of the dangers from HIV/AIDS has not penetrated because they think of themselves as different from "those" people whom they think get AIDS—namely, gay men, intravenous drug users, and hemophiliacs.[17] That heterosexual men frequent prostitutes was acknowledged in several recent Hollywood scandals. That middle-aged professional people with no drug arrest history may use illegal drugs is shown by several recent heroin deaths. Again, denial may cause women to assume that the men they sleep with are "clean."

In addition, there may be a higher percentage of older married men who are gay or bisexual and grew up in an era when they were more likely to deny or keep secret this aspect of their lives. Women whose male partners have sex with other men, especially those who may engage in anonymous sexual encounters, perhaps involving substance use, are at risk of HIV transmission from this partner/spouse. This risk exists across communities and is a risk for women of all cultural groups.

As the 1994 CDC Surveillance Report makes clear, most women initially reported without apparent risk are found to have become infected through heterosexual contact.[18] One medical review of such cases indicated that transmission risk to heterosexual women may be as high or higher from one HIV-positive partner as the risk to individuals classified as having "multiple partners" (meaning more than one partner within a certain time period—for example one year).[19] A more recent study from project AWARE in San Francisco confirms that women who think they are in a monogamous relationship, but are not, may be at greater risk than women who are not monogamous because these women (those who think they are monogamous) fail to protect themselves.[20]

Vaginal dryness is another risk factor for older women. In fact, any woman who has vaginal penetration is more susceptible if her vagina is dry. This can happen if intercourse is forced on a woman, if intercourse takes place before the adequate lubrication that comes with full arousal, or in those women whose vaginas are drier, thinner, or shorter. Rates of lubrication vary at any age. Some women experience vaginal dryness as they are going through menopause, some at an older age, and some never do. As women age, the walls of the vagina may thin and become more subject to tearing. In addition, the ability of the vagina to increase in length in response to sexual arousal may decrease, resulting in increased cervical abrasion during intercourse. Such tears and abrasions can create entrances for infection.

A variety of unsafe sexual practices contribute to the risk for HIV transmission. There is, however, little if any data to document sexual behaviors among older women, such as the extent of anal sex or the use of sex toys, both of which practices might present a risk factor for HIV transmission. Infection from the use of sex toys may present a risk to older women who have sex with women, and who may think they are not at risk for HIV.

Older people have rarely been included on the lists of people "at risk" for HIV/AIDS. We now know that it is not categories of people but rather the behavior of people that puts them "at risk." On the contrary, sexuality continues and its expression is often limited only by the unavailability of partners. Many progressive long-term care facilities are now allowing more privacy to residents and are acknowledging the sexual activities that often take place among residents. In addition, Dr. Jocelyn Elders' comment about masturbation being part of normal sexuality is just as fitting for old people as it is for adolescents.

Although myths and stereotypes may suggest that midlife and older women do not use drugs, this is not the case, and it is important to realize that midlife and older women continue with drug- and alcohol-related behavior that they began earlier in their life and that this poses a risk for them as it does for younger women. The threat of violence also remains a very real risk for older women and continues to affect their ability to protect themselves from HIV transmission.

While a body of literature is beginning to develop that recognizes the epidemiological, medical, and psychosocial issues of HIV/AIDS in the older adult, much of it is still focused on older gay men. Older women remain the most invisible of all groups in this epidemic. More research as well as provider and community education is needed to improve identification and treatment as well as to promote prevention among those at risk.

Aging is not a disease. There are many women in remarkably fit health well into very old age. There is far more diversity among a group of eighty-year-olds than among eight-year-olds because their life's experiences have shaped them differently and affected their health status. Education, income, nutrition, work and living environment, exposures to toxins, what money can buy and the stress that lack of money causes, one's acceptance and respect by society or lack thereof all create differences in the health status of older women.

Other Psychosocial Issues of Older Women

Discovering that you are infected with HIV is a shock to an individual at any age. However, for midlife and older women who may not have been aware of their risk, it can be particularly frightening and disorienting. These women may not know anyone like themselves and have no idea where to go for information and support.[21]

Women who become infected with HIV may not have known of a husband's or partner's use of IV drugs, his sexual activities with other women including prostitutes, or his bisexual activities until he is diagnosed. Older women who develop HIV/AIDS themselves must face the disapproval and discrimination of the many people who, as with any sexually transmitted disease or problem involving illegal substance use, judge women more harshly than men.

One problem for anyone with HIV/AIDS is the issue of disclosure. Women report that their sexuality often shuts down completely when they learn of the diagnosis.[22] When they begin to regain some feeling for their lives and for their sexuality, they are faced with the problem of when to tell a potential new partner. Do they tell a new acquaintance right away, perhaps embarrassing them both or ending a potential friendship, or do they wait and be criticized for leading someone on or even jeopardizing a partner through unprotected exposure? These women may also fear lack of support or even abandonment by friends or long-time sexual partners.

Midlife and older women may already be coping with changes in self-image and sexual functioning due to aging. HIV adds another dimension to this picture.

> Between HIV and menopause . . . my interest in sex has changed. . . . I don't want to be a cute little teenager but I do want to be a sexy older woman. I've had to realize there are changes and get used to them. . . . I used to dance all night long but I can't do that anymore.
>
> The same 51-year-old HIV + woman

Older women infected with HIV are at a different stage of life than younger adults who become infected. For those in midlife, the responsibilities of being a parent as well as the responsibilities to aging parents create a different set of stressors than found among younger or single adults. Children and parents will have to be among those individuals that midlife women will need to consider informing of their status. Some women in this age group have experienced rejection and loss from "both sides" of these generations.

> My older daughter has rejected me and my husband, who is also positive. She says we have "made her an orphan" and has refused to see us since we told her about the diagnosis. . . . My husband's parents are angry at losing the support they expected to have from us in their old age. . . . We also had to find a home for my younger daughter who had special needs. We finally found a place for her to live, but then we had to tell her that her Mom and Dad were going to die.   The same 48-year-old HIV + woman

However, not all families are rejecting and unsupportive to the positive older adult.

> My family has been very supportive. But I still worry about letting some of the kids know that I'm sick.   The same 51-year-old HIV + woman

Older women may be affected by HIV/AIDS even if they don't have or will not ever contract the disease themselves. As caregivers, as relatives and friends, as coworkers, they are affected by the illness and deaths of many others.[23]

Women have been and still are the traditional unpaid and poorly paid caregivers. Much of the care of the ill has always fallen on their shoulders, both in health care institutions and at home. In fact, the entire health care system is supported by the unpaid family workers and the underpaid health aides in hospitals and nursing homes, and the home care workers and home health aides in community services.

Many women have lost children and grandchildren to the disease. The loss of a child or grandchild is one of the saddest losses. As one woman said of the death of her 39-year-old son, "This is contrary to nature. I'm supposed to die before him." Parents have always died and grandmothers have always taken on the responsibilities of raising grandchildren when needed, but now many more face this task. By the year 2000 it is estimated that 100,000 children and teenagers will be orphaned because they lost a parent to AIDS. One-third to one-half of these children will go to live with their grandparents, and much of the burden will fall on older women.[24] Older people will need financial help and social support.

Women have worked energetically for public notice and awareness, for research, and for public education about HIV/AIDS from the very beginning when it was mistakenly labelled a "gay" disease. They worked with gay men to form hospices, meal delivery programs, and alternative systems for obtaining drugs and treatment. Now these same efforts need to be expanded to serve older women.

Socioeconomics, Culture, and Issues of Access

Because of the paucity of research on older women as a group, it is even more difficult than usual to address the complex way in which racial, cultural, and socioeconomic issues affect HIV transmission risk and the availability and acceptability of HIV-related services. It is clear that socioeconomic status is highly correlated with overall health status. For poor midlife and older women, the lack of access to health care may preclude opportunities to receive risk-assessment and prevention messages. Even for those women who may have insurance and receive regular health care, the lack of any HIV programs which cut across medical disciplines may require these women to seek a variety of providers, and reduce their chances of receiving integrated and coordinated care.

As noted earlier, for older women of color, actual or perceived racism on the part of health care providers may pose a barrier to care.[25] Women of some cultural groups—such as some members of the Asian community where sexuality may not be discussed outside of the family[26] or Latinas, for whom sexual innocence is highly valued[27]—may be less likely to use HIV-related services that are not sensitive to cultural issues. Such cultural issues may be even more salient for midlife and older women. One study of midlife and older Latinas documented that these women were apparently seeking care at later stages of HIV disease than their younger counterparts. This may have been caused by perceived cultural barriers to the use of these services.[28]

Economically and culturally accessible and acceptable prevention, education, and treatment services for older women of all cultures must be part of the women's health agenda.

Reaching Midlife and Older Women

We must encourage the distribution of materials and discussion about HIV/AIDS at all places and in all media reaching midlife and older women such as clubs, churches, libraries, print and broadcast news and feature stories, hospitals and health centers, and senior centers. Support the continuation of messages about HIV/AIDS prevention for all ages, and urge public health departments, AIDS committees, and other organizations to add messages and education for people over the age of forty.

Health care educators and providers can reach elders through the system of community-based services for the elderly.[29] Every state has a state agency designated as the elder authority and federal Area Agencies on Aging that have the responsibility for administering funds from the Older Americans Act. Elders can be reached through educational programs at senior centers[30] and senior housing, from which they are often able to spread what they learn to their friends. The use of peer leaders has been a successful model in health education among elders.[31] Don't assume elders are not computer literate. In addition to private ownership, senior centers and libraries are setting up computers available to the public so that information on the Internet will increasingly reach elders. SeniorNet, a service located on America Online, now has 18,000 subscribers and operates seventy-five computer learning centers. Additional thousands of elders are "surfing the net."

Reaching health care providers and policy makers requires education through different channels. Continuing education programs are required of all licensed professionals and are an excellent way to reach providers. Physicians and nurses should discuss HIV/AIDS with every patient, especially certain groups of women. For example, like women who are past menopause, women who have their uterus and/or ovaries removed (hysterectomy/oophorectomy) need information about condom use for STD protection.[32] A woman with any sexually transmitted disease also needs special instruction.

State public health departments and associations also provide educational programs and need to be alerted to HIV/AIDS among older people as a subject worth pursuing. Advocacy and educational organizations have worked extensively with gay men to organize, educate, change behavior, and reduce the rate of infection. Now it is women's turn to organize, and educational groups and agencies must work with women of all ages to slow the rate of infection among women—including older adult and elderly women.

Staff in hospitals, nursing homes, hospices, and home health and home care agencies need training not only in the medical aspects of HIV/AIDS but in dealing with their assumptions and attitudes toward people with HIV/AIDS, including older people. Universal precautions should be applied everywhere to protect against the transmission of many diseases. These precautions are not being followed everywhere, especially where old people are cared for, because of the false assumptions that the precautions are only for HIV and that old people couldn't have HIV.

In some instances, funding for educational programs for the elderly has been denied because of the assumption that the elderly are not at risk and are going to die anyway.[33] While there has been an increase in community-based services for people with AIDS, programs for the elderly are threatened by federal and state budget cuts. There is a need for more services for older adults living with HIV.[34]

The Need for Women-Focused Models of Care

Health research to date has focused primarily on white men and therefore the information and models of care which have developed do not fit the needs of women, including older women. Older women are the most invisible and underrecognized of those women living with HIV disease. Obtaining accurate information, testing, diagnosis, and informed respectful care remains problematic.

> Finding someone who is on your side is not an easy thing. . . . I will go to my grave angry, because HIV is just another area where women are discounted.   The same 48-year-old HIV + woman

NOTES

The authors would like to thank Carolyn Bottum; Andy Epstein, AIDS Bureau, Massachusetts Department of Public Health; Paula Minnihan; Carole Miselman; Evie Richardson; Jack Starmer, New England AIDS Education and Training Centers; and Sandy Warshaw, Older Women's League.

1. D. Scheurman, "Clinical Concerns: AIDS in the Elderly," *Journal of Gerontological Nursing* 20.7 (July 1994): 11–17.

2. S. M. Gordon and S. Thompson, "The Changing Epidemiology of Human Immunodeficiency Virus Infection in Older Persons," *Journal of the American Geriatric Society* 43.1 (January 1995): 7–9.

3. D. A. Hertogh, "Sexually Transmitted Diseases in the Elderly," *Infections in Medicine* (May 1994): 361–71.

4. F. L. Brisbane and M. Womble, *Working with African Americans*, HRDI (Chicago: International Press, 1990).

5. E. de la Vega, "Considerations for Reaching the Latino Population," *SIECUS Report* 18.3 (February–March 1990): 801–9.

6. P. E. Stevens, "Lesbians and HIV: Clinical, Research and Policy Issues," *American Journal of Orthopsychiatry* 63 (1993): 289–94.

7. W. El-Sadr and J. Gettler, "Unrecognized Human Immunodeficiency Virus Infection in the Elderly," *Archives of Internal Medicine* 155.2 (23 January 1995): 184–86.

8. E. E. Schoenbaum and M. P. Webber, "The Underrecognition of HIV infection in Women in an Inner-City Emergency Room," *American Journal of Public Health* 83 (1993): 363–68.

9. D. G. Sutin, D. N. Rose et al., "Survival of Elderly Patients with Transfusion-Related Acquired Immunodeficiency Syndrome," *Journal American Geriatric Society* 4.1 (1993): 214–16; N. Carre, C. Deveau, F. Belanger et al., "Effect of Age and Exposure Group on the Onset of AIDS in Heterosexual and Homosexual HIV-infected Patients," SEROCO Study Group, *AIDS* 8.6 (June 1994): 787–802.

10. Center for Women Policy Studies and American Association of Retired Persons (CWPS & AARP), *Midlife and Older Women and HIV/AIDS: Report on the Seminar, November 4–5, 1993* (Washington D.C., 1994), 11.

11. J. Piette, T. J. Wechtel et al., "The Impact of Age on the Quality of Life in Persons with HIV Infection," *Journal of Aging and Health* 7.2 (May 1995): 163–78.

12. CWPS & AARP, 17.

13. CWPS & AARP, 11; A. B. McCruden and W. H. Stimson, "Sex Hormones and Immune Function," in *Psychoneuroimmunology*, ed. R. Ader, D. L. Felten, and N. Cohen (San Diego: Academic Press, 1991), 475–93.

14. B. Doress-Worters and D. Laskin Siegal, *The New Ourselves, Growing Older: Women Aging with Knowledge and Power* (New York: Simon and Schuster, 1994), 31.

15. Conversation with CDC AIDS Clinical Trials Information Line, 12 September 1995.

16. D. Feldman, "Editorial: Sex, AIDS, and the Elderly." *Archives of Internal Medicine* 154.1 (10 January 1994): 19–20; R. Stall and J. Catania, "AIDS Risk Behaviors among Late Middle-Aged and Elderly Americans: The National AIDS Behavioral Surveys," *Archives of Internal Medicine* 154.1 (10 January 1994): 57–63.

17. G. Schiller, S. Crystal et al., "Risky Business: The Cultural Construction of AIDS Risk Groups," *Social Science and Medicine* 38.10 (May 1994): 1337–46.

18. SDHHS, PHS 5.

19. H. Clumeck, H. Tailman et al., "Cluster of HIV Infection among Heterosexual People without Apparent Risk Factors," *New England Journal of Medicine* 321.21 (November 1989): 1460–62.

20. CWPS & AARP, 7.

21. CWPS & AARP, 16.

22. R. Brown and J. R. Rundell, "A Prospective Study of Psychiatric Aspects of Early HIV Disease in Women," *General Hospital Psychiatry* 15 (1993): 139–47.

23. Sarah Brabant, "An Overlooked AIDS Affected Population: The Elderly Parent as Caregiver," *Journal of Gerontological Social Work* 22.1/2 (1994): 131–45.

24. L. Minkler and K. M. Roe, *Grandmothers as Caregivers: Raising Children in the Crack Cocaine Epidemic* (Newbury Park, Calif.: Sage Publications, 1993); C. Levine and G. L. Stein, *Orphans of the HIV Epidemic: Unmet Needs in Six U.S. Cities* (The Orphan Project, 121 Avenue of the Americas, 6th floor, New York, NY 10013, 1994).

25. Brisbane and Womble.

26. L. Chin, "Health Care Issues for Asian Americans," *Journal of Multicultural Community Health* 1.2 (Fall 1991): 17–22.

27. De la Vega.

28. CWPS & AARP, 15.

29. L. Balsam and C. Bottum. "Understanding Aging and Public Health Networks," in *Public Health and Aging,* ed. Tom Hickey (Baltimore: Johns Hopkins University Press, in press).

30. "Educating Elderly on AIDS: The Golden Years Can Also Be Risky," *New York Times,* 9 August 1994: A14. This article describes a program on AIDS given at the Eugenio Maria de Hostas Neighborhood Service Center in Miami, Fla.

31. L. Suarez, L. Lloyd, N. Weiss et al., "Effect of Social Networks on Cancer-Screening Behavior of Older Mexican-American Women, *Journal of the National Cancer Institute* 86.10 (18 May 1994): 775–79; I. Tessaro, E. Eng, and J. Smith, "Breast Cancer Screening in Older African-American Women: Qualitative Research Findings," *American Journal of Health Promotion* 8.4 (March/April 1994): 186–293; L. Rubenstein, *You Owe It to Yourself: Mammography Awareness Campaign for Older Women* (Washington, D.C.: American Association of Retired Persons, Health Advocacy Series, October 1991).

32. "Surgical Sterilization among Women and Use of Condoms," *Journal of the American Medical Association* 268.14 (14 October 1993): 1833.

33. *New York Times,* 9 August 1994.

34. C. Garvey, "AIDS Care for the Elderly: A Community-Based Approach," *AIDS Patient Care* 8.3 (1 June 1994): 118–20.

9

HIV/AIDS and Asian and Pacific Islander Women

Willy Wilkinson

Willy Wilkinson is an Asian/Pacific woman of mixed heritage and a long-time AIDS service provider to API communities. As the first API community health outreach worker (CHOW) in San Francisco, she conducted street-based AIDS education and ethnographic research in the Tenderloin, Chinatown, and South of Market neighborhoods. Pioneering an outreach model that she developed specifically for API communities, she accessed API drug users and their sexual partners, API women working in massage parlors, and the general API community.

While few women were infected with HIV a decade ago, they now represent 50 percent of all new infections. Of those with an Acquired Immune Deficiency Syndrome (AIDS) diagnosis, nearly one in five are women. Women of color account for a significant majority of these women.[1] As women of color whose needs have not been assessed, Asian and Pacific Islander (API) women are at an alarming risk for HIV/AIDS. Between 1992 and 1993, AIDS cases among API women escalated two-and-a-half—fold.[2] For many reasons, there is great cause for concern about future incidence as HIV continues to take hold in this community. There are enormous social, cultural, economic, and communicative barriers that make it difficult for API women to access HIV prevention messages and appropriate care.

In the United States, Asians and Pacific Islanders are the fastest growing population. Currently there are nearly ten million APIs nationwide, and these numbers are expected to quadruple by the year 2050.[3] While 37 percent of APIs are American-born,[4] nearly two-thirds of the population represents immigrants and refugees. According to the U.S. census, 35 percent of APIs over the age of five reside in linguistically isolated households.[5] Of those who speak an API language at home, 55 percent have limited or no English capability.[6] Due in part to linguistic and cultural isolation, APIs have traditionally had higher rates of HIV infection than any other ethnic group. Indeed, escalating rates of infection have reached a crisis point: In San Francisco, between 1992 and 1993, APIs were the only racial group with an increased percentage of reported AIDS cases.[7]

Impact of HIV/AIDS on Asian and Pacific Islander (API) Women

Nationally, API women account for nearly 10 percent of all API AIDS cases. Of these cases, 44 percent are documented under heterosexual contact and 17 percent are among injection drug users (IDUs). Of those cases classified as heterosexual contact, 31 percent are as a result of sexual contact with an injection drug user, 30 percent are sex with a bisexual male, and 28 percent are sex with an HIV-infected person, risk not specified.[8] There is no statistical compilation for sexual contact with another woman, nor are transgender people statistically recognized.

Though API women are 29.1 percent of the women's population in San Francisco,[9] limited behavioral or clinical research has been conducted on this population. Reliable seroprevalence estimates, as well as ethnographic research and data collection of such subpopulations as API sex workers, substance users, lesbian and bisexual women, and transgenders are minimal or nonexistent. Limited (if any) research has been conducted on the impact of HIV or treatment approaches on API women.

Social isolation, economic disadvantage, and cultural expectations create barriers that impede access to HIV prevention and direct services. Risk factors of API women include lack of education, limited language access, lack of familiarity and comfort with American institutions, no health insurance, work and family responsibilities that take precedence over health concerns, fear of police and the Immigration and Naturalization Service (INS), and cultural insensitivity of service providers.

Some of the behavioral risk factors of API women include denial, difficulty asserting protection from risk activities (such as negotiating condom use), and the fact that API women are not likely to seek services unless there is a crisis. Issues of shame and confidentiality that pervade matters of health, sexuality, and drug use within the API community make it difficult for API women to discuss risk behavior with service providers.

According to the 1990 U.S. Census, the category "Asian" encompasses twenty-nine distinct racial and ethnic groups, and the term "Pacific Islander" covers twenty. Within this Asian/Pacific Islander (API) category there is extraordinary diversity. For instance, there are over a hundred languages and dialects spoken among this population. Furthermore, there can be great cultural, social, economic, religious, and political differences between ethnic groups, as well as within specific ethnic groups.

As a broad category, APIs are the fastest-growing population in the United States, with annual growth rates exceeding 4 percent during the 1990s.[10] Birth rates are expected to triple from 4 percent to 11 percent by the year 2050.[11] Further, API immigration is projected to exceed the API birth rate over the next thirty years. As API immigrants flee political turmoil, seek economic betterment, or come to the U.S. for family reunification, over three million API immigrants and their descendants will be added to the U.S. population by the year 2000.[12] The total API population in the U.S. is estimated to reach 41 million by the middle of the twenty-first century.[13] Women comprise approximately half of this population.

It is important to note that 37 percent of APIs are American-born,[14] some of whom have been in this country for as many as six generations. The API population encompasses people who are not only varied ethnically, culturally, and linguistically; there is a range of skill levels with regard to English capability, educational level, economic status, access to services, and familiarity and comfort with American institutions and cultural expectations. Women within the API community, like women from other traditional cultures, are less likely to be in a position to access information and services (see risk factors). It is also important to note that even though people may have been in this country for many generations, it is probable that cultural behaviors and belief systems have been retained. Assumptions cannot be made either way.

While the API population in the United States has grown from 3.5 million in 1980 to 7.3 million in 1990 to 9.8 million in 1995,[15] APIs continue to be chronically underserved by our health care system. Health care services directed at the larger API community, when available, have traditionally focused on general health and prenatal care. Though the number of API AIDS cases has skyrocketed since the beginning of the epidemic, there is still alarmingly little emphasis on HIV and AIDS in health care delivery to this population.[16] API women in particular often view AIDS as a white, gay male disease that has little to do with them, and the lack of HIV prevention efforts targeting API women contributes to this misconception.

While current epidemiological data shows a lower incidence of AIDS cases among Asian/Pacific Islanders than African Americans, Latinos, and whites, these numbers can be misleading. Lower numbers, due in part to poor statistical accuracy, belie the fact that there is indeed great cause for concern about the future incidence of HIV infection among APIs. Throughout the course of the AIDS pandemic, APIs have traditionally had the highest rates of infection of any ethnic group. A recent San Francisco study indicates that between 1992 and 1993, APIs were the only racial group with an increased percentage of reported AIDS cases.[17]

Inaccurate statistical information on APIs has resulted, in large part, from underreporting and misclassification. Anecdotal reports suggest that significant numbers of APIs with AIDS have been undercounted. The stigma and shame associated with AIDS, as well as a lack of knowledge about Western medicine, have kept many APIs from seeking Western medical care. Fears of deportation, language inaccessibility, and general mistrust of American institutions are other factors associated with APIs "falling through the cracks." Misclassification refers to the fact that many APIs have been racially misclassified as Latino, white, Native American, or African American, or have simply fallen under "other" (many states have no statistical category for APIs).[18] Disease misclassification, opportunistic infection misclassification, or misdiagnosis have also contributed to poor statistical accuracy.

The *reported* AIDS cases among APIs in the United States totaled 2,991 as of December 1994. Of those, 9.7 percent are among women.[19]

Estimates

Heterosexual Women

Nationally, 44 percent of AIDS cases among API women are documented under the "heterosexual contact" exposure category. Among these cases, 31 percent occurred as a result of "sex with an injection drug user," 29.5 percent are "sex with a bisexual male," 27.9 percent are "sex with an HIV-infected person, risk not specified," 9.3 percent are "sex with a transfusion recipient with HIV infection," and 2.3 percent are "sex with a person with hemophilia."[20]

Injection Drug Users

Nationally, 17 percent of AIDS cases among API women are among injection drug users (IDUs). This figure represents only a slightly higher number of cases than those contracted via heterosexual contact with an injection drug user.[21] When combined, they represent 30.3 percent of all AIDS cases among API women. Clearly, API women needle users and their partners are contracting and developing AIDS.

Transgenders/Lesbian and Bisexual Women

The fact that there is no statistical compilation of transgender people or women who have sex with women in AIDS case data or other statistics pertaining to HIV-related concerns does not mean that there are no API people in either of these categories, nor that neither population is unaffected by HIV. The needs of both communities will be discussed later in this article.

Barriers to Prevention and Treatment

While the larger API population is at a cultural and linguistic disadvantage when seeking services, API women have far greater cultural, linguistic, social, and economic barriers that further impede access to services. For the larger API population, cultural and linguistic voids in service provision contribute to inappropriate, insufficient, and underutilized programming. For API women, the situation is exacerbated by enormous social isolation, economic disadvantage, and cultural expectations that make it harder for women to get care. For instance, service providers would be more effective if they enhanced their sensitivity to the issues of shame and confidentiality that pervade matters of health, sexuality, and drug use within the API community. For API women, there may be a particular reluctance to discuss such intimate matters with a stranger, if at all. Providers need to understand that these issues may need to be addressed in such a way as to provide clear prevention messages without necessarily assigning any obvious connections between the client and the risk behaviors. In many API cultures, high value is placed on politeness and listening skills. While the client may not admit to risk activities, she can receive the information, in a sense, as an anonymous audience member receiving a general health prevention message.

Language Barriers

First, there needs to be a common language between service provider and client. While most American-born API women are comfortable with conversational English, the majority of immigrant API women are much more isolated from opportunities to learn English than their male counterparts. They are often too busy with work and family responsibilities; issues of time, money, family, raising children, and limited access to educational opportunities can make a woman's ESL (English as a Second Language) education a low priority. In order to reach limited-English and monolingual API women, linguistic capability or interpretation services are essential in service delivery. Visual aids that include pictures of risk activities (as well as those activities that are *not* possible exposures to HIV), of precautionary measures, and of the human reproductive system are also helpful.

Denial

The first psychological barrier to getting the HIV prevention message across to API women is the denial that HIV and AIDS is something that warrants their concern. Even in 1995, AIDS is still largely perceived by many API women as a white, gay male disease that has nothing to do with them. Low numbers of reported AIDS cases (due in part to underreporting and misclassification) and denial about risk behavior within the API community contribute to the false sense that there is nothing to worry about. Misconceptions about HIV transmission further compound the attitude that AIDS is best prevented by staying away from possibly infected people rather than be taking necessary precautions.

Difficulty Asserting Protection from Risk Activities

When precautions are understood, cultural norms of politeness and not "making waves" make it very difficult for API women to assert themselves in condom and bleach negotiation. There have been many anecdotes of women having difficulty negotiating condom use with casual as well as steady partners, or "johns" (the customers of sex workers) who are willing to pay more for sex without a condom. One telling story involves an API woman injection drug user. When this woman spoke with an outreach worker, she recounted her difficulties negotiating bleach within her drug-using circle. Self-assertion in safer sex and needle hygiene can be very problematic for API women because it involves going against the grain of long-standing cultural behaviors. The situation is further compounded by the fact that sex or drug partners of API women engaging in high risk behavior are often non-APIs. There can be the sense, as was the case with this client, that these partners' needs and wants are more important than their own, or that they as API women have little or no power in the situation. Further, many API women face domestic violence when trying to assert the need for safer sex or needle hygiene. Many women just don't have the option of "forcing" their partners to use protection without being emotionally or physically abused.

API Women Do Not Seek Services

On the issue of direct services, another key issue for API women, as with all women, is "getting them to clinic." Whether because of a lack of awareness of services available to them, the inappropriateness of those services, lack of health insurance, or economic constraints, many APIs do not seek services until there is a crisis, thus making their first contact with service providers in the emergency room. API women, who are most often taking care of the needs of others, are most likely to take care of themselves last. API women clients often need to be encouraged to go for medical checkups even when symptoms persist. One example of the effectiveness of outreach programs targeting API women is the case of a Thai immigrant woman who, because of lack of information about STD clinics and limited English, had gone years without gynecological care. With the outreach worker's encouragement, helped by her ability to advocate and interpret for the client, the client got checked for STDs. A massage parlor worker, she had unknowingly contracted syphilis, which would have presented serious problems if left untreated.

No Time for Health Care

It is important to note that, as is the case for other women of color, AIDS is just one more issue in the lives of API women. There are many other survival issues that require attention. To begin, many API women are working very hard just to have enough money to get by. This could mean long hours doing exhausting work with little or no sick time. Some reasons for these long hours are lack of education and skills, language barriers, lack of access to jobs with better conditions, immigration status, and expectations of a family business. In addition, there may be intergenerational family responsibilities that API women are expected to handle, such as caring for a mother-in-law or caring for children.

Other Pressing Concerns

Immigrant and refugee women may have persistent legal matters pertaining to immigration, as well as general fear and stress about immigration policies. Women who work in massage parlors or other aspects of the sex industry, as well as those who use drugs, are often most concerned about the police. Massage parlor workers report frequent harassment by cops who have sex with them, then charge them with prostitution. (One woman swallowed the condom to get rid of the evidence.)[22] Fortunately, as of March 1995, condoms can no longer be used as evidence in prostitution-related offenses in San Francisco.[23] Still, for immigrant sex-industry workers, fears about the police and the Immigration and Naturalization Service (INS) take precedence over everything else. Finally, women who trade sex for money, food, drugs, a place to stay, or protection on the streets are not necessarily thinking about something (i.e., HIV infection) that could manifest itself much further in the future.

Domestic Violence

Women who are involved in abusive situations with their sexual partners or family members are trapped in a system of control and domination. Their personal freedom may be greatly limited, and they may live under constant threat of physical, emotional, psychological, or sexual abuse. Any deviation from what is expected may be met with violence as a means of controlling their behavior. In these circumstances it is very difficult for women to assert their needs, much less call attention to an issue that could ignite feelings of jealousy and questions of infidelity, such as in attempting to negotiate condom use. A woman involved in an abusive relationship may be in danger of exposure to HIV, particularly if her partner is involved in high-risk activities and refuses to take necessary precautions.

The Asian Women's Shelter reports that in 1994 it served 66 women and children and turned away 155 women and 174 children. Clearly it is at capacity, and it is now expanding to accommodate this increasing demand.[24]

Sexual Assault

Further, API women are at risk of exposure to HIV via sexual assault, whether committed by a known or an unknown perpetrator. This horrifying situation may be compounded by blame and the false assumptions of their families, communities, and other peers. The age-old questions may arise within the survivor's family and community: "What was she wearing? What did she do to bring this upon her?" Anecdotal reports from a Vietnamese outreach worker describe stories of newly-arrived Vietnamese women who have been sexually assaulted. One limited English woman in her forties was raped and told no one, not even her husband. After seeing an ad in a Vietnamese-language newspaper, she sought help from this outreach worker, who counseled her and provided the necessary interpretation to help her get tested for HIV and STDs. Another Vietnamese woman, in her thirties and mentally impaired, was repeatedly raped one night by three men. She too eventually made contact with this outreach worker, who helped her access the necessary health care services.

Often women are afraid to seek help for fear that they will be stigmatized and blamed for the sexual assault. This blame and assumption exists within the API community as well as the lesbian community. In a roundtable discussion among HIV+ women, a lesbian who contracted HIV through sexual assault stated, "I've met many, many women . . . who have gotten it through sexual abuse or rape. Some lesbians I know . . . just automatically assume that I was out fucking men."[25]

Subpopulations

Sex Workers

While heterosexual women as a group are undoubtedly at risk via unprotected sexual contact, women who make their living from the sale of sex are continually faced with possible exposure. In the world of prostitution, codes of behavior are dictated on the streets. Nowadays, those who are willing to forego safer sex precautions as a means of making more money are viewed with great contempt. On the other hand, those who refuse to comply with requests for unsafe sex acts are often "career hookers" who have years of experience and a perspective on their life and profession that goes beyond the next trick. No matter how "sick" from addiction or otherwise desperate they are, they will refuse this type of negotiation; for even in their darkest hours, they can recall the devastating face of AIDS that many of them have witnessed firsthand. Nonetheless, some sex workers desperate for the next hit, food, or rent will still accept offers of more money in exchange for sex without a condom. Those that negotiate unsafe sex acts are likely to be newer on the street, desperately drug-addicted, or occasional sex workers who are in denial about what they do. These are the people who are most at risk.

API women who work in the sex industry in this country are much less likely to work on the streets and more likely to work in the sheltered environment of a massage parlor. Those API women who are on the streets are usually American-born women or transgender women. Few immigrant women are familiar and comfortable enough with American society to work the streets; most are very concerned with advertising this type of behavior as well. A workplace where purportedly "only massage" takes place dignifies a "shameful" profession and plays into denial about what actually occurs. Massage parlors provide a more private environment from which to work that becomes its own world.

While there is the security that a massage parlor is much safer than the street, the isolation of this environment in fact creates a false sense of protection. Though an immigrant API woman with limited English skills can function within her own linguistic and cultural context (because there are others from her country in her environment), she stays isolated from most opportunities to better her English and thus enable her to make the transition out of sex work. She is also isolated from most opportunities to educate herself about the risks of unprotected sexual contact; while there is camaraderie among massage parlor workers, they are much more isolated from the information-sharing and outreach efforts available on the street.

Further, many women who work in massage parlors are "indentured" to work for owners who have paid their airfare and set them up in the U.S. These massage parlor owners are for the most part not interested in seeing that these women become educated about safer sex, legal issues, or health care access. Continual fear of police arrest or deportation is pervasive, so any strangers other than customers are viewed with great distrust. In this environment women are not only trapped into working off their debt; they are also in a situation where johns come to them. They cannot refuse the trick in the same way that a street hooker can refuse to get in a car. Anecdotal reports from outreach workers indicate that women in massage parlors are often confronted with johns who refuse to wear a condom, so they must devise ways to ingeniously sneak it on. Some women have been distressed to emerge from a sexual situation in which they could not see what was happening, only to find that the john had broken the condom to enhance his pleasure.

Outreach workers have found that many massage parlor workers are unfamiliar with the workings of their own bodies and the way that HIV and STDs are contracted. These sex workers have benefited from diagrams of female sexual organs and explanations of gynecological health in order to better understand HIV and STD precautions. Some women, particularly women who are younger and newer to prostitution, are accepting offers for more money for sex without a condom. Like their street counterparts, the older career massage parlor workers are enraged, for this makes their jobs harder when johns want the same deal from them. Some massage parlor owners (particularly male owners) will look the other way if it means better business. Anecdotal reports suggest that illness and drug addiction are rampant in some massage parlors that have not been accessed by outreach workers.

Many heterosexual and bisexual women working in massage parlors meet their boyfriends while at work. Sometimes these relationships can provide an escape opportunity or at least the fantasy of it, though they may further compound their risk. Often, condoms are seen as something worn while at work, but not between people in love; thus, though these men may continue to frequent sex workers, they do not wear condoms with their girlfriends. When these women try to negotiate condom use, they are often met with great resistance.

It bears mentioning that outreach workers have estimated that 25–50 percent of API women in massage parlors are lesbian or bisexual. While they may identify themselves as such, lack of information about resources, limited language skills, and unfamiliarity with American society has made it difficult for them to access lesbian/gay services.

Another problem that is ravaging massage parlors is gambling addictions. While this problem affects the API community at large, API women who work in massage parlors are more likely to be exposed to gambling opportunities and to have a disposable income with which to play. Some women are in debt for hundreds of thousands of dollars, and are thus trapped into continuing to work in the sex industry. Others *begin* working in massage parlors in order to pay off their gambling debts.

For many reasons, API massage parlor workers are not likely to seek health care. Some reasons are lack of familiarity with medical resources available to them, limited English, and shame and denial about the nature of their work. When they do seek out health care, it is usually to handle a particular health concern rather than as preventive medicine. Problems arise when service providers are not aware of a client's profession, and clients are unwilling to disclose this for fear of the stigma attached. Service providers need to devise ways to provide clients with general health information and prevention education without making such disclosure necessary.

Undoubtedly, API women who work in massage parlors are at great risk for HIV. There are many aspects of their situation that put them at risk: their immigration status, limited English, lack of education and familiarity with resources, a feeling of being trapped in their situation, denial about what they do, and sometimes, a newness to the profession.

Substance Users

While female API drug users do not necessarily "advertise" their behavior by hanging out high on the street, the reality is that there are significant numbers using injection and other drugs. National statistics indicate that 17 percent of AIDS cases among API women are among injection drug users.[26] Difficulty expressing feelings, cultural expectations, and family pressures are some of the reasons that API women "self-medicate" with drugs. Prevention Point Needle Exchange reports that during the period from January to June 1995, API women made 170 visits to exchange sites in San Francisco.[27] This figure accounts for 32.8 percent of the API total. Given the enormous stigma attached to drug use within the API community and the care that many API women drug users take to assure confidentiality about their drug habits, it is significant that this many API women are seeking such a high-profile service.

For various reasons, many API women do drugs with people who are not part of the API community. It affords them anonymity and allows departure from community and culture. Still, many API women are using drugs within API circles. (Anecdotal reports from outreach workers witnessing cogendered carloads of Vietnamese youth copping crack on Sixth

Street is one instance of visibility.) And when they hit bottom, API women substance users are often reluctant to seek treatment; the whole concept of treatment involves talking about feelings to strangers. Mainstream treatment facilities may not understand their culture, and they are afraid to "lose face" by enrolling in a treatment facility geared towards APIs. Also, API services are usually less prepared to handle their concerns as women. Women's services may require program participation that is not culturally accessible to them. Those API women who are reluctant to seek treatment are likely to "fall through the cracks" while turning their pain inward and spiraling further into addiction.

Furthermore, information about drug-paraphernalia hygiene has been slow to reach injection drug users as a whole. In a group interview with HIV+ women, one woman spoke to the need for better education about cleaning not just syringes, but all other paraphernalia as well:

> If we could have got some education about that, we could have known that that cooker was just as infectious as the needles. So it took us ten years to finally figure it out. Girl, and by that time we were all infected.[28]

In addition to the use of substances that involve injection practices, many API women are using other more easily administered substances, such as crack and crystal. These drugs give the false sense that they are not putting themselves at risk for HIV, while being "cool." Yet many drug-addicted women turn to survival sex for the next hit, for a place to use or stay, for protection, or for cash. Since drug-addicted people and people who are high when engaging in sexual behavior are less likely to use safer sex practices, these women are clearly putting themselves at risk.

Lesbian and Bisexual Women

Though documented HIV seroprevalence among lesbian and bisexual women has been considered low, there are many factors that put this population at risk. There is enormous pressure within the API community as well as within the larger society to conform to heterosexual expectations. API lesbian and bisexual women not only contend with racism, sexism, classism, anti-immigrant bias, language barriers, lack of access to education and jobs, economic constraints, etc.; they must battle the homophobia in their daily lives. If they are different in their gender presentation (i.e. "butch") they are also faced with discrimination based on gender identity or appearance. Such oppression has led to self-destructive behavior in some, such as drug use or unsafe sex. Some lesbian and bisexual women with drug habits have resorted to survival sex.

In general, the majority of lesbian and bisexual women with HIV became infected through the sharing of drug paraphernalia or through unprotected sex with a man. Yet evidence of woman-to-woman transmission is mounting. The CDC admits that while they are not documenting cases of woman-to-woman transmission, they consider oral sex a risk.[29] Anecdotal reports demonstrate that increasing numbers of women have contracted HIV through sexual contact with female partners. Though educational prevention efforts have begun to reach this community, the message is not being heeded; the majority of lesbians are still under the illusion that they are somehow immune. The 1993 HIV Seroprevalence survey among lesbian and bisexual women conducted by the San Francisco Department of Public Health reported 91.9 percent unprotected oral sex between women.[30]

When lesbian and bisexual women become infected, they are often met with hostility within the lesbian community and difficulties finding support services that meet their needs. In the case of a Pacific Islander lesbian/bisexual injection drug user with AIDS, questions arise: What services are available to her? Women's services may have a support group for her to attend, though service providers and clients may not be familiar with her cultural background and context. An API health service may also have a support group, though often the specific issues of Pacific Islanders are disregarded. The same is often true in drug prevention efforts for the API community. Though there is a Pacific Islander presence in Asian/Pacific lesbian and bisexual (APLB) groups and organizations, there has not been a concerted effort to outreach to and network with Pacific Islander women. Further, the APLB community may not be ready to embrace HIV-infected people as their own. Often, women in this situation must find their support from gay men and heterosexual women.

Transgender People

The term transgender is used to describe individuals, who, for various reasons, adopt a gender identity that is not congruent with their physical status. This group includes pre- and postoperative transsexuals, transvestites/cross-dressers, drag kings and queens, and men and women who pass as the "opposite" sex. While transgender individuals (TGs) all have significant psychological and emotional cross-gender identification, their behavior and sense of personal identity varies. Since sexual orientation is itself distinct from gender identity, TGs are lesbian, gay, bisexual, heterosexual, and asexual. For the purpose of this project, consideration is given specifically to API TGs who are preop FTM (female-to-male) and postop MTF (male-to-female). In particular, the issues of FTM individuals deserve focus, as they are rarely addressed.

Many female-to-male transgender people remain preoperative because, in the words of James Green, director of FTM International, "there's no such thing as a sex change operation, at least for FTMs."[31] Indeed there is, but the risks of surgery, the fact that the results are less than ideal, and prohibitive costs make surgery a less viable option for some. The first step is hormone treatment, which helps create a "male" appearance (facial hair, deepening of the voice, muscular strength, etc.) while diminishing "female" characteristics (gynecological functions, skin softness, distribution of body fat, etc.). Those wishing to transition to a male identity must continue with testosterone for life. Secondly, there is "top" surgery, a bilateral mastectomy and chest reconstruction. There are four primary techniques used for removal of the breast, all effective though with varying degrees of scarring, and ranging in price from $1,800 to $6,500.[32] "Bottom" surgery, or genital reconstruction, is less effective and much more complicated, and can range in price from $6,000 to $10,000 for metoidioplasty (enlarging the clitoris and severing suspensory ligaments to create a micropenis) and $50,000 to $150,000 for free tissue flap transfer phalloplasty (transferring skin and muscle tissue from the forearm, groin, or thigh).[33] To date, there is no surgery that will create a fully functional penis that looks "normal" in size and appearance. For this reason, and because of the astronomical expense, many FTM-identified people choose to take testosterone and get their breasts removed, but forgo genital reconstruction. It is often the case that FTMs are somewhere in the middle of this process, for this transition into a "male" physical body takes years.

Furthermore, many FTMs, while cross-living as a man, may not have undergone surgery to remove their uterus, ovaries, or vagina. This can present a problem when someone who presents as a man seeks services for "female" conditions. Whether a cancerous condition aggravated by testosterone or a simple yeast infection, the problem will not be treated competently if this individual is met with ridicule and disrespect. Indeed, whether FTMs physically pass as men or not, they may well be wary of seeking treatment for such matters. Such contact with services would invite difficult psychological issues as well as the possibility of disclosing one's "secret." Often, TGs are forced to revert to their original gender in order to obtain services.

Male-to-female transgendered individuals are also less likely to seek health care out of fears that they will experience ridicule or that their issues will not be understood. Though a low percentage of MTFs actually go through with sexual reassignment (approximately 5 percent of clients served by Asian AIDS Project's Transgender Program),[34] they have very specific gynecological needs once they have completed transition. Postop MTFs need annual gynecological checkups and a mammogram every other year. They also should have an annual blood workup to check hormone levels. Invariably it is difficult to find health care providers who are sensitive to and understanding of their particular health care needs; often transgendered people have had their surgery in other parts of the country or world and may not have an established provider relationship. Finally, the particular linguistic, cultural, immigration issues, and so forth relevant to APIs can create barriers to appropriate care.

For that portion of the transgender population that is API, there are various issues that contribute to limited access and potential risk for HIV infection. Since many API transgender people are English language— limited or monolingual immigrants, language access poses an additional barrier to profound gender identity discrimination, racism, and classism. Like American-born transgender people, many have difficulty securing mainstream employment and (particularly MTFs) resort to sex work, drug dealing, or other unconventional work for survival. Many API transgenders, especially those who have engaged in high risk activities, are reluctant to get tested for HIV. They are also less likely to receive adequate medical and social services, and may never obtain information about HIV that takes into account their physical situation or identification. (Anecdotal reports of discussion at the first FTM Conference of the Americas, held in San Francisco in August 1995, suggest that many FTMs are uninformed about HIV transmission or their risk while engaging in sexual activity.)

Like all people, TGs are at risk for HIV through unprotected sex with men or women. Those who may be particularly at risk via sexual behavior are gay- or bi-identified FTMs and MTFs who have sex with men, especially as sex work. Further, drug use and the sharing of syringes puts TGs at risk. The Transgender Program of Asian AIDS Project reports that speed is the drug of choice among the largely MTF transgender population that they serve. The use of this and other drugs, as well as the sharing of syringes for the injection of hormones or steroids, put TG people at risk for infection. Again, lack of acknowledgment and respect in the health care setting can greatly limit access to services that can meet their needs.

Barriers to Appropriate HIV Prevention and Direct Services for API Women

The following list highlights many of the client issues as well as provider issues that need to be addressed in order to achieve more effective service provision for API women:

- Misconceptions about HIV/AIDS—The perception that HIV/AIDS is a disease affecting white, gay men, therefore having nothing to do with them, or that HIV/AIDS is transmitted casually through sharing utensils, riding the bus or other casual contact, or through mosquitoes. Misunderstanding about appropriate precautions. Finally, the perception that AIDS is contracted "when God calls."
- Cultural barriers to discussing such personal matters as sexuality, drug use, illness, and death, particularly with a stranger. A misperception that the actual discussion will "bring illness into the family."
- Inadequate education about gynecological health, sexuality, and STDs.
- Cultural mores that encourage women to be nonassertive and to care for the needs of others before their own, causing difficulty to assert themselves in condom negotiation.
- Difficulty asserting themselves when negotiating needle hygiene (separate syringes or bleach between uses) or other precautions to avoid contamination from drug paraphernalia.
- Limited language access. There are thirty-two Asian/Pacific languages in the Bay Area. Current HIV education, prevention, and direct services in appropriate API languages are insufficient, as are translation and interpretation services. This is especially important given the social isolation of immigrant API women, who are much less likely to gain a working command of English than their male counterparts.
- Lack of understanding about the U.S. health care system, social service benefits, and lack of health insurance coverage. General mistrust and suspicion of health and social service providers.
- Current immigration policies and climate surrounding statewide Proposition 187 (an anti-immigrant bill endorsed by Governor Pete Wilson that discrimi-

nates against undocumented residents) that instill fear about jeopardizing immigration status if services are sought. Fears are raised in this population that service providers will turn their names in to the Immigration and Naturalization Service (INS) and that they will be deported. Additionally, there are fears that an HIV + status or AIDS diagnosis will lead to deportation.

- Police harassment of massage parlor workers and others in the sex industry continues making them reluctant to use condoms or have them in their possession for fear of arrest. (Until recently, the presence of condoms on the premises has been allowed as evidence of probable cause in prostitution-related arrests in San Francisco.)[35] A conviction on prostitution charges will most likely lead to deportation for noncitizens.

- Cultural insensitivity among service providers—Service providers not giving API women full services, mistreating them, not obtaining full medical consent and, treating them like they're stupid or ignorant. This is especially true for patients with accents.

- Limited outreach efforts educating API women about HIV *in their own neighborhoods,* informing them about existing services, and encouraging their participation in those services.

- Insufficient HIV education by service providers during gynecological and prenatal visits. There is a constant denial that sex work, drug use, S/M sexual practices, lesbian/bisexual women, STDs, and HIV/AIDS even exist in API communities.

- Limited opportunities to transition out of sex work. Unavailability of culturally and linguistically appropriate services to help with this transition.

- Lack of sensitivity among service providers to lesbian and bisexual women's health concerns, lifestyle, and risk practices.

- Limited availability of drug treatment. Insufficient culturally and linguistically appropriate drug programs and treatment staff.

- Limited outreach efforts and medical and social support for transgender APIs, both preoperative female-to-males (FTMs) and postoperative male-to-females (MTFs).

- Lack of research on the impact of HIV on API women and API transgender people.

- Limited (if any) AIDS clinical trials open to API women. This is generally an issue for all women, but given the invisibility of APIs and the myriad of cultural and language issues, there is undoubtedly a lack of recruitment of API women into clinical trials.

ACKNOWLEDGMENTS

Special thanks to my partner, Georgia Kolias, for her support, encouragement, and phenomenally inquiring mind.

NOTES

1. Information given by the Centers for Disease Control AIDS Information Hotline and the National AIDS Clearinghouse, December 11, 1995. U.S. estimates are derived by averaging wide-ranging figures produced by medical mathematicians for the CDC. Current AIDS statistics are through October, 1995.

2. Centers for Disease Control, U.S. Department of Health and Human Services, *Health United States, 1994,* 1995: 147.

3. U.S. Department of Commerce, *1990 Census of Population, Asians and Pacific Islanders in the U.S.,* 1990 CP-3–5.

4. U.S. Department of Commerce, 1990 CP-2–6, Section 1–4.

5. Dept. of Commerce, 1990 CP-2–6, Section 1–4: 199.

6. Dept. of Commerce, 1990 CP-2–6, Section 1–4: 199; and Dept. of Commerce, *Statistical Abstract of the United States 1994,* Bureau of the Census: 129.

7. HIV Prevention Planning Council, *1995 San Francisco HIV Prevention Plan:* 267.

8. Centers for Disease Control, U.S. Department of Health and Human Services, *1994 HIV/AIDS Surveillance Report,* 1995.

9. "Asians in America," 1990 Census, Classification by States, *Asian Week,* 1991: 45.

10. R. Chang, *HIV/AIDS in the Asian and Pacific Islander Communities* (Asian/Pacific AIDS Coalition, 1993), 3.

11. Chang.

12. Chang.

13. Dept. of Commerce, 1990 CP-3–5.

14. Dept. of Commerce, 1990 CP-2–6, Section 1–4.

15. Dept. of Commerce, 1990 CP-3–5.

16. Throughout the course of the AIDS pandemic, APIs have traditionally had higher rates of infection than any other racial group.

17. K. Whitlock, "Asian and Pacific Islander and Other People of Color Transgender Issues," *Transgender Outlook,* 1995: 7.

18. Chang, 5.

19. Centers for Disease Control, *1994 HIV/AIDS Surveillance Report,* 1995.

20. Ibid.

21. Ibid.

22. Conversation with Dawn Passar and Roe Johnson, Asian AIDS Project outreach workers, July 6, 1995.

23. D. Conkin, "D.A.: Condoms [do not equal] Prostitution," *Bay Area Reporter,* April 6, 1995.

24. Conversation with Mimi Kim of the Asian Women's Shelter, December 1, 1995.

25. Lyon-Martin Women's Health Services, The National Lesbian/Bisexual Women's HIV Prevention Network, *Woman to Woman,* June 1995, 9.

26. Centers for Disease Control, *1994 HIV/AIDS Surveillance Report,* 1995.

27. HIV Prevention Project, Prevention Point Needle Exchange, client contacts, January—June, 1995. Racial group was determined by "apparent ethnicity" and is thus subject to human error.

28. Lyon-Martin, 10.

29. Lyon-Martin, 7.

30. San Francisco Department of Public Health AIDS Office, *HIV Seroprevalence and Risk Behaviors among Lesbians and Bisexual Women: The 1993 San Francisco/Berkeley Women's Survey,* October 1993, 1.

31. James Green, "Getting Real about FTM Surgery," *Chrysalis: The Journal of Transgressive Gender Identities,* 1995: 27.

32. Green, 28.

33. Green, 30.

34. Conversation with Kiki Whitlock, Transgender Program Coordinator at Asian AIDS Project, November 1995.

35. Conkin.

10

Interpersonal Power and Women's HIV Risk

Kathryn Quina, Lisa L. Harlow, Patricia J. Morokoff, and Susan E. Saxon

All four authors are at the University of Rhode Island. *Kathryn Quina,* Ph.D., is Professor of Psychology and Women's Studies, specializing in long-terms effect of sexual abuse and HIV risk. *Lisa L. Harlow,* Ph.D., is Associate Professor of Psychology, teaching methodology and specializing in multivariate techniques, including structural modeling, and in psychosocial issues in women's health. *Patricia J. Morokoff,* Ph.D., is Professor of Psychology and Director of the Clinical Training Program, specializing in women's health and sexuality. *Susan E. Saxon,* A.M., is a Ph.D. candidate in clinical psychology and graduate research assistant with the Women's Health Research Project and the Cancer Prevention Research Center. The first three authors have worked together for the past seven years on issues of HIV risk for women, most recently supported by a grant from NIMII (Lisa Harlow, Principal Investigator; Kathryn Quina and Patricia Morokoff, Co-Principal Investigators).

Everywhere we look in our culture there are images of women's sexuality as powerful: from Harlequin romances to pornography, from ancient deities to contemporary idols such as Madonna. Their power is often portrayed as dangerous to men, as in Homer's sirens or Eve's original sin. Yet even in these dangerous forms, women's sexual power is usually limited to attracting (passively) or seducing men (indirectly active), usually because of the way they look. The roles of pursuer, sexual initiator, and more powerful partner remain firmly in the reins of men (e.g., Charlene Muehlenhard and Marsha McCoy 1991).

Clearly, the power to refuse unwanted sex and to make wanted sex safer are vital concerns for women's health. Transmission of HIV through heterosexual contact is on the rise (Centers for Disease Control (CDC) 1995), with particularly high risks from bisexual and injection drug using

men. More than a quarter of the men reported to the CDC as homosexu-
ally transmitted AIDS cases had recently engaged in sex with a woman
(Susan Chu et al. 1992). Ken Mayer and his colleagues in the Boston
Partners Study have observed that the practices of bisexual men were
particularly risky, as they were more likely than exclusively homosexual
men to have unprotected anal intercourse with their male partners and
were not protecting their women partners (1994, personal communication).
Various studies (reviewed by Patricia Morokoff, Lisa Harlow, and Kathryn
Quina 1995) have indicated that injection drug using (IDU) men are most
often having sex with non-IDU women, and often do not tell their non-
IDU partners about their drug practices.

In heterosexual relationships, the safest sex practices are abstinence, use
of a latex condom with spermicidal cream or jelly during intercourse, and
alternative sexual relationships in which ejaculate does not come in contact
with oral, vaginal, or anal areas. Therefore, any unprotected sexual activity
with a partner with a sexual or drug-use history at any time since 1980 puts
a woman at risk. Women cannot depend upon heterosexual partners to
disclose their serostatus or health risks, as men report they frequently
deceive their sex partners about their other relationships and behaviors
(Susan Cochran and Vickie Mays 1990).

While abstinence is possible for women, in relationships it is usually not
practiced nor desired. Nor are noncontact sexual alternatives. Thus for
many women the only solution is consistent condom use, a practice in
which the male partner must agree to, or be persuaded to, participate—at
least until the female condom becomes more effective and accepted (Institute of Medicine 1994, in Hortensia Amaro 1995; Morokoff, Harlow, and
Quina 1995).

Thus, in order to plan effective ways to reduce HIV risk to women, we
must understand the heterosexual relationships that underlie these risks. In
order to do that, we must understand interpersonal power. In this chapter
we will outline our multifaceted interpersonal power theory of women's
HIV-risky heterosexual behavior and offer supporting data collected by the
University of Rhode Island Women's Health Research Project. Our approach is informed by feminist theoretical perspectives, methodologies, and
processes.

The framework our research team has adopted presumes that the influ-
ences on sexual behavior among women in heterosexual relationships are
multifaceted, and include psychosocial/attitudinal, relational, and behav-

ioral factors. We have developed a comprehensive prediction and intervention approach which emphasizes variables which theoretically are associated with interpersonal power for women, some of which have not historically been associated with HIV research.[1] In doing so, we have considered relationship dynamics, gender role expectations, self-esteem and self-efficacy, the impact of violence, and sexual and condom mores.

We have adopted a rights-based focus to women's sexuality. Women have the right to refuse unwanted sexual attention, to initiate wanted sexual contact, and to experience sexual encounters as noncoercive and safe. To these ends, it is absolutely critical for women to feel confident and secure in choosing any sexual lifestyle, including condom use or abstinence from sexual intercourse on any occasion. Important consequences include whether the woman is effective in reaching her goal, how people feel about her, and most important, how she feels about herself. A rights-focused approach counteracts pressures on women to place the demands or needs of others, or the opinion others hold of them, as higher priorities than self-respect and self-protection.

Heterosexuality and Interpersonal Power

Despite high levels of knowledge about AIDS and its transmission, sexual behavior change has not occurred among heterosexual populations. In line with various national studies, we have found fewer than 20 percent of sexually active high school and college women use condoms (Harlow et al. 1993; Michelle Lang 1994; MaryAnn Paxson and Quina 1989). Thus it is clear that we must move beyond providing basic knowledge if we are to reduce HIV risk.

Prior research on HIV preventive behaviors has often focused on variables which presume personal control (e.g. health belief, self-efficacy) and group peer norms, such as those found in the gay community. As so eloquently discussed by Hortensia Amaro, applying the same methods and conclusions to women fails to take into account social, cultural, and intrapersonal variables which affect women's sexual and health-related behavior. For example, women have learned that taking an active role in initiating sex may result in negative attributions regarding their motives and personalities (Letitia Peplau, Zick Rubin, and Charles Hill 1977). As Naomi McCormick (1994) describes this dilemma,

> Women do not have a weaker, paler sexuality than men. . . . But, most
> women have not achieved the sexual empowerment advocated by many
> Liberal Feminists. . . . Traditional roles, culturally learned scripts for who
> does what to whom in a sexual relationship often hold us back (16).

One consequence of such persistent cultural beliefs is that many women
may have difficulty asserting themselves—positively or negatively—in intimate situations. Furthermore, they are often motivated by their concern for
others, even to their own detriment. Among college women, Miriam
Lewin (1985) found that the reason most often given for not refusing
undesired sex was concern about hurting their partners' feelings—more so
than shame or fear.

Research with young women indicates that a wide range of pressures to
engage in risky sexual behavior, from verbal persuasion through sexual
assault, are experienced within relationships (Janet Holland et al. 1990).
Both young men and young women list condom use as among the most
problematic issues in their sexual relationships (J. Noell et al. 1993). In one
study focusing on adolescents in inner-city schools, 60 percent of the
sample believed that "sex partners often disagree about whether or not to
use condoms" (David Siegel et al. 1991, 162). Men have been found to
evaluate the negative aspects of using contraceptives, in general, and for
using condoms, specifically, as higher than the positive aspects of their use
(Diane Grimley et al. 1993). Men also report more negative than positive
aspects of the practice of safer sex (HIV-avoidant) behaviors in general
(Colleen Redding 1993). Given such attitudes, it may be difficult for
women to feel comfortable asking men to use condoms. However, understanding and changing these attitudes is not a simple task.

Predicting HIV Risk-Related Behavior

In this section we will present our model of HIV risk and discuss the major
predictor variables that demonstrate the importance of interpersonal power
for women's sexual health, offering data from our various studies to support
each predictor in the model. Each predictor is measured with at least three
scales, allowing fairly stable measurement. In all, we have utilized over
thirty-five different measures for a range of independent/predictor and
dependent variables, some of which we have developed or adapted to HIV
risk research.

TABLE I
Predicting HIV Risk from Interpersonal Power

Interpersonal Power-Related Predictors	Risk/Risk-Related Dependent Variables
Sexual experience (common and diverse)	Number of occasions of unprotected vaginal
Substance use/abuse	sex weighted by partner risk
Sexual assertiveness (initiation, refusal, preg-	Number of sex partners
nancy/STD prevention, communication)	Percent of sexual contacts using condoms or
Sexual abuse	barriers
Interpersonal hostility (implicit and explicit)	Perceived HIV risk
Psychosocial attitudes (psychosocial well-be-	
ing, self-efficacy, psychosexual functioning)	
Demographics (race, relationship length, etc.)	

Table 1 outlines the interpersonal power model. In this model, we have identified eight interpersonal areas that predict HIV risky behavior, and three different measures of heterosexual HIV risk.

Gary Burkholder and Lisa Harlow (1995) reviewed the literature for methods of HIV risk assessment, and compared the effectiveness of five major measurement approaches using structural equation techniques. The results showed that weighting the number of occasions of unprotected vaginal intercourse by the partner risk on each occasion appears to be the most effective way to assess risk. Thus this variable is used as a dependent variable in much of our work. Other associated risk measures included in various analyses are frequencies of unprotected oral, vaginal, and anal sex; number of partners; perceived risk; AIDS-preventive behaviors; and percentage of contacts in which condoms were used.

Kathryn Quina et al. (n.d.) held a series of focus groups with two of the low-income groups targeted for the survey research (single mothers in a GED/literacy training program and older adults taking courses at a community-based college of continuing education), with two goals in mind: to learn more about them, and to enable them to help us design the most sensitive and effective research. Groups gave feedback on both the content and the process of filling out our survey, and raised important issues which were incorporated into the project. Psychometric values of our quantitative instruments, including internal reliabilities and factor structures, were not substantially altered or lowered, and in some cases improved, in spite of dramatic changes in wording of some items (Jennifer Rose et al., n.d.). Extensive opportunities for feedback from participants made it clear that for some of them the act of filling out the survey in itself was beneficial, as they had an opportunity to review and think about their sexual behavior and decision making.

Sexual Experience

Women who participate in diverse sexual activities have greater opportunities to be exposed to HIV than do others. On the one hand, as women increase their sexual experience (e.g., as their number of sex partners increases and they feel more comfortable experiencing sexual pleasure), they may take greater responsibility for their own sexual pleasure (Judith Long Laws and Pepper Schwartz 1977). On the other hand, increased sexual activity may signal indiscriminate activity, as occurs when a woman feels unable to refuse unwanted sex. Whether women initiate sexual encounters more readily as a means of defending against sexual force, or become indiscriminate as a result of sexual abuse, are chilling possibilities, but each has some support in the literature (e.g., Quina and Nancy Carlson 1989; Sally Zierler et al. 1991).

It appears from our research that women who are more sexually experienced are also engaging in more HIV-risky sexual behavior. Sexual experience was a predictor of HIV risk in college women (Harlow et al. 1993) and in women at some heterosexual risk living in the community (Harlow et al., n.d.). In this last sample, women in the highest-risk clusters had also had significantly more sexual experience than women in the lower-risk clusters.

Sexual experience also related significantly to some forms of sexual assertiveness in both college and community women. Common sexual experience was related to community women's assertiveness in communicating both information and preferences (Harlow et al. 1994), and to sexual-initiation assertiveness in college women (Grimley 1991). Morokoff et al. (n.d.) found that diverse sexual experience (multiple partners, engaging in practices that cause oneself or one's partner pain, etc.) was related to sexual-initiation assertiveness in community women. Positive experiences with sexual activity could be presumed to be associated with greater comfort with one's sexuality and greater willingness to initiate future sexual encounters and discussions about sexual interests. Among community women, for whom general levels of ("common") sexual experience were greater, higher scores on the diversity scale might indicate the individual had had more experience with more in-depth relationships that involved a wider range of sexual activity. On the other hand, the depth of those relationships may make it less likely that a woman will bother with safe practices, negating the advantages of initiation and communication assertiveness.

Substance Use/Abuse

The role of injection drug use (IDU) in HIV transmission to women is startlingly clear: 48 percent of HIV-positive women were infected through IDU, and another 20 percent are infected by sex with a man who is an injection drug user (CDC 1995). In addition to the risk to non-IDU women from IDU partners, discussed earlier, gender imbalances pervade drug practices. Women are more likely than men to share IDU equipment with their partners and to use the equipment after their partners (Hinden, Bigelow, Vickers-Lauti, Lewis, and McCusker 1992, and Clark, Calsyn, Saxon, Jackson, and Wrede 1992, cited by Kenneth Castro, Ronald Valiserri, and James Curran 1992; see Morokoff, Harlow, and Quina 1995 for a review).

Substance use can also interfere with a woman's ability to take responsibility for her sexual safety. Substance use may be particularly high in already vulnerable populations such as sexual abuse survivors (reviewed in Kathryn Quina and Nancy Carlson 1989) and battered women (e.g., Lenore Walker 1984).

We found that both college and community women who were engaged in alcohol or illicit drug use were more likely to engage in high-risk sexual behaviors (Harlow et al. 1993; n.d.). Michelle Lang (1994) found that a measure of potential substance abuse was a strong predictor of HIV risk for sexually active adolescent women, but not for men. For young women, alcohol and drug use was less frequent; anecdotal evidence also suggested it was more likely to be associated with social situations such as dates.

Sexual Assertiveness

Women have developed a variety of ways to signal sexual intentions. For example, women who are interested in attracting men are more likely to engage in flirting behaviors, and women who signal more frequently are more likely to be approached by men (Monica Moore and Diana Butler

1989). Timothy Perper and David Weis (1987) found extensive use of "proceptive behaviors" among women, such as smiling, touching, or gazing into a partner's eyes, behaviors which served to indicate women's interest in sex. But these same studies, and others, find a reluctance among women to use direct statements for initiating, refusing, or requiring contraceptive use.

Discussions with women suggested that there was a realm of sexual assertiveness behavior that was perhaps not related to general assertiveness. Unfortunately, there was little to work from in the literature about this construct. We developed a psychometrically sound measure, the Sexual Assertiveness Scale (SAS), which addresses three types of sexual assertiveness: initiation of desired sex, refusal of (noncoerced) unwanted sex, and pregnancy/STD prevention. Each behaves in distinct ways and each has been shown to be an important predictor of HIV-risk-related prevention behaviors (Harlow et al. 1993; n.d.).

With college women, Diane Grimley (1991) looked at predictors of initiation, refusal, and pregnancy/STD prevention sexual assertiveness. Self-reported ability to initiate wanted sexual activity was significantly associated with greater sexual experience, a history of sexual abuse, and higher self-efficacy for AIDS-preventive behaviors. Ability to refuse unwanted sexual activities was related to a lower anticipated partner negative response and a lower level of prior psychological victimization. Ability to assert contraceptive and condom use was associated with higher levels of self-efficacy, less prior psychological victimization, greater physical victimization, and greater sexual experience.

The results of two multivariate structural modeling analyses with a different sample of college women and with a community sample confirmed most of the specific relationships found in this study, and further indicated that the three SAS subscales tapped different aspects of the assertiveness construct (Morokoff et al., n.d.). For the community women, initiation assertiveness was predicted by greater sexual experience and better psychosexual attitudes; and both refusal and pregnancy/STD prevention assertiveness were predicted by greater condom self-efficacy and less anticipated partner negative reaction. Victimization predictors were not significant in these analyses.

Communication Assertiveness. A woman's ability to communicate effectively her desire for safe sex has been positively related to condom use (Joseph Catania et al. 1992). In a study of African American and Latina female clients of methadone clinics, condom use was demonstrated to be related to women's attitudes toward the negotiation of safer sex with a partner, and to their level of comfort with communication skills with that partner (R. F. Schilling et al. 1991).

Pamela Deiter (1994) introduced two new subscales to the Sexual Assertiveness Scale, focusing on requesting information about a partner's sexual history and asserting one's sexual preferences. Lang (1994) found that sexual communication assertiveness was one of the strongest predictors of HIV-risky behavior in adolescent women, but not men, suggesting that responses on this variable are strongly gender-based.

Harlow et al. (1994) examined ten sets of theoretically important predictors to these two sexual communication assertiveness measures, in three samples of community-based women at risk for HIV. Predictors of both types of communication assertiveness included high HIV prevention skills and refusal assertiveness. Information requesting was also predicted by low anticipated partner negative reaction, low condom use, low prior coerced adult sex, perception of low peer risk norms, and by more positive sexual attitudes, high sexual experience, more education, and high self-efficacy for condom use. Communicating preferences was also predicted by very high initiation sexual assertiveness and childhood sexual abuse.

Sexual Victimization

Being coerced or physically forced to engage in unwanted sexual activities may impact on an individual's relationships with future sex partners. It has been argued that some survivors attempt to maintain control in sexual situations, even engaging in undesired sex if necessary in order to avoid potential anger from, or loss of control to, a partner (e.g., Quina and Carlson 1989). In addition, for some women, sex becomes meaningless and is just another way of surviving. For example, Zierler et al. (1991) found that women at relative high HIV risk in the community who had experienced childhood sexual abuse had sex more frequently with casual sex partners, and were two times more likely to have multiple sex partners on an average yearly basis, when compared to individuals who reported no history of sexual abuse. Disproportionately high levels of childhood abuse was also observed among prostitutes, who were disproportionately likely to be HIV-seropositive.

The links from childhood victimization to adult risk may not be as direct for most individuals, however. Although community women in our highest risk clusters reported the highest levels of adult sexual victimization (Harlow et al. n.d.), Laura Johnsen (1995) found that in the same population, child sexual abuse did not directly predict HIV risk. However, child sexual abuse was significantly associated with mediating constructs of adult sexual victimization, psychosexual attitudes, sexual assertiveness, and adult relationship violence, each of which was significantly associated with HIV risk. Family of origin was also an associated predictor of HIV risk. In a similar vein, while sexual victimization did not directly predict any of the sexual assertiveness measures for community women, there were strong correlations between the SAS subscales and various predictor constructs which were associated with HIV risk (notably, anticipated negative partner reaction and psychosexual functioning) (Morokoff et al. n.d.).

Johnsen and Harlow (1996) also gave an idea of how this might work. They compared forty-two college women who reported a history of child sexual abuse to fifty-one women who did not report abuse. The survivor sample had more negative attitudes about sexuality, lower sexual assertiveness for pregnancy/STD prevention, less self-efficacy for HIV prevention, more anticipated negative partner reaction, and were more likely to have been sexually abused as a young adult. This is in line with findings by Deiter (1994), who found that among college women, prior victimization was negatively correlated with sexual assertiveness and self-efficacy. In a related study, community women who reported childhood sexual victimization were 1.2 times more likely to have experienced adult relationship violence, and five times more likely to report sexual victimization in adulthood, than women who did not report a history of childhood sexual abuse (Johnsen et al. 1995). Thus it may be that sexual victimization diminishes some women's ability to resist unwanted sex effectively, leading to further abuse (Diana Russell 1984).

Interpersonal Hostility

Research on violence against women indicates that "women's greatest risk of assault is from their intimates, particularly male partners" (Mary Koss et al. 1994, 41). In couples where physical violence has occurred, the balance of power and decision-making may be particularly inequitable. Murray Straus (1991, 26) has demonstrated that the amount of violence within a relationship is associated with the level of power dominance by the violent partner, with the least violence in egalitarian couples. Irene Frieze and Maureen McHugh (1992) found that using violence was one of the best predictors of a husband's decision-making power in marriages.

We found that physical violence from a partner was, indeed, associated with HIV risk, as measured by unprotected sex weighted by number of partners, for community women (Johnsen et al. 1995). In a canonical analysis, 12 percent of the variance was accounted for in one significant correlation with a victimization variate on which partner's physical violence loaded significantly. It appears that various forms of violence are interrelated for women: Ninety-five percent of the 139 women who reported higher levels of adult sexual victimization (calculated by average physical sexual victimization score) also reported some relationship violence, as compared to 51 percent of the 55 never-victimized women.

Anticipated Partner Response. It is reasonable to assume that violence does not have to be explicit in order to affect power in a relationship. Loretta and John Jemmott (1992) found that for their sample of African American women, responses of sexual partners were the most important normative influence against using condoms. Denise Stuntzner-Gibson (1991) reported that women often feel pressured to acquiesce to their partners' demands for unsafe sex, fearing angry or violent responses, rejection, or abandonment. She suggests that battered women may be at especially high risk of exposure to HIV because of their poor self-esteem and because of their inability to negotiate with their partners. Rudy Aguilar and Narina Nightengale (1994) found that women subjected to emotionally controlling abuse (e.g., being forbidden to work or see people outside the home) experienced significantly more feelings of powerlessness and hopelessness than nonbattered women or women subjected to other types of abuse.

In our college women, negative anticipated partner responses to requests to use contraceptives and condoms were a deterrent to assertion of safer sexual practices (Harlow et al. 1993). Among community women, Johnsen et al. (1995) found that implicit violence (exposure, touch without penetration, threat of abuse, coercive sexual experiences) and explicit violence (assault with sexual contact, physical abuse) were highly correlated with each other, and these victimization subscales together formed one canonical variate which was significantly correlated with the HIV risk variate. Anticipated partner response was also a significant predictor of pregnancy/STD prevention sexual assertiveness (Morokoff et al. n.d.), and of all forms of sexual assertiveness (Harlow et al. 1994).

Psychoattitudinal Variables

Psychosocial Well Being. Measures of meaning and purpose in life (or the lack thereof) have been found to be related negatively to drug use and suicidal behavior (e.g., Harlow, Michael Newcomb, and Peter Bentler 1986), and physical and psychological well-being (e.g., Gary Reker, Edward Peacock, and Paul Wong 1987). Harlow and Newcomb (1990) explored the factors associated with an individual's purpose and meaning in life among a community sample of 739 young adults. They found these constructs were highly interrelated with peer, family, and intimate relationships; perceived opportunity; and work and health satisfaction. They were negatively related to powerlessness. Interestingly, the strongest contributor to understanding the process and content of a meaningful and satisfying life was relationship satisfaction.

We found purpose and meaning in life were significant predictors of HIV-risky behaviors among college students, but perhaps not in the most obvious direction (Harlow et al. 1993). Overly optimistic attitudes about one's well-being were associated with greater risk behavior. We have suggested that this is due to a belief that one is not likely to acquire HIV, and this relationship might not hold among older, community-based women. Nevertheless, it is important to consider this possibility. Deiter's (1994) college women reported less self-confidence after intervention group meetings, suggesting that they were becoming more realistic about the difficulties in maintaining an assertive, rights-focused stance.

Self-efficacy. Among the various studies on both sexual intimacy and HIV prevention, self-efficacy often emerges as a significant psychosocial/attitudinal predictor. Albert Bandura (1989) has defined self-efficacy as the conviction that one can successfully execute the behavior required to produce a desired outcome. Social learning theory suggests that the more confident a woman feels regarding the discussion and use of contraceptives to prevent unintended pregnancies and condoms to prevent diseases, the more likely she will be to insist upon their use. A number of studies have shown that higher self-efficacy for birth control and condom use are associated with stronger intentions to engage consistently in their use (e.g., Judith Goldman and Harlow 1993; Jemmott and Jemmott 1992; Susan Kegeles, Nancy Adler, and Charles Irwin 1988). Our research has shown that self-efficacy for behaviors related to condom use and protection from HIV infection are significantly associated with less unprotected sex and choosing partners who have less sexual risk (Harlow et al. 1993).

Furthermore, self-efficacy is positively associated with initiation and pregnancy/STD prevention assertiveness (Grimley 1991). This relationship is understandable given the conceptual definition of self-efficacy as one's perceived ability to act on one's wishes. Among community women, self-efficacy was a very strong predictor of pregnancy/STD prevention assert-iveness, and in addition, self-efficacy was a significant predictor of self-reported refusal assertiveness (Morokoff et al., n.d.).

Psychosexual Functioning. Since Harlow et al. (1993) had observed higher risky sexual activity among women who were also higher in levels of initiation assertiveness, it was important to determine whether this was due to positive feelings about one's own sexuality or to more negative factors such as indiscriminate behavior. Thus a measure of psychosexual function-ing was added as a predictor construct. Initial analyses indicate that positive psychosexual attitudes are associated with less HIV risk. Perhaps women need to become specifically focused on their sexual attitudes before they begin to protect themselves.

Demographics: Ethnicity

Several researchers (e.g., Vickie Mays and James Jackson 1991; Gail Wyatt 1991) have expressed the need for HIV research to be culturally appropriate and sensitive. We felt particularly strongly about this issue, since the vast majority of women at risk locally as well as nationally are women of color. We made special efforts to recruit women of color, working with community agencies and leaders to ensure that we were carrying out an effective recruitment effort. The focus groups described above included groups of African-American women, whose feedback was valuable. After data collection, we compared subsamples of minority and nonminority women in two studies to ascertain whether there were any important statistical differences. In two separate cluster analyses, one of HIV risk (Harlow et al. n.d.) and one of communication assertiveness (Harlow et al.

1994), we found that the general patterns of predictors were comparable in the two groups of women, although women of color were significantly higher in levels of HIV risk-related behaviors and attitudes.

Implications of Interpersonal Power Theory

Feminist researchers have long pointed out that in order to understand women's lives, we must understand their experiences in a world of complex gender, cultural, and situational factors (e.g., Susan Brownmiller 1975; see also Bernice Lott and Diane Maluso 1995). More than a decade after the first alarms were sounded about women's heterosexual risk for AIDS, researchers are finally recognizing that this same complex of factors must be considered if we are to stem the pandemic in its new forms (Amaro 1995). To further these goals, researchers and practitioners should begin to explore new models and new variables such as the ones offered here. There is a wealth of feminist scholarship from which we can draw on women and power in relationships and relational behaviors, and much more to be pursued.

In this chapter we have provided a glimpse into the ways our research team has attempted to address interpersonal power-related HIV risk in a systematic, multifaceted way. Our model, now being tested with our community samples, has been shaped by our consistent findings that it is the interpersonal power behind a woman's decision that really counts. Whether that power is decreased temporarily by "voluntary" consumption of alcohol or drugs, or whether it has been excised from her repertoire by violent experiences, interpersonal power appears to influence women's options for safe and responsible sexuality.

Our next steps are already underway. We are exploring applications of these findings to interventions, taking both an interpersonal power-building approach with women and an integrated approach with men and women in relationships. We are examining in greater depth the other roles of victimization in women's lives and the complex relationship among forms of abuse. We are hopeful that our work will ultimately inform effective interventions to reduce HIV risk for women.

The variables that we find are important to HIV prevention may perhaps be applied in other realms to increase women's sexual safety. For example, if a woman wants to conform to her perceptions of the prevailing social norms, such as not wanting to appear promiscuous, she may initiate a "scripted refusal," even if she wants to have sex (Muehlenhard and McCoy 1991). In a scripted refusal, a woman's role is to refuse a man's sexual advances, and the man's role is to persist until the woman complies. Unfortunately, mixed messages such as these may have detrimental consequences. If a woman's real sexual refusal is not taken seriously by a man, and he persists according to what he mistakenly perceives to be a scripted refusal or an intentional sexual signal, unwanted sexual intercourse may occur. These applications are being evaluated in our ongoing work on sexual assertiveness and women's sexuality.

NOTES

1. Over the past seven years our research team, the University of Rhode Island Women's Health Research Project, has examined various aspects of HIV-risky heterosexual behavior in women, focusing on predictors of HIV risk with the long-term goal of developing effective interventions. For this research program, we have developed several scales, including the Sexual Assertiveness Scale, which has been developed and psychometrically assessed with over 1,600 women (Morokoff et al. n.d.). Lang (1994; n.d.) has surveyed over 200 adolescent women in four samples. Several studies have examined college women: Harlow et al. (1993) examined predictors of HIV-risky behavior among 497 women in relationships. Related studies have predicted sexual assertiveness (Grimley 1991; n = 234) and explored the role of childhood and adult sexual abuse (Johnsen and Harlow 1996, n = 591). Patricia Gallagher (1992) and Deiter (1994) conducted interventions to increase college women's safer sexual practices (n = 60) and their communication assertiveness for safer sex (n = 90), respectively. Eight hundred women living in the community, each meeting at least one heterosexual HIV risk criterion, have now been assessed at least one time point in a longitudinal three-wave study. From these data, Harlow et al. (n.d.) utilized cluster analysis to distinguish groups of women at differing levels of heterosexual risk; Johnsen (1995) utilized structural modeling to explored the role of child sexual abuse and family violence history on adult HIV risk; Johnsen et al. (1995) looked at connections between various forms of adult victimization and HIV risk; Harlow et al. (1994) examined communication assertiveness in greater depth in subsamples of this group; and Morokoff et al. (n.d.) analyzed predictors of sexual assertiveness.

Reprints of this work are available from the first author at the Department of Psychology, University of Rhode Island, Kingston, RI 02881, Internet KQUINA@uri-acc.uri.edu.

This research has been supported by Grant MH47233 from NIMH to Lisa L. Harlow, Principal Investigator, and by a grant from the URI Foundation to Kathryn Quina and Patricia J. Morokoff.

REFERENCES

Aguilar, Rudy J., and Narina N. Nightengale. The impact of specific battering experiences on the self-esteem of abused women. *Journal of Family Violence* 9 (1994): 35–45.

Amaro, Hortensia. Love, sex, power: Considering women's realities in HIV prevention. *American Psychologist* 50 (1995): 437–47.

Bandura, Albert J. Perceived self-efficacy in the exercise of control over AIDS infection. In Vickie M. Mays, George W. Albee, and S.F. Schneider (Eds.), *Primary prevention of AIDS: Psychological approaches*. London: Sage, 1989. 128–41.

Brownmiller, Susan. *Against our will: Men, women and rape*. New York: Simon and Schuster, 1975.

Burkholder, Gary J., and Lisa L. Harlow. "Using structural modeling techniques to develop appropriate HIV risk models." American Psychological Association meetings, New York, August 1995.

Castro, Kenneth G., Ronald O. Valdiserri, and James W. Curran. Commentary: Perspectives on HIV/AIDS epidemiology and prevention from the Eighth International Conference on AIDS. *American Journal of Public Health* 82 (1992): 1465–70.

Catania, Joseph A., Thomas J. Coates, Susan Kegeles, and Mindy T. Fullilove. Condom use in multi-ethnic neighborhoods of San Francisco: The population-based AMEN (AIDS in Multi-Ethnic Neighborhoods) study. *American Journal of Public Health* 82 (1992): 284–87.

Centers for Disease Control. Update: AIDS Among Women—United States, 1994. *Morbidity and Mortality Weekly Report* 44.5 (1995): 81–85.

Chu, Susan Y., Thomas A. Peterman, Lynda S. Doll, James W. Buehler, and James W. Curran. AIDS in bisexual men in the United States: Epidemiology and transmission to women. *American Journal of Public Health* 82 (1992): 220–24.

Cochran, Susan D., and Vickie M. Mays. Sex, lies, and HIV. *The New England Journal of Medicine* 322 (March 15, 1990): 774.

Deiter, Pamela J. "Sexual assertiveness training for college women: An intervention study." Unpublished doctoral dissertation, University of Rhode Island, 1994.

Frieze, Irene H., and Maureen M. McHugh. Power and influence strategies in violent and nonviolent marriages. *Psychology of Women Quarterly* 16 (1992): 449–65.

Gallagher, Patricia J. "AIDS risk reduction training among college women." Unpublished doctoral dissertation, University of Rhode Island, 1992.

Goldman, Judith A., and Lisa L. Harlow. Self-perception variables that mediate AIDS-preventive behavior in college students. *Health Psychology* 12 (1993): 489–98.

Grimley, Diane M. "Predicting sexual assertiveness in college age women: A model building approach." Unpublished master's thesis, University of Rhode Island, 1991.

Grimley, Diane M., Gabrielle E. Riley, Jeffrey M. Bellis, and James O. Prochaska. Assessing the stages of change and decision-making for contraceptive use for the prevention of pregnancy, STDs and AIDS. *Health Education Quarterly* 20 (1993): 455–70.

Harlow, Lisa L., and Michael D. Newcomb. Towards a general hierarchical model of meaning and satisfaction in life. *Multivariate Behavioral Research* 25 (1990): 387–405.

Harlow, Lisa L., Michael D. Newcomb, and Peter M. Bentler. Depression, self-derogation, substance use, and suicide ideation: Lack of purpose in life as a mediational factor. *Journal of Clinical Psychology* 42 (1986): 5–21.

Harlow, Lisa L., Patricia J. Morokoff, Kathryn Quina, and Pamela J. Deiter. "Communication sexual assertiveness and AIDS-related communication in women." American Psychological Association meetings, Los Angeles, Calif., 1994.

Harlow, Lisa L., Kathryn Quina, Patricia J. Morokoff, Jennifer S. Rose, and Diane M. Grimley. HIV risk in women: A multifaceted model. *Journal of Applied Biobehavioral Research* 1 (1993): 3–38.

Harlow, Lisa L., Jennifer S. Rose, Patricia J. Morokoff, and Kathryn Quina. Clusters of HIV risk takers: Related behaviors and attitudes. Manuscript under review.

Holland, Janet, Caroline Ramazanoglu, Sue Scott, Sue Sharpe, and Rachel Thomson. Sex, gender, and power: Young women's sexuality in the shadow of AIDS. *Sociology of Health and Illness* 12 (1990): 336–50.

Jemmott, Loretta Sweet, and John B. Jemmott III. Applying the theory of reasoned action to AIDS risk behavior: Condom use among Black women. *Nursing Research* 40 (1992): 228–38.

Johnsen, Laura W. The relationship between sexual victimization and HIV risk behavior and attitudes in a community sample of women. Unpublished doctoral dissertation, University of Rhode Island, 1995.

Johnsen, Laura W., and Lisa L. Harlow. Adult problems in living associated with childhood sexual abuse. *AIDS Education and Prevention* (1996).

Johnsen, Laura W., Kathryn Quina, Lisa L. Harlow, and Patricia J. Morokoff. "Role of victimizations in women's heterosexual HIV risk." American Psychological Association meetings, New York, August 1995.

Kegeles, Susan M., Nancy E. Adler, and Charles E. Irwin. Sexually active adolescents and condoms: Changes in one year in knowledge, attitudes and use. *American Journal of Public Health* 78 (1988): 460–61.

Koss, Mary P., Lisa A. Goodman, Angela Browne, Louise F. Fitzgerald, Gwendolyn Puryear Keita, and Nancy Felipe Russo. *No safe haven: Male violence against women at home, at work, and in the community.* Washington D.C.: American Psychological Association, 1994.

Lang, Michelle A. "An assessment of adolescent HIV-risk predictors." Dissertation-in-progress, University of Rhode Island.

———. "Cognitive, attitudinal and behavioral risk predictors for AIDS among heterosexual adolescents." Unpublished master's thesis, University of Rhode Island, 1994.

Laws, Judith Long, and Pepper Schwartz. *Sexual scripts: The social construction of female sexuality.* Hinsdale, Ill.: Dryden Press, 1977.

Lewin, Miriam. Unwanted intercourse: The difficulty of saying no. *Psychology of Women Quarterly* 9 (1985): 184–92.

Lott, Bernice, and Diane Maluso, Eds. *The social psychology of interpersonal attraction.* New York: Guilford, 1995.

Mays, Vickie M., and James Jackson. AIDS survey methodology with Black Americans. *Social Science Medicine* 33.1 (1991): 47–54.

McCormick, Naomi. *Sexual salvation: Affirming women's sexual rights and pleasures.* Westport, Conn.: Praeger, 1994.

Moore, Monica M., and Diana L. Butler. Predictive aspects of nonverbal courtship behavior in women. *Semiotica* 76 (1989): 205–15.

Morokoff, Patricia J., Lisa L. Harlow, and Kathryn Quina. Women and AIDS. In Annette L. Stanton and Sheryle J. Gallant (Eds.), *Psychology of women's health: Progress and challenges in research and application.* Washington D.C.: American Psychological Association, 1995. 117–69.

Morokoff, Patricia J., Kathryn Quina, Lisa L. Harlow, Pamela R. Gibson, Laura W. Johnsen, Diane M. Grimley, and Gary J. Burkholder. "Development of the Sexual Assertiveness Scale for women." Manuscript under review.

Muehlenhard, Charlene L., and Marsha L. McCoy. Double standard/double bind: The sexual double standard and women's communication about sex. *Psychology of Women Quarterly* 15 (1991): 447–61.

Noell, J., A. Biglan, J. Berendt, and L. Ochs. Problematic sexual situations for adolescents: Alcohol and unsafe sex. *Health Values: The Journal of Health Behavior, Education & Promotion* 17 (1993): 40–49.

Paxson, MaryAnn A., and Kathryn Quina. "Sexually active vs inactive women's attitudes and knowledge concerning contraceptive use." American Psychological Association meetings, New Orleans, 1989.

Peplau, Letitia, Zick Rubin, and Charles T. Hill. Sexual intimacy in dating relationships. *Journal of Social Issues* 33 (1977): 86–109.

Perper, Timothy, and David L. Weis. Proceptive and rejective strategies of US and Canadian college women. *Journal of Sex Research* 23 (1987): 455–80.

Quina, Kathryn, and Nancy L. Carlson. *Rape, incest, and sexual harassment: A guide for helping survivors.* Westport, Conn.: Praeger, 1989.

Quina, Kathryn, Lisa L. Harlow, Patricia J. Morokoff, Pamela J. Deiter, Michelle A. Lang, Jennifer S. Rose, Laura W. Johnsen, and Robbie Schnoll. "Women and HIV: Focus group model for increasing research effectiveness." Manuscript under review.

Redding, Colleen A. "The transtheoretical model applied to safer sex behavior among university students: A cross-sectional investigation." Unpublished doctoral dissertation, University of Rhode Island, 1993.

Reker, Gary T., Edward J. Peacock and T. Paul Wong. Meaning and purpose in life and well-being: A life-span perspective. *Journal of Gerontology* 42 (1987): 44–49.

Rose, Jennifer S., Lisa L. Harlow, Patricia J. Morokoff, Kathryn Quina, Michelle A. Lang, Laura W. Johnsen, and Pamela J. Deiter. "Survey revision: Improving readability and maintaining psychometrics." Manuscript under review.

Russell, Diana E. H. *Sexual exploitation.* Beverly Hills, Calif.: Sage, 1984.

Schilling, R. F., N. El-Bassel, L. Gilbert, and S. P. Schinke (1991). Correlates of drug use, sexual behavior, and attitude toward safer sex among African American and Hispanic women in methadone maintenance. *Journal of Drug Abuse* 21 (1991): 685–98.

Siegel, David, Nancy Lazarus, Flora Krasnovsky, Meg Durbin, and Margaret Chesney. AIDS knowledge, attitudes and behavior among inner city junior high school students. *Journal of School Health* 61 (1991): 160–64.

Straus, Murray A. Physical violence in American families: Incidence, rates, causes and trends. In Dean D. Knudson and JoAnn L. Miller (Eds.), *Abused and Battered: Social and legal responses to family violence.* New York: Aldine de Gruyter, 1991. 17–34.

Stuntzner-Gibson, Denise. Women and HIV disease: An emerging social crisis. *Social Work* 36 (1991): 22–27.

Walker, Lenore E. A. *The Battered Women's Syndrome.* New York: Springer, 1984.

Wyatt, Gail E. Examining ethnicity versus race in AIDS related research. *Social Science Medicine* 33 (1991): 37–45.

Zierler, Sally, L. Fiengold, Deborah Laufer, P. Velentgas, I. Kantrowitz-Gordon and Kenneth Mayer. Adult survivors of childhood sexual abuse and subsequent risk of HIV infection. *American Journal of Public Health* 81 (1991): 572–75.

11

Hitting Hard: HIV and Violence

Sally Zierler

Sally Zierler, DrPH, is an epidemiologist and professor in the Department of Community Health at Brown University School of Medicine. She has been an activist in the women's health movement since 1974. Her research focuses on social justice and its biologic expression.

Introduction

Two epidemics primarily affecting women 15–44 years of age are HIV infection and sexual partner violence. This chapter presents evidence for their concurrence in women's lives. In part, this is because social circumstances that lead to HIV exposure also put women at risk for violence. First, HIV is linked to injection drug use, a setting that carries its own risk for violence in sexual relationships, whether in a context of sex-for-drug-exchange, or of intimacy.[1–4] Second, HIV is most prevalent among women during their years of reproductive expression. Childbearing or childrearing is a frequent setting for women to learn of their own HIV infection, and pregnancy is also a time that spouses or boyfriends of women may be more violently reactive, such that a context of pregnancy may increase risk both for awareness of infection, as well as for partner violence.[5,6] And third, most women with HIV are living in poverty, a milieu associated with increased risk of partner violence. Yet economic dependence on sexual partners makes it hard for women to walk away from a violent relationship.[7–11] This may be particularly so after an HIV diagnosis.

An equally important fact is that HIV itself may provoke violence against women regardless of whether or not they have experienced violence in a given setting previously. In one scenario, violence may occur in a relationship context where women have already experienced partner violence and the fact of infection serves to escalate this violence. Or, the fact of HIV may precipitate violence or abandonment in settings where these had not occurred. Thus, the emphasis in this chapter is on partner violence against women who are currently infected.

To date, little empirical evidence exists to evaluate plausible links between HIV and violence in women's lives. A brief review of data on women with HIV and on women harmed by partner violence, however, makes presumptive connections between these two epidemics compelling.

Women and HIV

As of November 1995, the CDC reported that 72,828 girls and women had an AIDS diagnosis.[12] Their infections were linked overwhelmingly to injection drug use: the CDC attributes nearly half of infection to direct participation in drug injection, and another 20 percent to sexual encounters with men participating in drug injection.[13] Five years ago, among women 25–44, AIDS had become the sixth leading cause of death, and within two years it moved to number four. Nationally, for African-American women in this age range, AIDS tops all causes, and for Latinas is the third leading cause of death.[14] A recent study reporting on causes of death among women with HIV infection reported that women were dying at a faster rate than men despite comparability in disease progression. Among the reasons speculated for this finding were "lower socioeconomic status, homelessness, domestic violence, substance abuse, and the lack of social support."[15]

Women and Violence

Hinted at by this conjecture is the fact that young women also die from three other leading causes: accidents, homicides and suicides.[16] A recent survey from the Bureau of Justice Statistics[17] noted that 75 percent of women reporting intentional violence against them (defined as rape, sexual assault, aggravated assault, or simple assault) knew their perpetrator. In 29 percent of cases, the perpetrator was an "intimate partner," defined in this report as a former or current husband or boyfriend. Women most likely to report these incidents were 19–29 years old and living in households with annual incomes of less than $10,000. Compared with married women, women separated from husbands were twenty-five times more likely to report intimate partner violence. Of 3,454 murders of women in 1992 for whom the relationship to the murderer was identified to the Federal Bureau of Investigation, the Uniform Crime Reports noted that 41 percent were by a current or former boyfriend or spouse and 32 percent by an acquaintance or friend.[17] In Boston, during the first decade of the AIDS epidemic, a mortality study among women ages 15–44 showed homicide as the third leading cause of death.[18]

Physical Violence

Not included in the mortality statistics are annual estimates that four million women in the U.S. are severely assaulted by their male partners.[19] This figure, awful as it is, obscures the fact that some women are more at risk than others. For like HIV's distribution, partner violence against women follows social divisions marked by class position and race/ethnicity, creating strata of extreme vulnerability to violence victimization. In part, this vulnerability may manifest itself through sexual activities that are not expressions of shared desire, but strategies for economic survival, particularly among women who are homeless or dependent on men for economic support, whether through sex work or domestic partnerships.[20] For example, a recent Baltimore study of risk of partner violence among women during their most recent childbearing year revealed that women living in the poorest neighborhoods and with high unemployment were found to be most at risk for partner violence.[21] Another recent study reported a sixfold difference between black and white rates of domestic homicide. However, these differences were entirely explained by differences in socioeconomic conditions, measured in this study by the size of a household relative to the number of people occupying each room.[22]

Few surveys have been published on the prevalence of partner violence among community-based primary care patients. A recent report of nearly two thousand primarily middle-class, educated, and English-speaking women, of whom nearly 50 percent were over the age of forty-five and attending primary care internal medicine practices revealed that, overall, 5.5 percent of women had experienced being hit, slapped, kicked, or otherwise physically hurt by a husband, ex-husband, or boyfriend. Over a fifth of the women reported having been physically and/or sexually abused at some time during adulthood, and nearly a third at any time in their lives.[23] However, when analyses were limited to women aged 18 to 35, with annual family incomes less than $10,000, and who were receiving medical assistance or had no health insurance (thus more similar to women with HIV infection in the U.S.), 14–22 percent reported current partner abuse. Two other studies in primary care settings, also examining women generally more affluent than women with HIV infection, detected 12–14 percent of women to be in relationships with men who physically assaulted them.[24,25]

The modifier "partner" in these studies of physical and sexual violence typically was in relation to current or former husbands or boyfriends, referred to in the literature as "intimate partners." But intimate partners of women may be female, as well. Very little is known about lesbian couples, however. Although one study estimated that 37 percent of lesbian couples experienced physical battering in their relationship,[26] it is difficult to know what this means in comparison to heterosexual couples. Dynamics that prompt violence between couples, the nature of violence, and reporting of what is considered to be abusive may not be comparable in lesbian and heterosexual relationships.

Sexual Violence

Partner violence also occurs in relationships that are not necessarily emotionally intimate, such as sexual contacts through sex work. Because women with HIV infection are likely to be economically poor, sex may be sold or traded for material goods (including housing, clothing, or food for family members or for drugs). Commercial sexual contacts, tricks, clients, or johns[27–31] may create hazardous working conditions for women. Studies have reported that prostitute women with the greatest financial need were at greatest risk for violence victimization by their male clients.[27,31] Exchanging sex for drugs is also associated with heightened risk for violent encounters with sexual partners.[1,29,32] In a study of female prostitutes in Glasgow, the authors noted that "a typical female streetworking-prostitute in Glasgow was aged 25, unemployed, an injecting drug user and had commenced prostitution 4 years before. . . . Her main concern was likely to be violence from clients."[29] A particular form of violence commonly suffered by prostitute women is rape.[31–36] A recent Rhode Island study of mostly white, working-class adults found that over half of women reporting that they had sex for economic purposes had been raped in adulthood, twice the risk reported by women not doing sex work.[33]

Rape and other forms of sexual abuse are also not reflected in mortality data. These forms of violence are less frequently perpetrated by strangers than by men known to women, including relatives, husbands, and boy-friends. Based on data from the "Rape in America" survey, as well as an August 1995 report from the Bureau of Justice Statistics, somewhere be-tween a half a million and 700,000 rapes a year are inflicted on women and girl children each year in the U.S.[37] Other studies report even higher estimates: In one, 42 percent of six thousand college women reported forcible sexual contact or attempted rape; in another, 14 percent of women ever married reported rape by their current or former husbands;[38] and in yet another study among women reporting physical assault by their male partners, 33 to 46 percent described marital rape as part of this experi-ence.[39]

Linking Violence with HIV

Gendered dynamics that contribute to the incidence of violence against women also erupt more insidiously in sexual and drug-using practices that selectively expose women to HIV. In a recent study of women's tolerance to domestic abuse by their partners, "the main reasons [women stay in violent relationships] are economic and emotional dependency on their violent partner, guilt, low self-esteem, and the extreme difficulty, if not the impossibility of changing the situation."[40] In a remarkably similar vein, women reported comparable reasons for tolerating male partners not using condoms during sex. In a study of barriers to HIV risk reduction, 2,527 Latina women in the northeastern United States "expressed feelings of powerlessness, low self-esteem, isolation, lack of voice, and inability to affect risk reduction decisions or behaviors with their partners."[41] In a study of African-American women in Los Angeles, women who depended on their male partners for financial assistance for housing were more likely to have sex without condoms than women who did not depend on men for economic reasons.[42]

Thus, mortality data alone do not tell the story of how partner violence and HIV infection connect, for most women who experience partner violence are not killed, and most women diagnosed with HIV infection remain alive for many years. Living with HIV infection, women face considerable challenges that compound and exacerbate conditions of social and economic deprivation that typically informed their lives before their diagnosis. Even so, an event that may trigger violence is the fact of infection itself.

How can this be? First, as noted above, those women most likely to become infected are also those who are more likely to be with sexual partners who threaten or actually use violence to control them. Underscoring links between HIV and violence in women's lives, at a recent conference on women and HIV infection, reports of women in drug treatment programs and women sexual partners of IDUs in San Juan, Juarez, Boston, Los Angeles, and San Diego showed high rates of physical and sexual assault: 42 percent of women in drug treatment reported that their sexual partners physically hurt them; 45 percent reported that their partners threatened them with violence; 21 percent said they had sex with a partner because they were afraid they might be hurt if they refused.[43] In a Centers for Disease Control study of 1,104 women surveyed from three urban communities (New York, San Francisco, and Miami) not in drug treatment programs or the criminal justice system, 14 percent reported rape in the last year. Rape survivors were more likely than women not reporting recent rape to: smoke crack (89 vs. 57 percent, odds ratio = 5); be homeless (17 vs. 6 percent, odds ratio = 3.2); engage in sex work (85 vs. 50 percent odds ratio = 5.9).[44] In a New England study of 409 women who provided interviews on lifetime experiences of rape and HIV-related risk exposures, women with HIV infection tended to report a higher frequency of rape in their adult lives relative to women without HIV (35 vs. 22 percent; odds ratio = 1.9, 90 percent confidence interval = 1.0–3.6). Fifty-five percent of women reporting sex for drugs or income also reported rape as adults, compared with 23 percent of women not involved with sex work (odds ratio = 4.2, 90 percent confidence interval = 2.4–7.2), and this relation between rape and sex work was observed among women with HIV infection (odds ratio = 3.7) as well as without HIV (odds ratio = 4.4).[33]

Second, state-level policies of partner notification place women at the mercy of disclosure obligations that may do more harm than good.[45] Some ethicists have argued[46] that it is harmful for women to disclose their status to sexual partners who may be abusive as a result—that the harm women face (due to risk of violence) is greater than the harm their sexual partners face (due to risk of sexual transmission of HIV by women partners).[47,48] Historically, the phrase "partner notification" has referred to formal or informal strategies for bringing awareness to sexual partners of possible exposure to a sexually transmitted disease. A question raised in a recent health law and ethics article on partner notification (as a public health strategy to prevent HIV transmission) posed: "But can such efforts be effective when the HIV-infected patient is a woman who fears domestic violence and the partner to be notified is the man she fears?"[45]

Studies Linking Violence and HIV

What has been documented that directly links having HIV infection with increased vulnerability to violence in sexual relationships? To date, only one study and one abstract have appeared that directly address this question.[49,50] Although neither of these accounts quantified the occurrence of experiences of violence, threats of violence, or economic abandonment in women's lives, they document, either through women's health care providers, or through ethnographic studies of the women themselves, that this link is real and strong. The only extant published study was based on a mailed survey to Maryland health providers of women with HIV.[49] Of the 136 providers surveyed, 45 percent reported having at least one woman patient who stated that she was afraid that her partner would physically hurt her if he knew she was infected. Additionally, 56 percent of these providers said they had been told by women that they feared emotional abuse (defined as threat of violence or intimidation) and 66 percent reported fears of abandonment. Providers who reported these experiences estimated that 18 percent, 29 percent, and 35 percent of women in their practice feared, respectively, physical abuse, emotional abuse and abandonment. To quote from the article, providers reported that: "patients were hit, kicked, beaten, punched, or raped by partners; one woman was shot, one jumped from a third-floor window to escape being shot, and one received a knife wound to the face. 'One male became angry, throwing things in the hospital room and had to be removed by security.' . . . [P]atients were yelled at, harassed, intimidated, spit on, and called names such as 'sluts, no good, and bitches.' Both women and their children were threatened, 'If I am infected, I will kill you.' One woman had 'AIDS bitch' written on her door. . . ."

Violence in relation to disclosure of HIV infection was also a basis for fifty in-depth interviews about disclosure, reported in an abstract and presentation at an AIDS conference in 1995.[50] Although most women had discussed their infection immediately, about 25 percent delayed disclosure for periods ranging from a few days to three months. All but one woman disclosed her status to another person. Even so, nearly two-thirds reported being afraid to tell anyone because of rejection, discrimination, or violence. Violence was less frequent than the women feared, but 6 percent experienced violent responses by their partners.

Abandonment

Related to experiences of violence and threats of violence are threats of and actual abandonment. Although abandonment is not defined here as an act of violence, the effects of being deserted by partners on whom women with HIV were financially dependent may have serious consequences, including homelessness and potentially harmful strategies for economic survival. To quote providers' accounts, again, from Rothenberg's study, "women found their partners withdrawing physical, emotional, and financial support; two were left homeless; many lost their children, family and friends. 'One women came home to find the garbagemen loading what was left of her possessions into the back of a truck.' 'Most partners left within 72 hours and all left by three to four months.' "[49]

Other accounts of partner abandonment were described by a provider from a community health center in Massachusetts. She recited how women have expressed fears to her that no one else but their abusive partner will want them now that they have HIV; and a violent relationship is better than no relationship. Another woman told her that sex had become emotionally and physically painful since her disclosure to her partner—that there was such an absence of affection and abruptness that it felt like rape: "he would put on 16 condoms if he could—he comes into me and then is gone." And yet another twist on HIV as a stimulus for partner violence was revealed when the husband of an infected woman, while she was in the hospital for treatment of an opportunistic infection, was sexual with another woman. He became physically violent with this woman, prompting his arrest. When his wife was released from the hospital, he asked her to testify on his behalf. To add to the tragedy of this story, when the wife learned that her husband had been sexual with this woman he had battered, she confronted the woman about it. The woman said, "What difference does it make? You're going to die anyway."[51]

Recommendations for Research

The intersection of violence and HIV in women's lives requires careful study for several reasons. The first relates to policies of partner notification. In the case of HIV infection, some states have mandatory, and therefore involuntary notification procedures. Infected individuals who refuse to inform partners of possible exposure may be criminally liable. Almost all states have legislated that physicians are legally protected to disclose a known patient's infectious status to individuals with whom that patient may have transmitted the virus. Such notification may be done without the knowledge or consent of the patient.[45] The possibility that notification is a trigger for violence prompts reconsideration of these policies.

In addition to affecting policy on partner notification, empirical data on partner violence in the lives of women with HIV would potentially raise a number of concerns for programs and providers addressing women's personal and clinical experiences, and also for the women themselves. Given likely connections between HIV and violence in women's lives, it is important to document the need for screening for risk of violence victimization when women are tested for HIV, as well as when they are seeking HIV-related health care. Also, shelter programs and other resources that support battered women may be unaware that HIV infection may increase risk for partner violence, and thus may not have resources that address specific needs of women with HIV.

Additionally, women with HIV infection need social and economic support. Decisions to disclose the fact of infection to partners may be predicated on concerns about economic abandonment, sexual or physical violence, or informing others who might abuse the knowledge (such as getting fired from a job, or being socially shunned). A cost of disclosing is increasing isolation at a time when stability and support may be particularly needed. Furthermore, since one pattern of partner violence is to limit women's mobility,[38] disclosure of HIV may result in limiting women's access to health care services at a time when they are in particular need of care. Considering sexual partner violence in the lives of women with HIV infection also raises questions to which there currently are no answers. For example, does living within relationships that are emotionally and physically stressful burden immune functioning, affecting disease progression and susceptibility to HIV-related illnesses? Partner violence is associated with depression and suicidal ideation.[23] How do these comorbidities affect HIV disease progression in a context of relationship violence? Additionally, how does having a life-threatening illness affect women's relationship to violence? Does diagnosis with HIV alter women's perspective of what it means to be safe? More specifically, are women less or more likely to tolerate emotional and physical abuse in the context of having HIV infection?

Recommendations for Local Action

Clearly, there is much that medicine, public health, and social policy have yet to address in describing, and then attending to, the particular relationship dangers facing women who are living with HIV infection. Despite these shortcomings, there are grassroots strategies toward reduction of harm that may guide women to safety. One example comes from a volunteer for the Rhode Island Needle Exchange Program, who began including information on shelter programs and domestic violence hotline numbers with needle, syringe, and condom distribution. Immediately, women noticed the information. One said, "Oh yeah, this is how come I'm homeless."[53] Another form of action is to contact community-based organizations that work toward prevention of violence against women to suggest cross-training with HIV testing and counseling staff. Screening women for risk of violence in a context of HIV testing, or HIV-related care, implies a need for linkages between agencies that serve women with HIV and those that serve women living in battering and abusive relationships. Two models for intervention that have connected HIV and violence in women's lives are PROTOTYPES, in Los Angeles, California[43] and Casa Myrna Vazquez in Boston, Massachusetts.[52] These programs link AIDS and domestic violence staff to service women's needs in a context that reflects more realistically the profound challenges women are facing. A physician and a lawyer, Barbara Herbert and Lois Kanter, have described their linkage of medical and legal services in an emergency department of a large urban hospital where they treat one to three women every night as a result of acute injury by sexual partners.[54] Their program brings in law students and practicing lawyers to assist women in getting temporary restraining orders without women having to leave the hospital to get to a police station or courthouse. From anonymous interviews of women attending the emergency department, the program notes two major themes: "Many women have found restraining orders helpful in their successful attempts to leave battering relationships, and many women have physically fought back their batterers to preserve their safety or make possible an escape." Whatever action is undertaken, its agenda and expression must be informed by women most affected by these interlocking epidemics of violence and HIV.

But focusing on women alone leaves out all agency. Prevention has limited meaning without recognition and deliberate attention to the causes of violence. At the most proximal level, programs that work with batterers must be a conspicuous part of the response for sustainable and effective prevention of partner violence. In the context of HIV infection among women, the likelihood that their sexual partners are infected, as well, may affect partners' sense of powerlessness and subsequent expression of rage against their women partners. Furthermore, prospects of losing women as active, vibrant participants in their relationships may prompt responses from partners that include violence.

In considering private spaces that hold these links between HIV and partner violence, it is important to note that they are framed by something larger: public structures supporting multiple forms of social control forged by class, gender, and racially assigned positions. Seen in this light, a perversely logical connection emerges between HIV and partner violence, a connection of shared etiology because of institutionally sanctioned abuse of women, use of violence as legitimate expression of control, and gendered forms of economic deprivation. It is not by accident that the distribution of HIV in women inversely mirrors the distribution of political and economic power. And this disparity is likely to increase as a result of current legislative and economic initiatives, such as cuts in social welfare programs, reversal of affirmative action, political redistricting that effectively strips nonwhite communities of electoral control, and loss of jobs when U.S. industries relocate to pay lower wages for greater profits in needier areas. A net result is that women are forced into increasing economic dependence and potentially harmful strategies for survival.

These strangling forces of disenfranchisement are likely to include partners of women as well, given the class and racial/ethnic distribution of women most at risk for HIV and violence. People who are violent against women may have experienced assaults against their own humanity, through racial discrimination, economic impoverishment and the social alienation that accompanies it. Thus, the brutal and logical concurrence of violence and HIV happens within a private and public sphere created and controlled by people in power—principally men— whose institutions control social and economic resources and their distribution, and whose gender authority control women through intimidation and brute force.

Such control and its consequences are not inevitable. Connections of personal violence and public injustice lay bare some links of accountability for these epidemics of violence and HIV. Exposing who and what is accountable for these links is a necessary step to fuel people's vision and action for justice.

ACKNOWLEDGMENT

The author is grateful to Dr. Nancy Krieger for her thoughtful review and comments on multiple versions of this chapter.

REFERENCES

1. M.T. Fullilove, R. Fullilove, and G. Kennedy et al., "Trauma, crack and HIV risk," Paper: Eighth International Conference on AIDS, Amsterdam, Abstract PoD 5477, 1992.

2. E.S. Lake, "An exploration of the violent victim experiences of female offenders," *Violence and Victims* 8 (1993): 41–51.

3. R. Dembo, L. Williams, L. La Voie et al., "A longitudinal study of the relationship among alcohol use, marijuana/hashish use, cocaine use, and emotional/psychological functioning problems in a cohort of high risk youths," *International Journal of Addictions* 25, no. 11 (1990):1341–82.

4. S.K. Schwarcz, G.A. Bolan, M.T. Fullilove, J. McCright, R. Fullilove, R. Kohn, and R.I. Rolfs, "Crack cocaine and the exchange of sex for money or drugs." *Sexually Transmitted Diseases* 19 (1992): 7–13.

5. A.B. Berenson, N.J. Stiglich, G.S. Wilkinson, and G.D. Anderson, "Drug abuse and other risk factors for physical abuse in pregnancy among white non-Hispanic, black, and Hispanic women," *American Journal of Obstetrics and Gynecology* 164 (1991): 1491–99.

6. H. Amaro, L.E. Fried, H. Cabral, and B. Zukerman, "Violence during pregnancy and substance use," *American Journal of Public Health* 80, no. 5 (1990): 575–79.

7. Karim Q. Abdool, Karim S.S. Abdool, K. Soldan, and M. Zondi, "Reducing the risk of HIV infection among South African sex workers: Socioeconomic and gender barriers," *American Journal of Public Health* 85 (1995): 1521–25.

8. E. Reid and M. Baily M, *Young women: Silence, susceptibility and the HIV epidemic* (United Nations Development Program, 1992).

9. H. Amaro, "Love, Sex and Power," *American Psychologist* 50 (1995): 437–47.

10. D. Worth, "Sexual decision making and AIDS: Why condom promotion among vulnerable women is likely to fail," *Studies in Family Planning* 20 (1990): 297–307.

12. Z. Stein, "Editorial: More on women and the prevention of HIV infection," *American Journal of Public Health* 85 (1995): 1485–88.

12. Centers for Disease Control (CDC), "First 500,000 AIDS cases—United States, 1995," *Mortality and Morbidity Weekly Report (MMWR)* 44 (1995): 849–53.

13. CDC, "Update: AIDS among women—United States, 1994," *MMWR* 44 (1995): 81–84.

14. CDC, "US Public Health Service Recommendations for HIV Counseling and Voluntary Testing for Pregnant Women," *MMWR* 44, no. RR-7 (1995): 2.

15. S.L. Melnick, S. Renslow, T.A. Louis et al., "Survival and disease progression according to gender of patients with HIV infection," *Journal of the American Medical Association* 272 (1994): 1915–21.

16. "Cancer Statistics," *CA Cancer Journal for Clinicians* 44 (1994): 7–26.

17. R. Bachman and L.E. Saltzman, "Violence against women: Estimates from the redesigned survey," *Bureau of Justice Statistics* NCJ-154348 (1995): 1–8.

18. M. Katz, M. Holmes, K. Power, and P. Wise, "Mortality rates among 15–44 year old women in Boston," *American Journal of Public Health* 85 (1995): 1135.

19. American Medical Association, Council on Scientific Affairs, "Violence against women: Relevance for medical practitioners," *Journal of the American Medical Association* 267 (1992): 3184–89.

20. V. Mays and S.D. Cochran, "Acquired immunodeficiency syndrome and Black Americans: Special psychosocial issues," *Public Health Report* 102 (1987): 224–31.

21. P. O'Campo, A. Gilen, R. Faden, X. Xue, N. Kass, and M. Wang, "Violence by male partners against women during the childbearing year," *American Journal of Public Health* 85 (1995): 1092.

22. B.S. Centerwall, "Race, socioeconomic status, and domestic homicide," *Journal of the American Medical Association* 273 (1995): 1755–58.

23. J. McCauley, D.E. Kern, K. Kolodner, L. Dill, A.F. Schroeder, H.K. DeChant, J. Ryden, E.B. Bass, and L.R. Derogatis, "The 'battering syndrome': Prevalence and clinical characteristics of domestic violence in primary care internal medicine practices," *Annals of Internal Medicine* 123 (1995): 737–46.

24. N.E. Gin, L. Ruker, S. Frayne, R. Cygan, and F.A. Hubbell, "Prevalence of domestic violence among patients in three ambulatory care internal medicine clinics," *Journal of General Internal Medicine* 6 (1991): 317–22.

25. B.A. Elliott and M.M. Johnson, "Domestic violence in a primary care setting: Patterns and prevalence," *Archives of Family Medicine* 4 (1995): 113–19.

26. R. Schilit, G-Y Lie, and M. Montagne, "Substance use as a correlate of violence in intimate lesbian relationships," *Journal of Homosexuality* 19 (1990): 51–63.

27. I. Vanwesenbeeck, G. van Zessen, R. de Graaf, and C.J. Straver, "Contextual and interactional factors influencing condom use in heterosexual contacts," *Patient Education and Counseling* 24 (1994): 307–22.

28. M.G. Shedlin, "An ethnographic approach to understanding HIV high-risk behaviors: Prostitution and drug abuse," *NIDA Research Monograph* 93 (1990): 134–49.

29. S.T. Green, D.J. Goldberg, P.R. Christie, M. Frischer, A. Thomson, S.V. Carr,

and A. Taylor, "Female streetworkers—prostitutes in Glasgow: a descriptive study of their lifestyle," *AIDS Care* 5 (1993): 321–35.

30. F. Delacoste and P. Alexander, *Sex work: Writings by women in the sex industry.* Pittsburgh: Cleis Press, 1987.

31. S. Hatty, "Violence against prostitute women: Social and legal dilemmas," *Australian Journal of Social Issues* 24 (1989): 235–48.

32. S. Zierler, B. Annes, and K. Mayer, "Women, HIV and sexual violence," Abstract #3274, American Public Health Association Meetings, Washington, D.C., November 1994.

33. S. Zierler, B. Annes, and K. Mayer, "Sexual violence against women living with or at risk for HIV infection," *American Journal of Preventive Medicine* (solicited, in review), 1995.

34. J. Miller and M.D. Schwartz, "Rape myths and violence against street prostitutes," *Deviant Behavior* 16 (1995): 1–23.

35. J. Miller, " 'Your life is on the line every night you're on the streets': Victimization and the resistance among street prostitutes," *Humanity and Society* 17 (1993): 422–46.

36. M.H. Silbert and A.M. Pines, "Pornography and sexual abuse of women," *Sex Roles* 10 (1984): 857–68.

37. M.P. Koss and M. Harvey, *The rape victim: Clinical and community approaches to treatment* (Beverly Hills, Calif: Sage Publications, 1991); *Rape in America* (Arlington, Va.: National Victim Center, 1992).

38. American Medical Association, *Diagnostic and treatment guidelines on domestic violence* (Chicago: American Medical Association, 1992), 4–8.

39. I.H. Frieze and A. Browne, "Violence in marriage," in *Family Violence: Crime and Justice, A review of research,* ed. L. Ohlin and M. Tonry (Chicago: University of Chicago Press, 1989), 163–218.

40. Quebec Commission on Health and Social Services, 1987, cited in State of Health of Women and Children Victims of Domestic Violence. L. Chenard, H. Cadrin, and J. Loiselle, *Direction de la sante publique,* Rimouski, Quebec, 1993, 3.

41. H. Amaro, "AIDS/HIV among Hispanics in the Northeast and Puerto Rico: Report of findings and recommendations," *Migration-World-Magazine* 19 (1991): 23–29.

42. G.E. Wyatt, "Transaction sex and HIV risks: A woman's choice?" Session WA1–1, Women and HIV Infection Conference, Washington, D.C., February 22–24, 1995.

43. V.B. Brown, "HIV infection in women: Models of intervention for violence against women," Abstract TD2–122, Women and HIV Infection Conference, Washington, D.C., February 22–24, 1995.

44. K.L. Irwin, B.R. Edlin, L. Wong, S. Faruque, C. Word et al., and the Multicenter Crack Cocaine and HIV Study Team, CDC, "Urban rape survivors: Characteristics and prevalence of HIV, syphilis and genital herpes." Abstract TE1–104, Women and HIV Infection Conference, Washington, D.C., February 22–24, 1995.

45. K.H. Rothenberg and S.J. Paskey, "The risk of domestic violence and women with HIV infection: Implications for partner notification, public policy, and the law," *American Journal of Public Health* 85 (1995): 1569–76.

46. R.L. North and K.H. Rothenberg, "Partner notification and the threat of domestic violence against women with HIV infection," *New England Journal of Medicine* 329 (1993): 1194–96.

47. European Study Group on Heterosexual Transmission of HIV, "Comparison of female to male and male to female transmission of HIV in 563 stable couples," *British Medical Journal* 304 (1992): 809–13.

48. H.W. Haverkos and R.J. Battjes, "Female-to-male transmission of HIV," *Journal of the American Medical Association* 268 (1992): 1855–57.

49. K.H. Rothenberg, S.J. Paskey, M.M. Reuland, S.I. Zimmerman, and R.L. North, "Domestic violence and partner notification: Implications for treatment and counseling of women with HIV," *Journal of the American Medical Women's Association* 50 (1995): 87–93.

50. A.C. Gielen, P. O'Campo, R. Faden, and A. Eke, "Women with HIV: Disclosure concerns and experiences," Abstract no. TA1–88, Women and HIV Infection Conference, Washington, D.C., February 22–24, 1995.

51. Ellen Miller-Mack, personal communication, November 1995.

52. William Jesdale, personal communication, October 1995.

53. L. Rice and D. Robbin, " 'When your relationship puts you at risk' — A collaborative education campaign about the connection between HIV/AIDS and domestic violence," Abstract no. TD2–125, Women and HIV Infection Conference, Washington, D.C., February 22–24, 1995.

54. B. Herbert and L.H. Kanter, Letter to editor, *Journal of the American Medical Association* 274 (1995): 1508.

12

Put Her in a Cage: Childhood Sexual Abuse, Incarceration, and HIV Infection

Debi Cuccinelli and Anne S. De Groot

Debi Cuccinelli is an HIV seropositive woman who is incarcerated in a prison for women in Massachusetts. *Anne S. De Groot, M.D.,* is the head of the TB/HIV Research Laboratory at the International Health Institute at Brown University. She has been involved in HIV prevention through biomedical research on vaccines in her laboratory and in her clinical work at the Massachusetts Correctional Institute in Framingham. She has been directing the HIV Clinic for women since May 1992. Working with the women at Framingham has made a profound mark on her life and thinking.

De Groot is also Debi's HIV doctor at the prison. Debi began to write this story after Anne asked—during her first appointment at the prison HIV clinic—if Debi had been forced to have sex against her will when she was still a child. Debi had never been asked that question by a physician before. This chapter tells Debi's story. Both Anne and Debi believe that there is a link between Debi's HIV infection and her sexual abuse, beginning at age six, by her brother. Debi says that telling this story made her a free woman even though she remains behind bars. This story is also about the special vulnerability of women to HIV infection. We have written this chapter to speak out about sexual abuse and to give a name to this aspect of women's vulnerability to HIV infection so that we may reduce HIV's impact on women before it is too late.

DEBI: I knew no one would believe me if I ever told them about my brother, so I never did. When I was six maybe before that I'm not sure of my exact age my brother started to touch and kiss me different from my other brothers and I didn't understand but I loved him. I remember the first day he raped me as if it was today I was getting out of the tub and he was going pee no one was home he was sitting for me I put my robe on and went to my room he came too. I sat on my bed he pushed me down and pushed himself inside of me. It hurt so bad I was crying he said if I told Mom he would break my doll house and I would never be able to go to the park. I didn't understand. But he said I made him, and he loved me, and I loved him.

It became an all the time thing. He would touch me hold me rub me and hurt me. I didn't know it was wrong at that point well I didn't like it or maybe I didn't understand. He took me everywhere with him. I felt special 'cuz my little sisters couldn't go. There were six kids three older brothers and two little sisters. My Dad was a drunk and my mom just there. There was no love but what I got from my brother.

This went on for maybe four years. It was almost my tenth birthday and my brother had a girlfriend now so he didn't hurt me as much. I was mad 'cuz he never took me out anymore. I was acting out, I needed to tell, I guess. So I told my Mom how he touched me. She hit me and said to stop making up stories and sent me to my room. She said if I ever lied like that I would end up in bad girls school. That day was the first day I cut myself. I went in the bathroom and took my Dad's razor and cut my wrist. It felt good and I liked it 'cuz nothing else hurt but that cut, my head and heart were free.

My brother broke my doll house just like he said he would but I didn't care about anything else anymore I hated life and I knew life hated me. I was a brat, trouble. I ran away at 11. I ended up in court for not going to school. My Dad said what do you want me to do build a cage for her the judge said no and took me away to bad girls school.

ANNE: Debi first visited my HIV clinic at the Massachusetts Correctional Institute in Framingham in 1994. During my three years of practice at the women's prison in Massachusetts, I had come to believe that it was extremely important to understand the framework of my patients' lives, if I was to have any positive effect on their disease. I became convinced that they would not adhere to the medications or complicated regimens that I prescribed if they did not value themselves as human beings. I tried many different ways to improve their self-esteem, but none had the impact of simply naming the root cause of their suffering. That sorrow and suffering, in most cases, was due to childhood sexual and/or physical abuse. In investigations of prevalence of HIV risk behaviors and of histories of childhood sexual abuse among women incarcerated at MCI-Framingham[1,2] we have now established that most of the patients in my HIV clinic, and many HIV-seronegative incarcerated women who do not yet attend my clinic, are survivors of childhood sexual violence.

Debi experienced sexual abuse at age six in a family that neither recognized sexual abuse nor protected her from it. Her mother's response to Debi's first request for help was, unfortunately, typical. As Debi will tell us, following the denial of her abuse by her mother, and rejection by her abuser, she sought love in many terrible places, always believing that she was to blame, always believing that she deserved the worst outcome. She was only thirty-two years old when she arrived at my HIV clinic in the prison, but she had already lived several lifetimes. In the course of my medical history and examination for her first HIV clinic visit, I talked to her about the links between childhood sexual abuse, drug use, sex work, abusive relationships, and HIV infection. I also asked her about her childhood experiences.

Debi chose to tell me about her experience of repeated sexual abuse by her brother. This was the first time she had been asked about sexual abuse by a health practitioner: the first time she was able to unburden herself of the entire story. Telling the story served to put her life in focus. During her incarceration, she began writing her life story, parts of which we will share with you here. It is a story that illustrates why some women come to live at the margins of our culture, and how difficult living at the margins is for these women. This story speaks clearly about the nature of women's vulnerability to HIV infection—Debi tells us about childhood sexual abuse and verbal abuse, about many suicide attempts, about failed attempts to find a protector, about early pregnancy, about physical brutalization by her sexual partner, and about adult sexual slavery. Heroin and alcohol were the only "medications" to which she had access that effectively numbed the pain that she felt.

Childhood sexual abuse is often at the root of adolescent "misbehavior" and has been associated with later participation in illicit drug use and sex work. The relationship between childhood sexual or physical abuse, adult sexual and physical abuse, and many forms of self-abuse (including suicide attempts, depression, bulimia, poor self-image, drug use, recurrent exploitative relationships, and sex work) have been well documented and described.[3–9] Unfortunately, the link between childhood sexual or physical abuse and women's vulnerability to HIV infection remains under-reported by, and obscure to, most health practitioners and public health officials, with few exceptions.[10–13]

Childhood sexual abuse is a major contributor to the vulnerability of women to HIV infection. Women's disempowerment including poverty, class, race, and ethnicity is a second major contributor. Jonathan Mann has stated that the greatest risk for HIV infection is to belong to a group of individuals who are underprivileged, discriminated against, or marginalized in any culture even before HIV is introduced.[3] Thus, distribution of condoms to sex workers, provision of clean needles to drug addicts, and dissemination of HIV education programs will not have any effect on HIV infection rates if the members of these marginalized groups are not empowered to use the HIV protection resources that are provided to them. Condoms are the perfect example: Wearing a condom is simply not a *choice* for any woman.[4] Condom use is subject to negotiation between a woman and her partner. If the woman is disempowered in relation to her male partner, the outcome of the negotiations will be determined by the dominant partner. Furthermore, women are often the last person in a drug-sharing group to use a shared needle, increasing the likelihood that the women will be exposed to HIV through injection drug use.[5]

Sexual violence also determines HIV risk exposure for women and girls. Sexual violence puts women directly at risk for HIV infection, and the emotional and behavioral sequelae of sexual violence may indirectly escalate their risk of HIV infection. Women who are survivors of childhood sexual abuse are vulnerable to HIV infection because they may become involved in abusive relationships or may exchange sex for love, drugs, or money. And they often become addicted to the drugs they use to self-medicate as a means of escaping from the memories of abuse.[13] Women who have a history of childhood sexual abuse are also be more vulnerable to HIV infection because they are more likely to prepare themselves for sexual intimacy by drinking or drugging.

Working at the prison HIV clinic has made the connections between sexual abuse and HIV infection perfectly clear to me: The women who attend my clinic are often involved in relationships in which they are completely disempowered in relation to their sexual partners and in which sex occurs in conjunction with drug or alcohol use. Sex with abusive partners frequently evolves into sex in exchange for protection from physical abuse, sex for shelter and food, and sex for money or drugs. It is extremely rare for these women to be empowered to reduce HIV risk exposure in any of these situations. Women who do exchange sex for money often tell us that they are able to insist on condom use with their clients; however, they remain at risk of HIV infection from their intimate partners, in relation to whom they are disempowered. Lastly, it is not uncommon for these women to be put at risk of HIV infection through rape. One woman offered her rapist a condom when it was clear to her that she was going to be overpowered by a man she knew to be HIV infected. The rapist took off the condom during the act, infecting her and ultimately infecting the child that was born nine months later.

The connections between sexual abuse and incarceration are also clear: Women who are engaged in drug use or solicitation of money in exchange for sex are more likely to become incarcerated than women who do not pursue these activities. The more often women use drugs and do sex work, the more often they become entangled with the law, and the more often they come into contact with HIV. Because the link between sexual abuse and drug use or sex work is rarely addressed in the context of law enforcement, these women resume high-risk behaviors as soon as they are released from any temporary restraint. The higher the number of exposures to HIV and to law enforcement, the higher the likelihood that these women will end up attending my HIV clinic inside prison walls.

DEBI: I was almost eleven and school was a joke. I was hanging with my brother's friends and sleeping with them to be accepted. I was sent to a bad girls school. I cried for days but not so much for my family but for the boys I was sleeping with. They cared I thought. I stayed in that school for six months and I was full of anger. I knew more now about sex drugs and men than I ever knew. I went home and ran away. All my life my father said I was a whore a pig a tramp. That I would never be anything I was stupid ugly fat god the list goes on.

When I left this time I went to Lynn. I was almost 12 I believe. I met a man I thought loved me. He bought me clothes told me I was beautiful and took me to bars. I was important! I thought. Before I knew it I was put on the street to sell my body and make money. The man was a pimp and I was his girl. I worked the streets of Lynn and found the more money I made the more he loved me. Until one night when I went with a girlfriend and spent some money on drugs and drinks.

He beat me and beat me bad. I didn't care it was better than going home. I walked the streets long hours at night and the men loved me! I liked what I did because it made me feel important. I got pregnant and I wasn't sure if it was a trick's baby or my pimp's. When I told him he beat me worse this time. He called me everything I knew I already was—my Dad had already told me. I snuck to the phone and called my Mother she came to get me. I was taken to my brother's in New Hampshire where I had my abortion.

I went back home after a few weeks. I tried school again but I just didn't fit in and again I ran away. This time they put me in a foster home. A older woman who I smoked pot with. I would watch her kids and she would let me have men over. This is when my drug addiction really kicked in. She would bring home older men. They would feed me drugs and drinks and I would sleep with them. She was very dirty. The kids and I didn't eat sometimes for days. I used to go to my family's house and steal food for us. Every dish in the house used to be dirty and a few times I had to do a bath tub of dishes.

I was in trouble all the time I hated school I did drugs and I was with people in their twenties and thirties now. Sex was fun but dirty after sex I would wash sometimes for hours. One night I was having a party and the kids were in their rooms the black lights were on the house full of pot, beer, and a fire started. The woman happened to come home and the flames coming out the floor. I ran for the kids she ran for her stereo.

The cops took us all away. I ran again. This time to all her [foster mother's] friends. I was turned on to speed and a needle. I loved it. I was now about 15. I drank in bars ran with the Hells Angels and was now having what I thought was fun. I was dating and living with a man 11 years older than me. Speed was my life—up for days weeks playing cards drinking and dancing at the corner bar. I was a stripper. I got enjoyment out of it because I was the center of attention and no one called me bad names. One morning I woke up very sick. Leo was at work I called my old foster mother to take me to the doctors. I was pregnant.

I wanted this baby. The doctor told me if I didn't stop doing drugs I would kill the baby. I wondered how he knew. From that day on I stopped the speed, pot, coke and drinking. I told Leo I was pregnant. He wanted me to abort the baby. I said no, he beat me like always. One day my Father paid a visit to Leo and told him to marry me or die. I was married April 10 1976 and my son was born October 14 1976. I was 16.

The day my son was born is still clear to me. I almost lost him and they had to do a C-section. That night Leo took one of his other girl friends home to our bed and bragged about it openly in the bar. When I was told I became very angry and I took Leo's gun and threatened to kill him. The cops came to my house and thanks to God my uncle Paul saved Leo and my son. Nothing was done. The gun was taken and I was taken to my mother's with the baby. I stayed at my mother's for about six months.

I hated my son. When I touched him he would cry and not stop. I had no idea how to be a parent. My mother had to teach me. And so I went home to Leo. My life was a mess. I didn't like this man anymore. He beat me and cheated on me all the time. I began to drink again smoke pot then the coke no needles yet. I lived this way for a year and a half and one day Leo left and moved to another state. I was lost! I had never been alone only when I was locked up years before.

My friend introduced me to a man about three months after. Ricky became my night mare. He moved in quickly and took to my son all was roses at first. Before I knew it my life was a prison. I couldn't go out unless he took me to the store. I was not allowed to have friends, the house had to be so clean you could eat off the floors. I was to iron his underclothes as well as get beat daily for a hair on the floor the music too loud not cooking right my son crying the phone rang and some one hung up it so must have been my boyfriend. He would come home at any time during the day he drove a truck. I would hear him coming and I would shake.

But he was good to my son. He did things with him and we lived in a beautiful house. When he would come home he would make me have sex with him and he would beat me and call me names just like my father did to my mother. Some times my son would cry outside the door and I would get angry 'cuz it would take Ricky longer to get off me. I became pregnant and I was afraid to tell him. So one night I got up the nerve to tell him. I wish I never had he beat me bad and I was running down the stairs he pushed me from behind. I was rushed by Ambulance to the hospital I lost the baby two days later. You can't imagine the guilt. He called me a murderer a baby killer and the beatings got worse and worse. He would never bruise my face but this time he broke my nose. I said I fell.

Once again I got pregnant. I was told to get pregnant by him so I thought it would be safe. It was Christmas eve I was five months pregnant. He came home drunk I was on the phone with my sister and didn't hear him come home he used to sneak in and try and catch me doing things. He began to beat me. My sister drove over with her husband to find me curled up in a ball trying to protect the baby. My son was screaming Linda broke a chair over Ricky's back there was blood everywhere the guys started fighting. I was screaming don't hurt him. Linda took my boy. I wouldn't leave. That night I ended up in the hospital for a week. I lost the baby and had broken ribs. My family got involved and Ricky moved out.

That wasn't the end. I started to drink in the morning sometimes all day. I would drink till I would pass out then start over. I loved him and I wanted him home. I knew all he and my father said was true I was a pig a whore would never be any good no one wants used meat. Ricky would say you're fat. I was 100 pounds. I began to cut myself again. I lived in my house my son would go on the bus to school and come home to me and I be still in pajamas shades down drunk. Ricky would come over for sex and then soon he was home. He stopped beating me for awhile but then things became the same again.

I couldn't take it. I became pregnant again this time no one would kill my baby. I told my father and he told Ricky if he beat me again he would be beat. Life was worse than ever, I was pregnant and not allowed out at all now. Ricky and my son did the shopping I cleaned and cooked and had sex whenever he said.

My daughter was born January 15 1982. She was beautiful. My home and children were my whole world. No one baby sat 'cuz I never went out. But life with Ricky was still the same. I was allowed one friend now a friend of Ricky 'cuz she was gay. She was allowed to take me and the kids out to the park and shopping. It was great. I would cry when she left 'cuz I was alone again. Our friendship grew and Judy had talked with Ricky about beating me and expressed her feeling on how it was affecting the children. It seemed to have worked except when Ricky would get drunk and bring all the guys home at two and three in the morning. I would get up and cook for them then it would be I was a whore and I was looking at his friends.

Judy and I became closer as the years passed and I fell in love with her. I told her one day of my feeling and she felt the same way. One day the children were at school and Judy and I slept together it was beautiful! I felt beautiful for the first time in my life. This went on and one day Ricky pulled an old habit and snuck in the house and found Judy and I in bed together my God he went crazy. Judy got away and called the cops. When they got to me I had 42 multiple contusions and lacerations just on my face and head my ribs were broke my face and neck what a mess. I woke up in ICU with my mother standing over me crying. I almost died that day.

Ricky went to jail for 6 months and then my father and brothers ran him out of town, out of state, he moved to Florida. That was 1984. I stayed with Judy and for the very first time I was happy! Maybe I was too happy.

I started going out with Judy and met new friends. I began to drink and before long I was doing coke. I learned to smoke it now and I loved it. I met a man who was a dealer. I slept with him for drugs and I saw Judy when I felt like it. She was always there for me. She would watch the kids and let me run and have fun. This man turned me on to the drug heroin. I went on a trip with him to Holland to bring drugs back. When I returned I was hooked on heroin and a slave once again only to something much worse than Ricky. I began to use a needle just like ten years before this.

I tried to care for my children which were once all I lived for but now I lived for heroin. I couldn't care for my kids work the streets and get high. It was all too much for me. Sometimes I would spend all my money and I would have to call my mother for food. Judy was getting madder and sick of the life I was leading. She left and I didn't care. I called my mother and asked her to take my kids for a few weeks while I went to detox. She did. I went to detox but left early.

The streets were hot and I had spent many a night in jail. I was working my way up to a real commitment, to the Framingham Prison for women. I needed a new way to make money jumping in and out of cars for $20 was just not making enough money for me. I began to rob houses. I made a lot more money and my habit began to get a lot bigger. I got busted in 1986 and that was my first trip to the prison.

I spent a year at MCI-Framingham and as crazy as this sounds it was like vacation. Judy would visit three times a week. I was involved in relationships with different women and for once in my life I felt like I fit in. My parents now had custody of my children and when I left in 1987 I went home to try to start over. Within weeks I was working the streets again with a needle in my arm day and night. I had no fear of death it seemed. I had been stabbed raped beaten yet I kept working the streets living on the edge.

This time was worse than ever. If I had $100 I would not spend it on a room. I would sleep in hallways, in a abandoned building, a car, not eating for days because every cent was for heroin. I would some times not shower for days then I would go to the beach house and rinse my body—or go with a trick to his house and shower. I went to New York with a friend, drugs were cheap but life was harder. I slept in cardboard boxes, crack houses full of bugs and rats. I remember one night shooting coke in a cold building somewhere on the lower east side. Candles were the lights and I sat watching the mice come out of the holes in the floors for hours. Thinking back makes me sad.

I returned to Boston after a three night stay in a jail in New York. Prison was no joke there and I felt lucky to get out alive. In Boston, the streets were full of girls and money was hard to make. Once again I turned to robbing houses. I was back at MCI-Framingham before I knew it.

This time people were being tested for AIDS, and a lot of girls I knew had tested positive. I began to wonder if I had it. Penny, a woman that grew up with me, came back positive. It was because of her I got the test at the prison. I remember feeling scared and waiting for the test to come back felt like months. Women who had the test would be called to the small clinic area, taken into a room and given the news. The ones that came out crying we all knew had tested positive. My day came and I could not go alone. I grabbed my girlfriend and went in shaking. I sat down and everything seemed to stop. The nurse's lips seemed to move in slow motion. I remember I wouldn't leave the room 'cuz I feared people would know. I didn't cry not yet I was in shock. One nurse told me I was going to die—sat with me for a few seconds asked me if I was going to hurt myself then said "Okay, next!"

There was no psychiatrist—no doctor—no support. Just a gut wrenching feeling that no words could explain. I left that room with a smile. My friend was happy for me. I went to my unit and took off all my clothes and went in the shower and cried like a baby. On my knees in a shower stall I asked God to take my life. I must have stayed in there for hours.

When I returned to my room I felt like people knew. I felt dirtier than ever before. My brother never made me feel this dirty. I couldn't shake the feeling for days I was living a secret greater than any and I couldn't hold it in. I would no longer let my lover touch me and she was getting angry thinking there was someone else. I only had a few months left before going home so I wanted no one to know, not in prison anyways because the people who knew others had it treated them like they had the plague, saying real crazy mean things.

I had put my test paper in my drawer and I came back into my room a few days later to find my lover with it in her hands. I went crazy with anger and fear. She knew and she was crying. I tried to lie but it didn't work. She held me and told me she loved me and it would be okay. I felt relief but still very scared other people would find out. She promised never to tell. I believed her. Judy was still in my life and I told her. She took it very hard and still does to this day.

My friends Penny and Judy came to visit every week. The visits were long and painful. Word had leaked out that I had it. I stayed in my room a lot and had a lot less friends. My lover had left and I felt very much alone. It was a week or so before I was to leave and my room mate came in the room with another girl. They said they had to talk to me about something. I sat down and this woman I had shared a room with for over six months told me I smelled. She said I had an odor about me! Not a body odor not a vaginal odor—but an odor. A odor like this other girl who was very sick with AIDS. I got so mad I said a what, an AIDS odor? They said yes!

I told them they were sick and why now did I have this sudden odor. I tried to laugh it off but I couldn't. I went across the hall to a women I had done time with since 1986, a lifer. I yelled at her and cried "Why didn't you tell me I smelled." She held me and laughed and cried with me trying her best to reassure me I didn't smell. I didn't believe her or any one I knew I smelled like AIDS. That night I took a shower and washed my body with a steel wool pad crying trying to get my skin clean and odor free. I ended up in a cage (in the Health Service Unit under observation) in a paper robe. I left from that cage to go home two days later.

I was full of rage at everyone in the world. I got home and I told my parents that we needed to talk. I slapped the piece of paper on the table and said good-bye. My mother was crying and begging me to wait. My Father called me a pig, whore, tramp, looser, bum, stupid, god the words went on.

I returned to the streets and once the warmth of that first shot of heroin ran through my body I was pain free. Nothing mattered to me. I had unsafe sex and I hoped each trick got it. The world owed me I thought! HIV was widespread by now like a wild fire out of control. I was ignorant and knew nothing about this disease because it seemed to kill fast. Some faster than others. I wanted to go fast.

I was living with a dealer and once in awhile I'd sneak out to make extra money for coke. The man I was living with got busted and when I came home the door was broken down and I knew my free high and roof over my head was gone. I began to rob houses again. I was forewarned that if I got caught again I would be in jail for a long time. I didn't care. I was living on the edge with AIDS so nothing could hurt me! Hallways, cars, abandoned buildings became my life once again. I would use rain water snow beer anything to shoot my drugs. Cleaning needles took time and was not for me.

I was on the run from the police for a string of robberies so I left Lynn and headed to Boston. I would steal and sell my body by day to get my drugs. It was September 20, 1990 and I got arrested and sent back to Framingham. I was sentenced to six to ten years with two years to serve. People were not as ignorant about the disease but it was still hard. Being drug free meant facing and failing everything.

The medical staff was getting a little better. But women were dying due to poor medical treatment. I began to talk openly about my disease. The death of my friend Penny's baby really opened my eyes and heart. I started to read about HIV and AIDS. I wanted to learn. There was little support for us women here at MCI-Framingham at that time but those of us that were infected seemed to stick together.

It was a long two years before I was released. I had changed somehow, somewhere along the line, and treatment was recommended. I refused it out of fear. There was too much pain in my life and too many secrets for me to risk that chance of others finding out about my childhood and my past.

Once again I returned home. The house so beautiful on the outside and so damn ugly within. I was full of resentment towards my mother because she was raising my children and being the mother I once wanted to be. I felt out of place around my own children. They loved me still but I had lost their respect and parental love. I was just there. My father had built a small apartment in the attic of the house. It was beautiful and mine. But my family would say put the addict in the attic and after awhile it got to me. I couldn't take the name calling and the jokes about my disease. I knew in my heart my father built me that apartment out of fear, fear if I used his bathrooms or his dishes he would get sick. My mother would fight with him, saying she's our daughter, as I listened and cried. After some time I left once again. I was tired of hearing how bad I was from my father. After all, I had become all he had said, and more.

It seemed that the streets were all I knew and I was accepted as one of the girls now. One night I was working the streets and a trick had given me heroin in exchange for sex. When I shot those bags I don't remember what happened. I woke tied to a bed with doctors all around me. I had overdosed and was found lying on the main street dead. The doctors explained I was lucky to be alive. I was mad that they saved me.

I was on probation for the rest of that six to ten year sentence, and by getting high I had violated and was sent back to MCI-Framingham. This time something had changed. I was unsure what but it was there, a change. There were programs now to help learn about addiction, people who specialized in HIV and AIDS. A clinic and doctor just for us. In four short months I was parole eligible. I was working closely with Women and AIDS Project in the prison. My counselor was a women I had gotten high with and done time with years ago.

I began to have hope! She was my inspiration and I looked up to her. We talked about a program and as scared as I was I decided to give it a try. I was released to Spectrum house in Westboro Mass. I remember driving up to this big white house on a hill, people were smiling and I was shaking. As I walked in the door people stuck their hands out and welcomed me sharing words of comfort. I remained in that program for six months working hard and learning about both my diseases; addiction and HIV. I became very active in groups but I never spoke of my brother my brother. I painted a picture of a beautiful family life.

When I left Spectrum I was afraid to go home. I wanted to remain drug free and something inside said it wouldn't last at home. I went on to another treatment program in the town where I used to work the streets and do my drugs. I thought if I don't run from there I'll be fine at home.

The day before Christmas of 1993 I returned home. Life was great. I still lived in the attic and my father was still the same but I had changed. I went to meetings, sometimes three times a day and I had started to date a woman I was in treatment with. I was on parole and would be until 2001.

I was becoming a parent again and I was very much involved with my children's lives. I was the happiest I have ever been—maybe too happy! I had one relapse but quickly picked myself up and started back to my meetings asking for help. I was clean and doing well. I went to parole like I did every week to give urine to be checked for drugs. One day, the urine test became a nightmare. My test came back positive for narcotics. I demanded that my parole officer test it again and then again. I couldn't understand what was going on! I hadn't used drugs, and this test said I did. I was going back to jail for something I had not done and I was very angry to say the least.

I was allowed a hearing a week later. My lawyer and I walked in fearful of the outcome. I was to be given another chance if this urine test was clean. I gave it knowing it was. My parole officer was not in so the test was done in my absence. The phone rang later that day and the voice on the other end told me to pack my bags I was to return to MCI-Framingham the next morning.

I lay in my Mother's arms for some time that night crying and wishing I was dead. Death would have been better than returning to prison. After many tears from my mother, my daughter, and myself, I locked myself up in the attic and tried to take my life with pills of every kind.

Once again I woke up in a strange place, this time locked in a psychiatric ward. I could not leave for a week and upon release I was to report to my parole officer in my lawyer's presence. It was Monday morning and my mind was racing with fear.

I left that hospital and at a stop light jumped out of the car and ran for my life. In a matter of an hour I had a needle in my arm and all I had worked so hard for seemed to be gone. I knew at this point that this was my destiny. A whore on the streets with a needle in her arms carrying a deadly virus HIV.

I got high for four days stealing, working the streets, running from the law. On the fourth day I just couldn't run anymore. Something was different and no matter how much drugs I did the pain and anger remained. I called my parole officer and asked him to come get me on a corner in Lynn. With my head down I entered this prison six months ago. Full of anger at the world. Those dirty urines I found out later were from my son's cough medicine that had codeine in it. I had been taking it for a cough I couldn't shake.

I needed to see the psychiatrist and I also needed to see a doctor for the HIV. I had neglected my health for a long time. Going to the doctor clean and sober meant accepting I had HIV. I was not willing to ever accept that deadly disease. I saw a psychiatrist and I was not stable at that point. Finally, on a Friday, I went to the HIV clinic here at the prison. It was new to me to have a doctor here for HIV but things had changed.

When I walked in a beautiful woman with short hair put her hand out and introduced herself. She was warm and very caring. I liked her right away. I felt relaxed and for some reason I trusted her. I became very sick after I saw her that day and when I saw her again I believe the following week, remembering that I had meet this Doctor and she had sent me to the hospital in Boston for tests, I knew I was in good hands and it was safe to trust her with my life. I wanted to talk more with her. One day while in her office, sexual abuse came up and before I knew it I cried and told my secret of my brother, my dad, my life. She held me and felt my pain and told me it was okay and not my fault I was just a young child who didn't know better.

I felt all kinds of pain that day, but I also felt a million pounds lighter. I was asked to write about my brother and though it was one of the hardest things I've ever done, I wrote it for her to help others as well as myself. At first it hurt too much to read or really talk about. But each time it got easier and easier. I blamed God, my father, my mother, myself and life for what my brother did to me. Today I blame my brother!

I've been in jail for six months and though there's a fence around me to keep me locked in, I am free. There are no more secrets that keep me a prisoner inside of my own body. My parents know I didn't lie, though they don't accept it yet. The truth has been told.

ANNE: Every time I read this story, I cannot believe that Debi survived. I feel amazed and honored that she is in my life, and that she has the strength to tell this story to the world. Every time I see her, I can tell how much she has grown with each telling of the story. She is still in prison as we write this chapter, but I know, as she said, that she is free. As she says, the real truth has been told, and Debi is free of her cage. The connection between her six-year-old self and her thirty-two-year-old self is her own discovery. These images come through so clear: Debi as a six year old child who is in love with her older brother. Debi as a confused ten-year-old asking for help, getting dismissed, and not knowing where to turn. Ten-year-old Debi cutting her wrist with her father's razor and feeling relief because the razor takes away her emotional pain. Debi finding substitutes for the love she felt she was too terrible to deserve. Debi's father blaming her, and Debi blaming herself. Debi subjecting herself to abusive, angry, destructive men because she believed that she deserved no better.

Writing this chapter together has been redemptive for me and for Debi because there is teaching in this telling. Our goal is to tell her story, and to ask all women who wish to speak about the unspeakable to tell their stories, so as to bring about healing for themselves and for all women. Naming the unspeakable—past trauma—naming women's vulnerability to HIV, will begin the change we are seeking. We aim to continue this work together, to bring about change, to stop the epidemic of HIV among women, and to make a difference in women's lives.

The reason I am driven to do this work is that Debi's story is just one variation on a tragic theme that I have heard too many times in my clinic: childhood sexual abuse, early and frequent sex in exchange for temporary emotional support, drug use as self-medication, and drug use to make intimacy more tolerable and to diminish their emotional pain, drug dependency, abusive relationships, sex work, and eventually incarceration. Many of the women I see in clinic are still enmeshed in this vicious cycle, are still involved with abusive men, and cannot find their way out. Part of the work I do in clinic is to help these women rebuild their self-esteem, to learn to treasure themselves, and to find a new life when they get out of prison. I rely on the drug treatment programs that are available at the prison, and I depend on a small group of dedicated and compassionate coworkers who help set up discharge planning, but none of these services will help these women find new lives if they do not first hold themselves to be worthy of our efforts. Nor will these women adhere to the regimens of antiviral therapy and opportunistic infection prophylaxis that health practitioners prescribe if they have no self-esteem. Thus this work, of building self-esteem and engaging women in caring for themselves, is an essential part of providing HIV care in a women's prison and cannot be set aside.

I did not need to participate in research studies to convince myself that this tragic theme of childhood sexual abuse, continued involvement with abusive sexual partners, drug addiction, sex work, and incarceration is being repeated over and over in the lives of many of these women. Over three thousand women are incarcerated at the prison where I work every year. Approximately 90 percent of these women are injection drug users.[2] I have engaged in research about HIV risk at MCI-Framingham in order to bring the problems affecting these women to the attention of my medical colleagues and public health officials. Our research studies, which I will summarize here, have now proved conclusively that HIV infection is linked to childhood sexual abuse, and that AIDS is becoming one more tragic outcome for women incarcerated at MCI-Framingham.

Given the interrelationship between sexual abuse, drug use, sex work, and HIV, it should not be surprising that the HIV seroprevalence rate among incarcerated women is consistently higher than the rate among incarcerated men. At MCI-Framingham, the prison where Debi is incarcerated and where I have been practicing HIV care for four years, one in five women is HIV-seropositive. Read that sentence again and imagine yourself living at MCI-Framingham: One in five of the women at your dinner table is HIV-seropositive. One in five women walking in the prison yard with you is HIV-seropositive. At least one in five women at the prison Alcoholics Anonymous meeting or the prison Narcotics Anonymous meeting is HIV seropositive. More and more of the women you know are testing positive for the HIV virus every day.

In fact, the HIV seroconversion rate among women who are incarcerated at MCI-Framingham exceeds 6 percent (six per one hundred woman-years). That such a seroconversion rate should be observed in the United States is simply staggering: it is a seroconversion rate matched only by the seroconversion rate among women sex workers in Zaire, at the epicenter of the HIV epidemic.

Why should MCI-Framingham be at the center of an epidemic of HIV infection among women in Massachusetts? I and my Brown University colleagues have confirmed that childhood sexual abuse is a common experience among HIV-seropositive and HIV-seronegative women at MCI-Framingham, and that it contributes to the vulnerability of these women to HIV infection. One in two of the HIV-infected women interviewed for a 1994 study reported a history of childhood sexual abuse, as did one in four HIV-seronegative women.[2] This study also demonstrated that women who reported a history of childhood sexual abuse were at higher risk of HIV infection: they were 4.6 times as likely to participate in three behaviors that put them at risk for HIV infection (intravenous drug use, sex work, and not using a condom) and 2.8 times as likely to be HIV infected than women who did not report childhood sexual abuse.[1,2]

Overall participation in behaviors associated with HIV infection was very high among the group of 167 women we have surveyed for the two studies carried out at the prison: Ninety one percent of the HIV-seropositive women and 41 percent of the HIV-seronegative women reported injection drug use. Fifty-eight percent of the HIV-seropositive women reported having performed sex work (defined as exchange of sex for drugs or money), as did 41 percent of the HIV-seronegative women. Fifty-one percent of the HIV-seropositive women and 69 percent of the HIV-seronegative women reported that their male partners never used or infrequently used condoms.

The prevalence of a prior history of sexual abuse among the incarcerated women we studied is higher than the Bureau of Justice Statistics' report that 41 percent of women in prison and 44 percent of women in jail have been sexually or physically abused.[6,7] According to an American Correctional Association survey, over half of female inmates had a history of physical abuse, but only 36 percent had a prior history of sexual abuse.[8] Our estimates are more consistent with an earlier study of female offenders in Massachusetts, in which it was reported that 88 percent had experienced sexual and or physical abuse.[9] Our findings are also consistent with a study by Singer and Petchers: Forty-eight percent of women incarcerated in Cleveland reported childhood sexual abuse and 68 percent reported forced sexual activity as adults.[10] Our estimates may be more accurate than some institutional surveys; our study interviews were conducted by the patients' primary health care providers. However, we believe many incarcerated women cannot bear the emotional strain of discussing childhood sexual abuse, even with their primary health care providers. Thus all of these reports, including ours, may underestimate the true prevalence of histories of abuse among incarcerated women.

The connection between sexual abuse, physical abuse, and HIV risk behaviors has been made clear in these studies and in other published reports. Interventions to reduce HIV risk behavior among recently incarcerated women are desperately needed. Counseling should be provided for incarcerated survivors of sexual and physical abuse as a formal component of their rehabilitation. Drug treatment programs, HIV/AIDS risk reduction and education programs, and psychological and other support services that address adult and childhood physical and sexual violence and the low self-esteem that accompanies this abuse must be provided if HIV risk exposures are to be reduced among incarcerated women. The effect of such interventions on the reduction of HIV risk-taking behavior should be evaluated.

As we have shown in this chapter, childhood sexual abuse is a major contributor to HIV infection among incarcerated women; however, there are many other contributing factors. For example, Hispanic women are 1.5 times as likely than white women to be living with HIV at MCI-Framingham. Ethnicity, race, and poverty all contribute to the disempowerment of any woman and increase her risk of HIV infection. Poverty, race, and ethnicity must also be addressed by individuals and organizations wishing to impact the HIV epidemic: Why are women of color disproportionately affected by the epidemic? Why are women of color also disproportionately represented among incarcerated populations?

Debi and I believe that the key to prevention of HIV infection among women is to address the roots of their disempowerment. Physicians must ask in earnest about childhood experiences, including sexual and physical abuse. Health care practitioners must be aware of barriers to safer sex, to safer drug use, and to recovery from drug addiction. Physicians, health professionals, and public health officials must work to make women's lives safer. Interventions to reduce HIV risk among women, particularly among women who are in prison or have been incarcerated, must address women's disempowerment in our culture and the events that lead to that disempowerment. The general public, the departments of corrections, and federal and state officials need to be made aware of the high HIV infection prevalence and the high rate of HIV seroconversion among incarcerated and recently incarcerated women. Women who are incarcerated or recently released from prison *deserve* our attention. Debi's story is but one testimony: I have heard too many stories like this one from my patients. We must work to reduce HIV risk for these women before AIDS claims one more woman's life.

NOTES

1. Jessica Stevens, Sally Zierler, Virginia Cram, Diane Dean, Ken Mayer, and Anne S. De Groot, "Risks for HIV Infection in Incarcerated Women," in press, *Journal of Women's Health,* Summer 1995.

2. Jessica Stevens, Sally Zierler, Diane Dean, Ann Kathryn Goodman, M. Elizabeth Chalfen, and Anne S. De Groot, "Prevalence of Prior Sexual Abuse and HIV Risk-Taking Behaviors in Incarcerated Women in Massachusetts," in press, *Journal of Correctional Health Care* 2, no. 2 (1995).

3. J.M. Mann, D.J.M. Tarantola, and T.W. Netter, eds., *AIDS in the World* (Cambridge, Mass.: Harvard University Press, 1992), 579.

4. William Rodriguez, Paul Farmer, and Sally Zierler, "Socioeconomic Factors Influencing Access to Care and Survival in Women with HIV," Abstract TF3 161 at the Conference on HIV Infection in Women, Washington, D.C., February 1995.

5. P.C. Stephens, R. Jeimer, B. Griffith, B. Jariwala-Freeman, and E. Kaplan, "HIV Type 1 Survival and Load in Injection Equipment: Policy and Prevention Implications for Women," Abstract FE2–220 at the Conference on HIV Infection in Women, Washington, D.C., February 1995.

6. L.A. Greenfield and S. Minor-Harper, "Women in Prison," *Bureau of Justice Statistics Special Report,* U.S. Department of Justice, Washington, D.C., 1991.

7. T. Snell, "Women in Jail," *Bureau of Justice Statistics Special Report,* U.S. Department of Justice, Washington, D.C., 1992.

8. American Correctional Association, *The Female Offender: What Does the Future Hold?* (Washington, D.C.: St. Mary's Presses, 1990).

9. M.E. Gilfus, "Seasoned by Violence/Tempered by Law: A Qualitative Study of Women and Crime," doctoral dissertation presented to the faculty of the Florence

Heller School for Advanced Studies in Social Welfare, Brandeis University, Waltham, Mass., 1988.

10. M.I. Singer and M.K. Petchers, "The Relationship between Sexual Abuse and Substance Abuse among Psychiatrically Hospitalized Adolescents," *Child Abuse and Neglect* 13 (1989): 319–25.

11. D. Paone and P. Friedmann, "Sexual Abuse as a Risk Factor for HIV Infection," abstract TE1–102 at the Conference on HIV Infection in Women, Washington, D.C., February 1995.

12. B.K. Jordan, J.M. Caddell, J.A. Fairbank, and W.E. Schlenger, "Engaging in HIV Risk Behaviors, Another Outcome of Abuse and Violence," abstract TE1–103 presented at the Conference on HIV Infection in Women, Washington, D.C., February 1995.

13. M. Danovsky, L. Brown, H. Ford, K. Kessel, and L. Lipsitt, "Psychiatrically Hospitalized Adolescents: Sexual Abuse as a Co-factor in HIV Risk," abstract TE1–1–3 presented at the Conference on HIV Infection in Women, Washington, D.C., February 1995.

13

Women, Violence, and HIV/AIDS

Diane Monti-Catania

Diane Monti-Catania is the founder and director of the Advocacy Institute, a consulting firm dedicated to improving institutional and community response to violence against women, to poverty, and to HIV/AIDS. She is a nationally recognized training specialist in the area of violence against women and has been a leader in Connecticut's battered women's movement for the past eleven years. Ms. Monti-Catania has worked as a consultant to the National Resource Center on Domestic Violence, the Connecticut AIDS Residence Coalition to End Homelessness, and to many other state and community-based organizations. She is the vice president of the Board of AIDS Project Greater Danbury and is currently developing support groups for women with HIV. She coauthored, with Jill Davies, "Women, Domestic Violence and HIV/AIDs," a resource packet for the National Resource Center on Domestic Violence. In addition, she is the author of several training curricula on domestic violence and sexual assault and currently offers a workshop integrating the issues of violence against women and HIV/AIDS.

Belinda is thirty-seven years old. She is African-American. She is poor. She is a recovering addict and a survivor of childhood sexual assault. She is a mother, a partner, and a friend. She has lived on the streets and she has lived in shelters. She has been beaten up by her lovers and hurt by strangers. She is strong and courageous, and sometimes scared. She is infected with HIV and she will die quickly. She spends her free time speaking to junior high school students about understanding HIV/AIDS and how to prevent it. She is one woman who represents thousands of women who are struggling each day to get help and support from a system that has failed to recognize and understand the complexity of their lives. This chapter will address the relationship between violence in the lives of women and risks for HIV infection, and will explore how the institutional system has failed and what types of changes need to occur to reduce violence against women and the spread of HIV/AIDS.

Women and HIV cannot be discussed apart from the interrelated issues of poverty, addiction, women's health and violence. Recent statistics on these issues present a grim picture for women:

- One out of every three adult women will be victims of domestic violence in their lives.[1]
- Up to 50 percent of homeless families are homeless as a result of domestic violence, making domestic violence the leading cause of homelessness among women.[2]
- Homeless women report childhood physical or sexual abuse, rape or physical assault more often than housed women.[3]
- In the coming years, 90 percent of new HIV infections will occur through unprotected sexual intercourse.[4]
- The fastest-growing category of homeless people are families, most often women-headed families with one or two children.[5]
- Thirteen percent of women in this country report that they fail to receive the medical care they need in a given year. Among uninsured women, more than one-third (36 percent) fail to receive necessary care.[6]

These facts, taken separately, represent a challenge to the advocacy community to work to improve the lives of women. Taken collectively, which is how many women actually experience them, these facts illustrate that current efforts to prevent HIV infection or to reduce violence against women, although well-intentioned, have been largely irrelevant in the lives of many women. For example, a battered woman who has a history of substance abuse would not be eligible for shelter at many battered women's shelters because eligibility criteria prohibits any woman from using the shelter if she has any history of substance abuse. The same woman may also be denied access to a residential substance abuse treatment program because her violent partner is perceived as a threat to the other people in the program. While these rules may have some justification in terms of managing programs, they serve to exclude many women from getting the help that they may need. Women's experiences are not always crisis-oriented and their need for supportive services may not be focused on what programs or institutions would identify as their priorities or primary risk. For many women, understanding their choices, or lack thereof, is the first step to planning for managing their health, creating safety for themselves and their children, and sometimes changing their lives in dramatic ways. For advocates, understanding how limited women's choices often are is a first step toward effective intervention.

Violence against Women

There is no one clear definition of violence against women. Domestic violence is defined as controlling behavior of one partner toward another using a complex combination of physical, sexual, and emotional behaviors and assaults to maintain that control.[7] Domestic violence happens in all socioeconomic and cultural settings and in all types of relationships, whether heterosexual or homosexual. Rape is the term used most often by the public and media to describe a range of sexually assaultive and abusive behaviors, but it does not always include incest, child sexual assault, date rape, and spousal/partner rape. Society has created language to describe the horrors that most often men perpetuate against women, but much of that language is legal and dilutes the reality of women's experiences. Women are at risk of violence throughout their lives. Even prior to being born, children of battered women are at risk of being harmed if their mother is assaulted during the pregnancy. The *Journal of the American Medical Association* reported a study which documented that 17 percent of all pregnant women are battered during pregnancy.[8] As young girls grow up they are at risk of sexual assault. The National Victim Center's *Rape In America* study found that 32 percent of the women they surveyed had been sexually assaulted between the ages of eleven and seventeen, and 29 percent had been assaulted before the age of eleven.[9]

As girls move through adolescence their risk of interpersonal violence increases with the advent of dating. Reports of dating violence, including physical assault, sexual assault, and emotional assault are well documented.[10] In addition, young women are considered a particularly vulnerable population at risk for stranger assault. The risk to adult women does not diminish as they age. The U.S. Justice Department reports that adult women are just as likely to experience a violent victimization by an intimate partner (33 percent) as they were to be victimized by an acquaintance (35 percent) or a stranger (31 percent).[11] Violence continues in the lives of women through old age, with a recent American Association of Retired People report finding that elder abuse is disproportionately husbands against wives, as opposed to caretaker abuse, which has historically received more attention.[12] From birth until death, women live daily with violence or the threat of violence. Each episode changes the way they deal with and react to future events and the ways in which they relate to the people in their lives and the world around them.

A number of theories have been generated over the years regarding women's experience with violence.[13] Although these help to understand the complex nature of violence and its effect on women, each woman will experience and respond to the violence in a different way. A woman's experience of violence will be interpreted through her own individualized analysis of her risks, her options, and her resources.[14]

HIV/AIDS

Much of the early information that emerged regarding HIV and the transmission of the virus focused on gay men. Women were not seen as being at particularly high-risk unless they participated in what were defined as high-risk behaviors. Unfortunately, the routes of transmission for HIV are such that women are often unaware of or unable to control those risks. The main points of preventative messages have been: (1) practice safe sex, defined as either using a condom or limiting the number of sexual partners; (2) do not share needles if you are an intravenous drug user; and (3) know who you are having sex with: Ask them to be tested if you are not sure they are HIV-negative. Let's look at each one of these messages in the context of the women's lives as described earlier.

Practice safe sex. A woman who is a victim of violence, whether it was a one-time sexual assault or ongoing forced sex by her partner, rarely has an opportunity to request that a condom be used. Such a request, in either situation, may increase her risk of injury. Given the choice of immediate serious injury or the gamble of contracting HIV, many women have been forced to choose the latter. In addition, some women adopt a safety strategy of engaging in sexual behaviors that they believe present a lower risk for HIV infection. For example, a woman may decide that she will go along with her partner and have sex, but she will engage only in oral sex, believing that her chance of HIV infection will be lower than if she has vaginal intercourse. This strategy may work some of the time, but many women do not have accurate information regarding the continuum of safest to riskiest sex practices. Children who are victims of sexual assault will lack not only the opportunity but most certainly the knowledge to be able to protect themselves from HIV infection. In regard to the possibility of limiting the number of one's sex partners, many women are forced by a violent partner to have sex with multiple partners as part of their victimization. The freedom to choose partners, or limit the number of partners, is not always part of a battered woman's reality. Violence limits women's choices—and the more severe the circumstances, the more limited the choices.

One recent study found a definitive connection between childhood sexual assault and high-risk behaviors for HIV among the female partners of intravenous drug users.[15] Klein and Chao report in their study that 36 percent of their respondents had been sexually assaulted during childhood and 34 percent sexually assaulted during adolescence; 18 percent reported abuse during both childhood and adolescence. They found that these women differed significantly from nonabused women when predicting high-risk behavior for HIV infection, which was defined as having multiple sex partners, having sex while high, having sex with drug users, and trading sex for money. When controlled for race, they found that childhood sexual assault for African-American women was consistently predictive of HIV risk behaviors as adults.

What all this means, essentially, is that any prevention strategy that focuses on a woman, or a girl, requesting that her partner use a condom is essentially irrelevant to this entire population of women at risk.

Don't share needles. For women who are active drug users, the likelihood of violence in their lives is very high. Battered women often use drugs, though not exclusively intravenous drugs, as a way of coping with violence, and some women will share drugs with a partner as a way of maintaining some control. Again, the choices for women are often limited and their ability to say yes or no in any given situation fluctuates. Another fundamentally problematic aspect of this prevention strategy is that women are being infected largely by heterosexual contact, not by needle sharing; although clean needles will prevent some women from getting infected, this is not a strategy that will speak to the majority of women.

Know your sex partner. Ask him to be tested if you are unsure: This prevention strategy is based on a presumption of communication that is clear and honest. Unfortunately, that does not reflect the reality for most battered women (and many nonbattered women as well). HIV is transmitted by sex and drugs—two things that people feel shame and guilt about and about which they lie. To presume that someone will unequivocally know everything about their partner is unrealistic, and to assume that a battered woman could ask her partner about his sexual history, current sex partners or practices, or drug use is unfair. This area represents the highest risk to women. As the epidemic of HIV spreads, it is women's lack of knowledge about their partners' behavior and their inability, due to fear or socialization, to ask questions, that poses the greatest risk. As with condom use, many women feel that it is a better strategy to gamble on HIV infection than to raise these issues with their partners.

Asking that a partner get tested, or telling a woman to get an HIV test herself, often presents a risk for battered women. Many women believe that their partners would not tell them the truth if they were tested, and many also feel that they would rather not know. We must give women that choice, even if we believe it to be a dangerous one. Only the women herself will fully understand the risks that her violent partner may pose to her, and her decisions about her care and safety strategies must be her own.

In addition, when those prevention strategies fail, people who are infected with HIV have been encouraged to access good medical care early and regularly. For women this is rarely possible. As noted earlier, the Commonwealth Fund report on women's health clearly documented that women do not have access to the type of health care they need, and often they do not access what they do have for preventative medicine or regular checkups. And at this point in time, HIV is disproportionately affecting women of color who, as the report states, "are more likely to be poor, uninsured and to lack needed medical care than white women."[16] In short, the hope that women who are HIV-positive will access early and regular health care is unrealistic, given the facts.

Women, HIV, and Violence

It is likely that violence will emerge as the primary factor for the transmission of HIV to women over the next decade. The threat of becoming infected, as well as the threat of actually infecting someone, will be a tactic embraced by violent men and used against women. Institutional response to this particular set of circumstances must fully address this situation. We are being challenged to design prevention and treatment strategies that are based on the reality of women's lives. These strategies must include the following:

Access to care. Women are routinely asked to prioritize their needs to access care, but the more we learn about the particulars of women's lives, the more we understand the need to expand, diversify, and *combine* the services currently available. For example, a woman who is HIV-positive, battered, homeless and has two children may need a safe place to go, medical care, child care and help with legal issues regarding her children's future when she is too sick to care for them. This woman would, in all likelihood, have to go to a hospital, a battered women's program, an AIDS program, a child welfare agency, legal services, a homeless shelter, and possibly court to piece together the type of support that she needs. In order to help women in a way that meets their needs, we must facilitate institutional change that acknowledges that women need to address more than one resource at a time. This includes the cross-training of professionals so that there is a widespread understanding of the relationship between many of these issues and knowledge of resources in their communities.

Recognition of women's commitment to their children. Women, whether battered, HIV-positive, poor, homeless or all of the above, are usually committed to the well-being of their children. Some women, due to addiction, mental illness, or fear may be unable to care for their children or to make decisions that others think are in the children's best interest, but most women can and do care about their children. Access to services that allow women to remain connected to their children must be a priority of program planning over the next decade. A battered woman who needs substance abuse treatment should not be forced to make a decision between her own safety and health care and the safety and well-being of her children. However, most current systems would force this woman to give up her children during the period of time that she is in drug rehabilitation. Her choices will often be to leave the children with her violent partner, turn them over to child welfare, or split them up among relatives and friends. In addition, if she separates from her children she may lose her entitlement to housing assistance, thereby losing her housing. Once children have been surrendered to another's care and housing is lost, both are difficult to regain. This is not a choice that women can easily make, and often the choice will be to forgo treatment altogether. HIV/AIDS service organizations must also recognize that increasingly the women they are seeing with HIV/AIDS will have children. Planning for and including those children in women's programs will ensure that women are not being asked to choose between supportive housing and being with their children.

Long-term supportive programming. Crisis intervention programs are usually short-term, but women's lives and the challenges they face are ongoing. For example, most domestic violence intervention programs are designed to provide emergency shelter for short periods of thirty to sixty days. Most homeless programs have similar restrictions regarding ongoing use of a facility. HIV/AIDS housing programs, though seen as longer-term, have historically been designed for people who have converted from HIV infection to symptomatic AIDS and often do not allow people with active substance abuse problems or histories of violence. In order to provide women with the ongoing support they may need to plan for their own safety and that of their children, to access ongoing medical care, and to have long-term, safe, decent housing, the criteria for services must be revised. Services that are available to women on an ongoing basis will often be the most effective in providing help for women when they need it. For example, a woman with AIDS calls a hotline for battered women and reports that her husband is getting increasingly violent as she is getting increasingly weak, and she doesn't know what to do. The hotline counselor urges her to leave her partner so that she will be safe from his violence. The woman says she cannot possibly leave him: her children need their father because she, their mother, is going to die. The counselor says that when she is ready to leave, the battered women's program will be able to help her. This woman is most likely looking for ongoing support to be able to stay in her relationship and plan for the safety and well-being of her children. She may not require anything more than contact with the battered women's program over the next few months as they help her to think through her strategies for keeping the children safe while maintaining a semblance of family for the remaining time she may have with them.[17]

Conclusion

Violence against women has historically been addressed in terms of separate issues—domestic violence, adult sexual assault, and childhood sexual assault—while HIV/AIDS has been addressed first as a gay male issue and then as an issue for women without children. But the reality of women's lives includes violence throughout life, the threat of or presence of HIV infection, mental illness, addiction, poverty, racism, sexism, classism, and homophobia. To reduce the incidence of violence against women or reduce the risk of HIV infection to thousands of women, the institutional and social service communities must come together and bring resources to bear that are adequate to impact two major health pandemics threatening the lives of women. We must encourage the women to lead, listening to them and understanding what they want from the service community. We must develop the ability to change our institutions to respond to the reality of women's lives in a way that is supportive, effective, and relevant. We must be willing to abandon practices and programs that have not worked and redesign them so that we can confront this incredible threat to women's lives. Violence against women is eroding our sense of community and family, and HIV is killing our sisters and the mothers of our communities' children. If the enemy were foreign, we would bring all of the economic, military, and intellectual forces of the country to bear. The enemy, however, is within, and we must design a strategy that will eliminate both violence against women and children and HIV/AIDS from our future.

NOTES

1. Anne H. Flitcraft, Susan M. Hadley, Marybeth K. Hendricks-Matthews, Susan V. McLeer, and Carol Warshaw, *Diagnostic and Treatment Guidelines on Domestic Violence* (Chicago: American Medical Association, 1992).

2. *Domestic Violence—A Leading Cause of Homelessness,* Fact Sheet #10, National Coalition for the Homeless, Washington, D.C., 1994 (quoted from research conducted by Elizabeth Schneider in 1990 for the Ford Foundation).

3. Angela Browne, "Family Violence and Homelessness: The Relevance of Trauma Histories in the Lives of Homeless Women," *American Journal of Orthopsychiatry* 63, no. 3 (July 1993): 370–84.

4. Marge Berer with Sunanda Ray, *Women and HIV/AIDS: An International Resource Book* (London: Pandora, 1993), 6.

5. *The Connecticut Initiative on Homelessness and Family Violence* (Newton, Mass.: The Better Homes Fund, 1994).

6. *First Comprehensive National Health Survey of American Women Finds them at Significant Risk* (New York: Commonwealth Fund, 1993), 2.

7. Ann Jones and Susan Schechter, *When Love Goes Wrong* (New York: HarperCollins, 1992), 12.

8. Judith McFarlane, Barbara Parker, Karen Soeken, and Linda Bullock, "Assessing for Abuse during Pregnancy," *Journal of American Medical Association* 267.23 (June 17, 1992): 3177–78.

9. *Rape in America* (Arlington, Va.: National Victim Center, 1992), 3.

10. Robin Warshaw, *I Never Called It Rape: The MS Report on Recognizing, Fighting and Surviving Date and Acquaintance Rape* (New York: Harper and Row, 1988).

11. Ronet Bachman, *Violence against Women: A National Crime Victimization Survey Report* (Washington, D.C.: U.S. Department of Justice, 1994), 6.

12. *Abused Elders or Older Battered Women?* Report on the AARP Forum, October 29–30, 1992 (Washington, D.C.: American Association of Retired Persons, 1992).

13. Angela Browne, *When Battered Women Kill* (New York: Free Press, 1987); Judith Lewis Herman, *Trauma and Recovery* (New York: Basic Books, 1992); Susan Schechter, *Women and Male Violence: The Visions and Struggles of the Battered Women's Movement* (Boston: South End Press, 1982); Lenore Walker, *The Battered Woman* (New York: Harper and Row, 1979).

14. See Jill Davies, *Using Safety Planning as an Approach to Woman-Defined Advocacy* (Hartford, Conn.: Legal Aid Society of Hartford County, 1995).

15. *Homelessness and Family Violence* (Newton, Mass.: Better Homes Fund, 1994); H. Klein and B. Chao, "Sexual Abuse during Childhood and Adolescence as Predictors of HIV-Related Sexual Risk during Adulthood Among Female Sexual Partners of Injection Drug Users," in *Violence Against Women* 1 (Sage Periodicals Press, March 1995).

16. *First Comprehensive National Health Survey of American Women Finds Them at Significant Risk* (New York: Commonwealth Fund, 1993), 10.

17. For more information, see Jill Davies and Diane Monti-Catania, *Women, Domestic Violence and HIV/AIDS* (Harrisburg, Pa.: National Resource Center for Domestic Violence, 1995), 3.

14

Social Context and HIV: Testing and Treatment Issues among Commercial Street Sex Workers

Kim Blankenship

Kim Blankenship is a sociologist and an Associate Research Scientist at Yale University in the AIDS Program and the Institution for Social and Policy Studies. For the past five years she has been studying the relationships of gender, class, and race inequality with health, in general, and with AIDS risk in particular. She also works hard to conduct research that simultaneously addresses important intellectual debates and enhances the community in which it occurs. Thus, she has conducted a good share of her field work in the course of helping other community activists to organize and then to carry out the work of a collective organization of street-working women and other women advocating on their behalf aimed at HIV prevention and outreach.

My interest in this topic began in the spring of 1992 when the New Haven Mayor's Task Force on AIDS sought to develop an early treatment campaign to encourage testing of those at risk and thereby both prevent transmission of HIV and delay disease progression in infected individuals. It was a time when there was considerable talk of developing and promoting a standard of care for infected individuals, a time when a variety of treatments that appeared to delay the onset of symptoms and increase the quality of life of infected persons had become available. Indeed, HIV testing had come to be viewed as the first step in the clinical management of HIV, and early intervention had come to be viewed as central to prolonging health and survival.[1] In addition, HIV counseling and testing was becoming a health intervention in and of itself, providing individuals with an assessment of their personal risk, extensive HIV/AIDS education, and risk-reduction information.[2] It was also at this time that the state of Connecticut began to consider mandatory testing laws under the rationale that those identified as seropositive could be channeled more quickly into appropriate services.

The Task Force was particularly interested in learning more about the understanding of and experiences with testing and treatment among specific subgroups of infected individuals and those considered to be at greatest risk for contracting the virus. They were hoping to learn what people knew and did not know about, and subsequently to develop an educational campaign to promote testing and early treatment. As with most approaches to AIDS prevention, this increased attention to early detection and treatment of the HIV virus was premised on the view that people who the scientific community deems at risk consider themselves at risk and subsequently seek testing. It also assumes that they will make behavioral changes and follow advised therapeutic regimens when found to be positive. In this chapter, I evaluate these assumptions through an examination of early treatment issues among commercial street sex workers. Specifically, I address the questions: Are HIV+ street-working women being tested for HIV? Do HIV+ street-working women know the various ways in which they can lengthen and increase the quality of their lives? What factors facilitate or prevent street-working women from seeking or obtaining early treatment?

Methods

For insight into the circumstances of HIV testing and treatment among commercial sex workers, this discussion draws from my ongoing research with drug-using female street sex workers in New Haven. In December 1991 I joined two other community activists in the city to develop an AIDS prevention and education program for street sex workers. We were committed to creating a collective organization run by and for women on the streets, and we began by conducting street outreach and identifying local organizers from within the community. By the spring of 1992 the women had named our group Streets Incorporated and we were all—street sex workers and other activists—meeting weekly to discuss issues facing women on the streets that put them at risk for HIV and strategies for addressing them. At the same time, this activity became part of my field work among the women, through which I began to learn about the social organization of their community and the characteristics of their lives and work. I have been engaged in both the activist work and the research ever since.

In addition to hundreds of hours of field work and hundreds of pages of field notes, this paper draws from a number of other sources. For the first year we met, between spring 1992 and 1993, we recorded our weekly meetings. From then on we frequently kept minutes of the meetings. I draw from these sources as well. Finally, I have convened a total of seven focus groups relevant to the issue of testing and treatment over the three-year period from March 1992 through May 1995, two addressing AIDS risk—related behaviors, one focusing on early treatment, another on legal issues, one addressing housing concerns, and two that focused on access to and utilization of health care services. Of the forty-two street-working women attending these focus group discussions, one-third (fourteen) were African American, two were Puerto Rican, and the remainder white. They ranged in age from twenty to forty-eight, and all had a history of injection drug use and had engaged in commercial sex work at some point in their lives.

In the course of the following analysis I will draw from these materials, frequently representing the issues through the words of the women themselves. The names used in this analysis are pseudonyms.

AIDS Risk, Testing, and Behavioral Change

Numerous studies have demonstrated that, in general, HIV-risk behaviors are quite persistent even in the face of growing public awareness of the threat of the virus and even after the individuals in question have received the benefits of an AIDS intervention (although the persistence of behaviors varies somewhat depending on the targeted group).[3] What most of these studies show is that knowledge alone has had little impact on behavior. Similarly, an expanding body of research on testing shows that it too has little impact on post-testing behavior, particular among those who test negative.[4] Yet early intervention campaigns such as the one planned by the New Haven Mayor's Task Force are premised on the view that the spread of the virus can be curbed through testing and the quality of life among infected individuals extended by encouraging treatment, including drug therapies (such as AZT), outpatient care, dietary modifications, and other lifestyle changes, such as rest, exercise, and the ending of illicit drug use (particularly cocaine).

Is there reason to think that knowledge of available testing and treatment options will impact behaviors when knowledge of risk factors has had such limited effect? Perhaps. Some research suggests that knowledge of risk factors does not always promote behavioral change because individuals have not internalized the risk: While they are aware of the behaviors that place people at risk for HIV, they do not identify *themselves* to be at risk.[5] It may be that people who decide to get tested have done so because they identify themselves to be at risk, just as those who test positive will recognize not only the risk they pose to others if they persist with unprotected sex and needle sharing, but also the risk these behaviors pose to their own health. Indeed, studies do show that perception of their own risk and sense of responsibility to others are two frequently cited reasons for getting tested.[6] Research also suggests that individuals who are motivated to reduce their risk for HIV are more likely than those who simply possess information of their risk to change their behaviors (although behavioral change will be greatest when individuals also have the skills to act to reduce their risk).[7] It may be, then, that those who test positive will possess the motivation they require to change behavior and pursue their treatment. On the other hand, neither of these models accounts for the way social context affects individual behavior and may shape and constrain an individual's risk-taking and treatment-seeking activity even when she is seropositive.

To begin to address some of these questions I focus here on a group of female commercial street sex workers in New Haven. In general, commercial sex workers are considered to be at high risk for HIV, especially when they inject drugs. Data from one CDC study indicates that rates of HIV infection in this population range from zero to 47.5 percent.[8] One study of women at risk in the New Haven area shows a self-reported seroprevalence rate of 52 percent among women who have ever traded sex for money or drugs.[9] Estimates from my field work, based on self-reporting and the reporting of informed others indicate a seroprevalence rate of about 50 percent overall and 75 percent among women who inject. Given these high rates of HIV infection, it is at least as important to know about this group of women's testing and treatment behaviors as it is to know about their risk-taking activities. Although one study of compliance with zidovudine (ZDV, formerly AZT) showed that having a history of female prostitution reduced compliance rates, it offered no explanation for the finding.[10]

In what follows, I describe some of the social contextual factors operating to shape the testing and treatment-seeking behaviors of women on the street. In particular, this discussion will focus on three aspects of this context: AIDS-related knowledge and research, poverty and homelessness, and social isolation. I want to emphasize from the start, however, that to acknowledge social context and structure is not to deny women's agency and the power of individual initiative. While systems of inequality oppress and marginalize women on the street, the same women actively struggle against these systems and assert incredible will and effort to take care of themselves.

Testing, Treatment, and New Haven Street Sex Workers

Do women working in the street sex trade in New Haven get tested for HIV? All of the street working women who have participated in focus group discussions that I have run claim to have been tested at least once. But they all state that they know other women who work on the street who do not know their HIV status.

Most of the women who *do* know they are positive also have been told that they can extend the length and quality of their lives by making lifestyle changes and taking antiretroviral drugs such as AZT. Nevertheless, their first response to the devastation that they feel when informed of a positive test is often to turn to street drugs. Rose is a typical case in this regard. After many years of testing negative, her results came back positive last month. "When did you find out?" I asked her. "Friday. She called me over on Friday and showed me the results. She said I had to take another test because this one was inconclusive, but it was positive. Man, I felt so bad. And I got all this clean time, squeaky clean [she's been struggling to stay clean for the past several months and had her most recent relapse about two weeks before] but I left the program and I went out and got high. Like that. Fuck it. Man, but I gotta stop. I know I really need to stay clean, the drugs'll bring me down. My T-cell count is high, 1,600 so I got a long time. I gotta stay healthy, I know it's really important to take care of myself now."

If Rose is like most drug-using women on New Haven streets in her response to the news that she is positive, she is also like them in her knowledge that taking care of herself, which may include taking antiretroviral drugs, and regularly visiting the doctor can prolong the quality of her life. Nevertheless, most of these women's use of AZT and other HIV-related medications and the regularity with which they have visited doctors have fluctuated vastly over the three years that I have known them. To a large degree, both their initial willingness to get tested, visit doctors, and use drug therapies, as well as their fluctuating engagement with treatment has to do with matters of gender, class, and race inequality.

AIDS-Related Knowledge and Research

One part of the social context in which women live and work that is rarely examined as a factor affecting their AIDS-related behaviors is the huge enterprise that has developed around expanding and proliferating AIDS-related research and knowledge, which, at least in a city like New Haven with a major research university and several hospitals, has become almost an institution in itself. The information that is passed down from this enterprise has a tremendous impact on women working the streets of New Haven, many of whom have actually participated in at least one AIDS-related study or project. One such impact relates to their assessment of their own risk for HIV. Although many of the female street sex workers in New Haven have been tested, others have not, sometimes because they are afraid to know, but more typically because they do not perceive themselves to be at risk. And it is not because they are misinformed, uninformed, or in denial. Instead, it is, at least in part, because they have taken seriously the commonly accepted practice in the AIDS research enterprise of ranking risk. For example, at one focus group the following conversation ensued when I commented that it seemed as if everybody on the streets knew who had and did not have HIV.

> Sara: They think and assume. You don't know unless someone tells you.
> Grace: No, they assume now that because you're out on the streets and you shoot drugs, automatically you got AIDS. Which there's a lot of them that do. Listen you think about the shooting galleries and stuff that everybody had that we didn't know about drugs back then.
> Sara: Can you tell I'm positive? I want to lose some [pointing to her hips].
> Johnelle: There's a woman out there and she says, "I don't shoot I just snort so I don't have AIDS." I love that.
> Sara: That's bullshit.
> Grace: Oh yeah, yeah [adamant].
> Johnelle: And they've never been tested, you know.
> Grace: Do you know, I had to turn around and say to somebody one time, they think they couldn't get this, they wasn't in danger because they smoked the pipe. Are you insane? There are a lot of girls that turn around and have sores in their mouth. And that can pass it.

Sara: Yep. If you got a cut in your mouth or somethin, they got sores and you smoking the same pipe and it gets in that cut, you got AIDS.

Grace: You are not safe with this.

KMB: What about sex too, are they using condoms?

Johnelle: No.

Grace: Well it's supposed to be a sexually transmitted disease.

Lois: There's a lot of people don't know how it's passed. They just think it's passed in the drugs.

Johnelle: I'm out on the street. I just can't believe that mentality.

Grace: I know it.

Johnelle: Because they don't shoot drugs, they're not in danger of having AIDS.

These observations confirm two important aspects of sex workers' perceptions of their risk. First, among the women on the streets, injection drug users are far more likely to define themselves at risk than noninjectors. Furthermore, though most of the women on the street claim to have been tested at least once, those who have not been tested are invariably noninjectors. These field notes are typical of encounters of this kind:

As we walk up Ferry St. Lori and I see a young looking woman watching cars by the pizza place. . . . She watches us approach. "Hi, I'm Kim and this is Lori," I say. "We're with a group called Streets, Inc. that does HIV prevention and helps women on the streets. Would you like one of our goodie bags?" "Oh, I don't have to worry about AIDS. I don't shoot that stuff, smoking's my problem." "Well, do you know for sure? Have you been tested?" "Nah, but this is a great thing you know. There's women out here doin all kinds of stupid stuff. Not me, I don't give this away [she points to her crotch]. It's blow jobs for me." "Well, we have some kiss-of-mint condoms here if you want." She takes them, but she removes the syringe from the bag. . . . (9/14/94)

Not only is injection drug use viewed as more risky than noninjection drug use, but both groups view it as more risky than sex. And according to experts, who consistently rank risk behaviors in a similar way, they are not wrong. Unfortunately however, this knowledge affects sex workers' assessment of their risk and partly contributes to their unsafe sex practices, especially but not exclusively with personal partners. Liz explains this to me one day when we are talking about the period in her life when she knew about AIDS but before she had tested positive. She explained why she sometimes did not use condoms even though she knew that unprotected sex put her at risk for HIV: "I figured if I'm gonna get it, I'm gonna get it from the needle. I know that's not the only way, but that's just what I figured." Rose, quoted before, may be an even better example.

> Rose told me today she's positive. I feel so awful I don't want to believe it. "How could this be?" I ask. "I knew I was, this time. I just had a feeling." "But you've been so careful with your needles," I say. "Yeah, it's not the needle. It's the unsafe sex, man. There was the pills and the black outs, and plus, it seemed like I wouldn't get it like that, like all those years of sharing behind people who are dead, before we knew about it. I didn't get it then so I thought I was protected." (8/95)

Those women on the street who *do* know that they are HIV-positive struggle to maintain their health in a context that is rarely conducive to doing so. Consider their inconsistent use of AZT and other antiretroviral drugs. Grace recently passed away from AIDS related causes, but in the three years that I knew her, she went back and forth from periods where she adamantly advocated the use of AZT to periods where she refused all medications and medical help. She explained to me once the effort she put into taking her medications:

> I remember turning around and walkin around with it, didn't I? [she turns to Johnelle] I wouldn't throw it away. Right in my pocket. That was when I had to take it so much. I never went without. I used to set my watch every four hours cause that's how often I had to take it. My watch, "beep," I'd be sittin there and "beep, beep, beep," and I'd go off and go take it.

Yet, she told me months later about how she had

> kind of messed up. . . . I take AZT. I haven't taken it for a while. I gotta go get it. I haven't taken it in about two months, but I turn around and I know, the way I look, that I'm killin myself. See you don't think, you're told this in the beginning. You don't think it could really happen to you. Then when you start fadin and what not, then you get scared.

Grace's words powerfully convey her desire to live and take care of herself, and at many points in her life she put enormous energy into doing just that. At other times, she, like many other women like her, was unable to do so.

Although in the discussion referred to above, Grace associates her non-adherence to AZT with "killing" herself, other conversations that we have had suggest to me that she is not always certain that drug therapies are the best thing for her. Indeed, the fluctuating use of AZT among many women on the street is partly explained by their changing understanding of and experiences with AIDS-related research, and at times with their deep suspicion of this research. She did not associate the two things, but one of the times Grace was emerging from a period of nonadherence and disengagement from medical care of any kind, she told some friends, "AZT, it's been on the news. They're giving AZT that's made, it's not really AZT, it's made. They got a scam going on." "Who's giving it?" I asked. "The pharmacies, I guess."

In general, there is considerable confusion over the effects of AZT, particularly as it relates to other drugs. Common street wisdom is that cocaine speeds up the progress of the HIV virus, but women are unsure of what, if any, impact it has on AZT and other treatment regimens. Even more confusing is the relationship between methadone and AZT. As for the long-term impact of AZT and, by association, other antiretrovirals, the perception is that after more than a year, their persistent use will actually promote the onset of AIDS.

To the extent that the women's confusion reflects the status of current research, it is difficult to address. More difficult still to challenge is their tremendous suspicion that the available drugs are poisonous, experimental, and exacerbating the problem, and that the doctors are often using women for their own professional and financial gain. Furthermore, these suspicions are not the product of irrational fears or misinformation. They are deeply rooted in experiences of a class, race, and gender-divided world.

For example, I have been a part of, or privy to, many conversations like the following that took place at one of our meetings in August 1993 among a group of eight street-working women. We had been talking about the tendency of police to arrest women for prostitution and let the johns go.

Mary: It's like, why do they always arrest the women. We get arrested and they let the drug dealers go. Can you explain that to me?

Grace: 'Cause we be the ones that won't be hurtin them. We don't carry guns.

Brenda: Well, it's no different from anything else. They always experimenting on our bodies.

Mary: Yeah, we got a problem, cut em out. You know how many women in Puerto Rico they got, you know, sterilized?

Tracy: Why don't they sterilize men?

Brenda: Shit, can you imagine? [laughter] "Get away from my thing man." [more laughter]

Mary: I'd like to see that. All the doctors are boys. They don't want to be cuttin on themselves.

Women of color feel particularly expendable. In one focus group discussion in March 1995, on access to medical care, Yvonne echoed the words of others when I asked what her greatest health related worry was: "I'm worried they aren't tellin me that I'm positive. They're just figurin 'what does she need to know for? It's just another Black woman. Go ahead and let her die.' " One of her Black friends agreed but said: "It's race, yeah. But it's also cause we're drug users and we're poor too."

In a focus group in February 1992 women talked about AZT and other antiretrovirals in these terms.

> *Johnelle:* Well, how about the fact that because you're in the lower economic bracket that they offer all these experimental programs to the people that are you know, poverty level, they think they can offer a little bit of money. Do you think that they use you like guinea pigs?
>
> *Sara:* Yes.
>
> *Grace:* I would. I do.
>
> *Sara:* I do too.
>
> *Grace:* I wouldn't. . . . None of them experiments? You can't come to me with them. You know, cause I feel like if I'm goin. . . .
>
> *Sara:* People get killed like that. They put cocaine in them.
>
> *Grace:* You bring in all these experiments, makin people sicker. I see em, they're makin people sicker. Oh no, don't bring me that. I'll take my AZT and that's it. Do not bring me nothin else.

And a little later in the interview:

> *Paula:* That shit's toxic [AZT]. I don't believe in any kind of toxic. I don't. I watched my parents die from cancer.
>
> *Grace:* Well what's the difference? You turn around and puttin something, takin AZT? You turnin around and puttin drugs in your system?

It is clear that whether women working on the streets of New Haven are tested for HIV, and whether those who test positive receive treatment is in part shaped by their understanding of and experience with AIDS research. Furthermore, they view this research enterprise as imbued with gender, race, and class politics.

Poverty

Poverty is another important part of the social context that affects street-working women's access to and utilization of treatment. Many women on the street are not on any form of public assistance, but instead rely on sex and other forms of street work for all of their income. When Paula told me that she thought AZT was toxic, I asked if that was why she was not on it. Her friend answered for her: "She's not even on city welfare. She's got no money." "I just do what I have to do to get by," added Paula. "I gotta support a dope habit." Similarly, those women who do not receive public assistance, and even some who do, do not get regular medical care. Instead, they often rely on their stays in the women's prison for physical and gynecological exams.

Drugs such as AZT are not the only methods of caring for HIV infection. Good nutrition, reduced stress, rest, and generally healthy life-styles are also believed to enhance the quality of life for those with HIV. Women know this, but they frequently acknowledge that life on the streets makes these standards difficult to achieve. This is clearly revealed at one focus group discussion after a woman has told how she deals with the hurt of HIV by turning to the cooker.

> *Sara:* Every time you do that though, you're makin yourself sicker.
> *Grace:* Right? This is what I'm sayin.
> *Sara:* If you take AZT like you're supposed to. You get your proper rest and you eat right, you can live for a long time.
> *Grace:* How do you think I gained all that weight? I was takin care of myself. Now I'm killin myself, right?
> *Johnelle:* But if you don't have money then you can't get the kind of care. All right, cause the stress that's involved. To have a place to live.
> *Sara:* Right.
> *Johnelle:* It's just the everyday worries that come up.
> *Paula:* Big worries. Very big worries.
> *KMB:* Does that make it hard to take care of yourself?
> *Paula:* When you're out on the street. Like, I'm out on the street. And some-times I don't sleep cause their ain't nowhere to lay my head. And the places that are, man you don't want to lay down. You want to sleep with one eye open.

Later, Paula remarked: "Money would make a big difference. That's the biggest issue. You gotta choose, AZT or food." Grace agreed: "If I could turn around and work it would make me feel a lot different. I'd want to live. I'd *want* to live, you know?"

Similarly, the rigors of homelessness, which often accompanies street life, make it difficult to follow a regular drug therapy regimen, as this excerpt from my field notes reveals.

Liz tells us, "my doctor told me to try to take it [AZT] right after I got my methadone. That seems to help. Now I only throw up once every week or so instead of every day. So that's not too bad. Well, I mean, it's kind of embarrassing to be walking down the street throwing up. But hey, I've done a lot more embarrassing stuff than that in my life. And what am I gonna do?" This stops me short. I've never thought about it before but this is clearly a way that homelessness can affect your ability to take medication. Liz has to walk the streets from 7:00 in the morning until 4:30 because the shelter isn't open. So where can she get sick? (9/16/93)

She tells us that she takes her AZT twice a day. She worked this out herself. She tried different things and this works best. She can't take it all at once but if she spreads it out four times a day like they say she should, she tells us, she feels like her whole life is spent thinking about it. "I mean, every time I take one of these pills it reminds me that I have a deadly disease. I'm gonna die from this disease. And who the hell wants to think about that all the time?" she asks.

I have another insight. It's the homeless thing again. She's got to carry all of these pills around with her. She's got to find some water to take them with. She's got to remember or find out the time. It's easy for someone like me to do this. I can have a set time for these things. But what kind of a routine does Liz have?

Clearly the conditions and organization of her life made it difficult to reconcile with the requirements of early treatment, although Liz did the best that she could.

As numerous researchers have noted, poverty disproportionately affects women, particularly women of color.[11] Furthermore, feminist scholars have demonstrated both the existence of a dual welfare system, whereby women rely on AFDC and men on unemployment compensation for relief from poverty,[12] and the gender bias in the social security system, which disadvantages women for breaks in their work history and typically lower earnings than men.[13] While the women on the street have not read this work, they clearly have a similar understanding of the welfare and social security systems, as is revealed in the following discussion.

Johnelle: How about men that get SSI? Is it easier for men to get SSI?
Grace: I don't think so.
Johnelle: I know more men that got it than women, that's why I asked that.
Grace: Well, I think what it is, Johnelle, if there's more men that get it than women it's because it's more women that are not. . . .
Johnelle: I know one thing, there's a lot more groups for men than for women.

Sara: Another thing too, a lot of men have worked for years and women aren't. A lot more men are eligible. It's not exactly like SSI like we get. But SSI from where they work.

KMB: Social security?

Sara: Yeah. From where they work. That's why a lot of men get it. That's why they get their retros too. City welfare took $7,200 from me. Did they take yours?

Grace: City? Yeah. I don't even know what they took. I don't, I just let it go.

Sara: Well I know. They sent me a letter.

Grace: You know, I notice a couple of people, now that you mention it, do, they're gettin a lot of retroactive money back. A lot.

Sara: But that's because they had worked. See I said [to her male housemate], "Well how come you get your retro and I don't?" But they had worked enough where they're gettin a different type of SSI.

Grace: Yeah, it's a different one, it's a speedy one. I forgot what it's called.

The housing situation in New Haven is also gendered. More than a year ago, the only single women's shelter closed. Now there is only one shelter in the city where single women can go directly from the street, and that is a seventy-seven-bed facility with fourteen beds available to women. The other shelters in the area available to women either require a referral from a social worker or are reserved for women with children. When a grassroots organization opened a drop-in center for the homeless a few years ago, women hoped it would provide them with a place to go during the day. Although the drop-in center has been an important resource for many of the city's homeless, women on the streets do not view it as a place for them, exchanging stories with one another about feeling "oggled" and "undressed" by the men who hang out there.

In addition, the local YWCA, which housed a variety of residential programs for women and children, and where the Streets, Inc., office was located, closed down suddenly in April. Women who were in residence there talk of being thrown out on the streets. One night in June, I was doing outreach with two other women and we encountered Gerry. She has a long history of housing problems but had been working at the Y at the time it was closed. I asked her about it. "Hell yes, girl, I'm out of a job. But you'll never guess what program they saved. You'll never guess [her voice is getting louder]." "The men's program," says Liz, who is with me. "Shiiiiiit. Yes. That's it. They fuckin saved the men's program [she waves her finger for emphasis]. We wouldn't want them to be without no place to go now, would we? Shiiiiit."

It is clear women on the street understand the gendered nature of poverty and homelessness because they experience it daily. It is also clear that even as they struggle to maintain their health, their ability to do so is constrained by these conditions.

Social Isolation

HIV-positive street-working women's engagement with treatment and use of the health care system is not only determined by their ability to pay, or their experiences with the system. It also appears to depend on the degree to which they are socially connected. Grace is a good example of this. I had not known her very long in February 1992 when she commented at a focus group:

> I want to tell you somethin. I was doin good when I was hanging around and being around Johnelle and them, bein around Lois. When I stopped bein around them. When I started stayin home, I started gettin high. People started comin to my home they didn't care about all this. They didn't care about what they were doin. They come to my house, let me know they were HIV and then turn around and get off. And I wanted to say to them, "do you know what you're doing?" Course at the same time, I'm doin the same thing but I'm not lettin them know.

In the following years I got to know her well. During some periods she would do street outreach. It seemed there was not anyone on the street who didn't know her and stop to talk. One night she was too tired to come out, but as Chris and I walked around, Chris told me about a conversation they had a few days earlier in which she asked Grace why she gave so much to the group. "Well, it's like this Chris," she said. "I like feeling like I'm needed, like I have a place, a purpose." During other periods however, sometimes for several weeks, she would lock herself away in her small apartment and visit with no one. These were the times when she would miss medical appointments, stop taking her medications, and pay little attention to her own care. One night in late 1993 she emerged from such a period. This time, when we knocked on her door she opened it and gave us a warm greeting. She explained that she'd been keeping to herself but wanted to get out tonight. In the next breath, she boasted that she had been to the primary health care clinic each day that week and had two more visits scheduled in the remainder of the week. Her words recalled my experiences with Liz earlier in the summer.

Liz, who is also HIV-positive, had been living on and off the streets for about ten years. For the past several years she had not been on any form of public assistance, although she was eligible. After several months of keeping to herself, she showed up at the spot where we picked women up for meetings. She was full of energy and explained that she was coming out of "hiding" to get her life together. Her first step was to sign up for city welfare. She wanted me to get her into a women's shelter for the night so that she would be sure to make her morning meeting at the welfare office. When the shelter turned her away she was crushed. It took the hard work of several people over many more weeks to get her on welfare and subsequently enrolled in a drug treatment program.

Like Grace and Liz, there are many women on the street for whom fluctuations in their use of HIV-related medications and treatment are related to fluctuations in their degree of social connectedness. As Grace explained, when they are socially engaged they feel needed. At a meeting one time, when we were brainstorming about the kind of HIV prevention program we might develop for women on the street I asked, "What if we got money to send some street-working women to a training workshop so you could do the counseling yourselves. Would that be effective?" Sara answered, "It would educate us and make us feel we were doing something for ourselves and others." Someone else added, "If you're on your own, you ain't got nobody to care ["You don't care," Paula interrupts]. You live on the street, whatever. You might not eat for two or three days. You might not sleep for two or three days, you know? That's life." "Yeah," Sara adds, "the girls, they just don't care. What they got to live for, who they got that cares, it just don't matter, they've given up."

Conclusions

This discussion has sought to contextualize early treatment issues among women on the streets of New Haven who are considered at high risk for HIV. It suggests that many of these women have been tested for the virus and are aware that if they are positive, they can extend the length and quality of their lives by getting regular care, adopting healthy lifestyles, and taking antiretroviral drugs. Most of the women indicate that they have received this information in various pamphlets distributed at AIDS programs and other places throughout the city as well as in the counseling and testing process. This implies that educational campaigns such as those contemplated by the Task Force have already been fairly effective at getting out information and probably will continue to be so.

On the other hand, knowing what they should do does not always mean that women seek and obtain early treatment. It would be easy to attribute this to a sense of hopelessness and despair among these women. While they do express such feelings, they also show an incredible will and ability to survive. Ironically, it has sometimes been this desire to live that has kept them from seeking early treatment, as became clear to me when I first started talking about early treatment issues to women three years ago. Grace told me: "See, Kim, one time there was, when they turn around and it first came up about AIDS, it was AIDS and AIDS-Related Complex (ARC). That's all we knew about. And they showed on television, not people with HIV, they showed people with AIDS crumpled up in bed. That's all they showed. So therefore, 'I'm gonna look like that? I wanna die. I wanna die. Bring me the drugs and let me kill myself. Cause I don't want to walk around the streets. I'm a woman. I don't want to look like that walkin around.' I mean, you see people with big sores on their face and like I said, all crumbled up in the bed. That's all we knew about." Later, her words were confirmed in a discussion with Sara.

> *Sara:* A lot of people have it in their mind that it's [AZT] not going to help anyway.
> *Grace:* It's not gonna help. They might feel like I did in the beginning that "Hey, I'm playing the guinea pig and this is being prolonged and I don't want to prolong it."
> Sara: And I'm gonna die anyways.
> *Johnelle:* I remember when you were saying that. Yep.
> *Lois:* [emphatically] Oh Lord, I want to live as long as I can.
> *Grace:* I hear you.

As women have become aware of the distinction between HIV and AIDS, their desire to live and get treated has increased as well. Nevertheless, this analysis has suggested that their ability to do so is shaped by the social context of gender, class, and race inequality in which they live. In particular, this paper has discussed three aspects of this context that shape treatment-related behaviors of women on the street: the enterprise of producing AIDS research and knowledge, conditions of street life and poverty, and social isolation.

The policy implications of these findings should be clear. AIDS related research must be conducted responsibly and AIDS researchers should be responsive and accountable to the communities about and in which they study. Indeed, researchers should develop research priorities that are consistent with the priorities of those affected by the virus. Although educational campaigns might form one component of an early treatment intervention, they must be supplemented with programs that build on and expand connections among women and provide them with the resources and opportunities they need to be able to better act on their knowledge of the advantages of early treatment.

NOTES

1. Karolynn Seigel, Martin P. Levine, Charles Brooks, and Rochelle Kern, "The Motives of Gay Men for Taking or Not Taking the HIV Antibody Test," *Social Problems* 36, no. 4 (October 1989): 368–83; "Report of an Expert Panel on the Public Health Laboratory Role in Early Intervention and Treatment of Human Immunodeficiency Virus Infections," *Public Health Reports* 106, no. 1 (January-February 1991): 27–31.

2. Jeanette R. Ickovics, Allison C. Morrill, Susan E. Beren, Unjali Walsh, and Judith Rodin, "Limited Effects of HIV Counseling and Testing for Women: A Prospective Study of Behavioral and Psychological Consequences," *Journal of the American Medical Association* 272, no. 6 (August 1994): 443–48.

3. For reviews of this literature see Marshall H. Becker and Jill G. Joseph, "AIDS and Behavioral Change to Reduce Risk: A Review," *American Journal of Public Health* 78, no. 4 (April 1988): 394–410; and Jeffrey D. Fisher and William A. Fisher, "Changing AIDS-Risk Behavior," *Psychological Bulletin* 111, no. 3 (1992): 455–74.

4. For reviews see Donna L. Higgins, Christine Galavotti, Kevin R. O'Reilly, Daniel J. Schnell, Melinda Moore, Deborah Rugg, and Robert Johnson, "Evidence for the Effects of HIV Antibody Counseling and Testing on Risk Behaviors," *Journal of the American Medical Association* 266, no. 17 (November 1991): 2419–29; Ickovics et al.; and Donald A. Calsyn, Andrew J. Saxon, George Freeman, Jr., and Stephen Whittaker, "Ineffectiveness of AIDS Education and HIV Antibody Testing in Reducing High-Risk Behaviors among Injection Drug Users," *American Journal of Public Health* 82, no. 4 (April 1992): 573–75.

5. Eleanor Maticka-Tyndale, "Social Construction of HIV Transmission and Prevention among Heterosexual Young Adults," *Social Problems* 39, no. 3 (August 1992): 238–52.

6. Ickovics et al.; Seigel et al.; Ted Myers, Kevin W. Orr, David Locker, and Edward A. Jackson, "Factors Affecting Gay and Bisexual Men's Decisions and Intentions to Seek HIV Testing," *American Journal of Public Health* 83, no. 5 (May 1993): 701–4.

7. Fisher and Fisher.

8. Cited in Heather G. Miller, Charles F. Turner, and Lincoln E. Moses, eds., *AIDS: The Second Decade* (Washington, D.C.: National Academy Press, 1990).

9. A. Siobhan Thompson, Kim M. Blankenship, Jerre Winfrey, Frederick A. Altice, and Peter A. Selwyn, "Improving Health Care Utilization and Access for Drug-Using Women with or at Risk for HIV Infection in a Correctional Facility and at Needle Exchange Sites," HIV Infection in Women Conference: Setting a New Agenda, Washington, D.C., Abstract no. WB3–68, 1995.

10. Jeffrey H. Samet, Howard Libman, Kathleen A. Steger, Rajeev K. Dhawan, John Chen, Abby H. Shevitz, Rebecca Dewees-Dunk, Suzette Levenson, Donald Kufe, and Donald E. Craven, "Compliance with Zidovudine Therapy in Patients Infected with Human Immunodeficiency Virus, Type 1: A Cross-Sectional Study in a Municipal Hospital Clinic," *American Journal of Medicine* 92 (May 1992): 495–502.

11. Diana Pearce, "Welfare Is Not *for* Women: Why the War on Poverty Cannot Conquer the Feminization of Poverty," in *Women, the State and Welfare,* ed. Linda Gordon (Madison: University of Wisconsin Press, 1990); Ruth Sidel, *Women and Children Last: The Plight of Poor Women in Affluent America* (New York: Viking, 1986); Maxine Baca Zinn, "Family, Race, and Poverty in the Eighties," *SIGNS: Journal of Women in Culture and Society* 14, no. 4 (Summer 1989): 856–74.

12. Diana Pearce, 1990.

13. Dorothy C. Miller, *Women and Social Welfare: A Feminist Analysis* (New York: Praeger, 1992).

Part III

Working (through) Solutions

15

Healing from Within: Women, HIV/AIDS, and the African-American Church

Reverend Carol Johnson

Reverend Carol Johnson founded Harvard AIDS Ministries in 1992 while a student at Harvard Divinity School. Since its inception, Harvard AIDS Ministries has served 11,000 people by creating forums where partnerships might emerge between religiously, culturally, linguistically, sexually, spiritually, and intellectually diverse groups of people. Reverend Johnson has used curriculum development, AIDS prevention and education training, and HIV/AIDS training of trainers to include youth and other peer/affinity groups. Reverend Johnson brings to her work significant expertise in curriculum development and facilitation of training on issues of diversity, sex education, and dismantling homophobia, sexism, and other internalized oppression. She has been a sex educator (for 20+ years), a gay/lesbian/bisexual advocate (for 17+ years), and an HIV/AIDS educator and advocate (for 12+ years). Recently she helped create the national forum for African-American religious leaders, which is preparing churches in five pilot cities for the first National Black Week of Prayer for the Healing of AIDS. She has also expanded her efforts to include human rights advocacy for lesbians, women with HIV/AIDS, and adolescents. She is currently working on a master of divinity degree at Harvard Divinity School, where she has been a William Fellow.

I am an African-American woman who has been working on issues related to women's reproductive health since 1973, sexuality and sexual orientation since 1977, and HIV/AIDS since 1983. I began my studies at Harvard Divinity School (HDS) in 1991 to learn how to do ministry in the age of AIDS. At that time, there was one course which addressed AIDS directly (which was largely focused on the issues of men): an exhaustive search of our course catalogue and that of the Boston Theological Institute quickly revealed that it was, in fact, the only act in town.

Little about HIV/AIDS, let alone women and HIV/AIDS, had been incorporated into the standard curricula governing theological preparation for ministers, despite the fact that the pandemic was raging and that increasing numbers of women on both sides of the pulpit were begin to feel the impact of AIDS in their congregations, their communities, and their personal lives. I, along with a small handful of other students and administrators, responded by founding Harvard AIDS Ministries in 1992. We began to undertake some of the responsibility for identifying the gaps, assessing which tools, skills, and discourses were needed, and fashioning training for ourselves and other seminary students. I also served, and continue to serve, as a resource person who provides curriculum development, training and research, and other services for churches and other religious institutions locally, nationally, and internationally.

My decision to focus on African-American women in this chapter and to address it to the African-American church is based on a number of factors. I refer here not only to the disproportionate numbers of African-American women who are represented in AIDS statistics, where they are currently estimated to account for 50–55 percent of all women in the U.S. with HIV, but also to a revelation I had some years ago.

Shortly after I began studying at HDS I had the opportunity to be one of several facilitators at an HIV/AIDS prevention training for African-American women. While the standard safer-sex dialogue common to HIV/AIDS prevention and education tends to presume relational dynamics which are equitable, communicative, and free of any of the difficulty or embarrassment that often characterizes our actual efforts to negotiate sex, it became increasingly clear that the women in this training did not necessarily link the experience of safety with sexuality. Moreover, this point came home not only in this particular training, but in other subsequent training with women participants as well. In fact, it became clear whenever and wherever the full spectrum of women's experiences was acknowledged.

On this first occasion, we began a dialogue to try to explore our discomfort with the linkage of these terms by asking a simple question: What reasons did we and other women have for having sex? The brainstorming session that followed produced a series of discoveries about the complexity of the development of our sexual lives that rendered standard safer-sex dialogue moot. While safe sex presumes consensuality, our actual sexual experiences tended to run along a continuum from consensual to coerced sexual encounters. Sometimes women reported having sex for pleasure, companionship, to make babies, and for love. Far too often, however, women reported having sex for economic survival (survival sex), for status, to avoid being labeled a lesbian, for drugs, to prevent a partner from becoming violent with them or their children, or as a result of rape or incest.

As these conversations evolved it became apparent to me that churches and other religious institutions intending to develop AIDS ministries for African-American women infected with or affected by HIV/AIDS needed to sensitize themselves to issues around gender, power, and sexuality; moreover, I could see that if they were really intent on lessening the reality of women's vulnerability to HIV infection, they needed to attempt to grapple with the issues of drug abuse, incest, family and community violence, and child abuse. Despite the enormity of these needs, ministries are faced with a real dearth of theological reflection on the moral, ethical, and social justice issues which attend to African-American women and HIV/AIDS. My intention here is not only to alert readers to some of these specific issues, but to point out how an AIDS ministry can be developed which takes into account the continuum of experiences and needs of people infected with and affected by HIV/AIDS.

The African-American Christian church, along with other significant religious institutions (i.e., Islam) has long had a foundational role in the black community regardless of whether community members are churched or not. Traditionally it has been at the forefront of efforts for social justice and compassionate healing responses to a variety of issues and crises: These include dismantling Jim Crow, organizing the civil rights movement, securing the rights of African-Americans to vote, working on behalf of African-American economic development, inaugurating literacy programs and other educational initiatives, and countering the devastating impact of the Contract "with" America.

Thus the silences in our churches around HIV/AIDS seemed peculiar to many of us and appalling to most of us. Whereas the leadership body of the primary African-American religious institutions have been slow to respond to AIDS, other Black organizations have more readily responded to the challenges of the pandemic: Witness New York City's Harlem Week of Prayer for the Healing of AIDS (the initiative of The Balm in Gilead, which does educational programs and brochures around AIDS). Witness Ark of Refuge, Inc., in San Francisco and H.E.A.L., Inc., in Virginia, both AIDS ministries that developed in response to the pandemic. The Southern

Christian Leadership Conference not only implemented an AIDS program, but also formed a special initiative for African-American women with HIV/AIDS.

Other initiatives that respond to the HIV/AIDS pandemic specifically as it affects the African-American community, but which are not specifically religious or spiritual in intent and focus include the National Black Women's Health Project, Atlanta's Sisterlove Inc., and Diana Diana's Beauty Salon Project in South Carolina (where the local beauty shop functions as a center for the dissemination of information, educational materials, and protection). What is significant about all of these organizations is that they are spiritually focused or have a spiritual context, and that they attempt to acknowledge in culturally sensitive, appropriate, and significant ways the necessity of tailoring their education and prevention efforts to African-American women and their significant others.

We as African-American community are forever indebted to people such as Rev. René McCoy and Rev. Carl Beam (now Bishop Beam), the founders and elders in the Unity Fellowship Church. As AIDS began its devastating impact in the African-American and other communities of color, they valiantly led the development of powerful AIDS ministerial responses in Harlem and in San Francisco. During these early days, these two and others also joined with organizations such as the National Coalition of Black Lesbians and Gays, which created forums with public health officials and sought to beseech and engage our reluctant African-American church bodies to fashion active and compassionate responses to the emerging HIV/AIDS epidemic in the United States and the pandemic among Africans all over the Diaspora.

Thankfully, African-American religious institutions in the nineties have begun to come together to create a unified response to HIV/AIDS. Witness again the remarkable progress that has been made. In early 1994, under the leadership of a remarkable women, Pernessa Seele, fifty-one African-American religious leaders were invited to meet at a White House summit to sign an African-American Clergy's Declaration of War on HIV/AIDS.

This African-American National Clergy Summit brought together the leaders of every religious denomination, and represented 22 million Black Americans. Additionally, there have since been two national Black church training institutes and conferences around HIV/AIDS, and there is an annual Black Church Day of Prayer for the Healing of AIDS on the first

Sunday of March. I offer these few examples because the prevailing myths hold that African-Americans, and particularly our religious institutions, have failed to respond to HIV/AIDS in our communities. But the last decade in particular has produced a number of resources that are available for individuals, organizations and seminarians.

Many people going into the ministry, and many of those who are already ordained, think they know about AIDS. But what's understood—the cultural agreement—is that AIDS is a disease, when actually it's not: AIDS is a syndrome, and that means that there's a continuum of needs and experiences within that syndrome—people, both infected and affected, waiting all along that line with different and sometimes overlapping needs and experiences. For example, in the early stages of Acquired Immune Deficiency Syndrome, the "worried well" (women who have not been diagnosed but who know that they may have put themselves at risk) may need pastoral counseling and education, while those who acknowledge that they may have been exposed to someone who was (or possibly was) HIV+ may need to explore the possibilities of taking the HIV antibody test. Women who have been diagnosed and who have begun experiencing opportunistic infections may need pastoral visits, food, and advocacy for everything from health care to housing. At every point along the spectrum, women need pastoral acknowledgment from the pulpit and spiritual support around a variety of issues: grieving, death, shame, renewal. They also need support for their families and acknowledgment of their significant relationships, whether they be with men, women, or both.

This chapter is not intended as an exhaustive or comprehensive accounting of the complexity of issues that must be addressed. Rather, it is my intent to suggest that there are as many forms of AIDS ministries as there are people to design them. The most important thing is that those of us preparing for ministry begin to educate ourselves about the basic scientific facts, think through what our compassionate and ministerial responses might be (whatever our points of theological departure may be), and most importantly, that we start somewhere, however small. Starting where we are and building what we can will both hearten us and help to fuel the critical development of theological systems that provide the connective and cohesive bond that is so desperately needed. Our efforts will not only help us to minister to those infected with and affected by HIV/AIDS in our congregations and communities; it will also allow us to adopt a more active voice in the policy development and political processes which drive AIDS funding, research, medical services, and support initiatives.

In closing, I would like to acknowledge the difficulty in broaching these questions in communities which have traditionally maintained many silences, particularly around sex, sexuality, homosexuality, and gender issues. Further, the communities we serve, and the women who are impacted by HIV and AIDS, are already overwhelmed with critical health, medical, economic, educational, public health, and criminal justice challenges that also require our immediate and focused attention.

The most important fact about HIV is that it is preventable. And the most effective "vaccine" with which we can lessen the vulnerability of women to HIV infection is education, especially that which occurs within a context that recognizes and takes advantage of our rich spiritual heritage, our historical experiences in mobilizing our communities through our religious institutions, and a shift in consciousness and paradigm that disman-tles the disparate treatment that we as African-American women experience almost everywhere.

Despite the challenges—and there are many—HIV/AIDS is not greater than God, and our faith communities can be powerful bridges to healing for women infected with and affected by HIV/AIDS. There are effective models for prevention and spiritually based education that cover a range of perspectives and skill levels, and which are readily available. I have developed a model for thinking about and developing AIDS ministries (see figure 1).

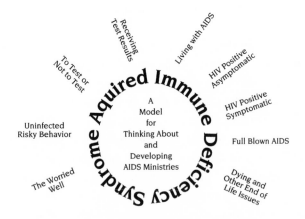

After AIDS: Families, Caregivers, and Communities
"A Model for Thinking About and Developing AIDS Ministries"©1992 Harvard AIDS Ministries

This model, "A Model for Thinking About and Developing AIDS Ministries," is designed to effectively acknowledge and speak to a wide range of perspectives and skill levels. The model is very flexible, and we have effectively utilized it to create training and other forums in environments as diverse as HIV/AIDS education at the George Meany Center of Labor Union Studies, the United Nations Fourth World Conference of Women in Beijing, China (AIDS/HIV and Women Track), and the State of New Mexico's HIV/AIDS and Spiritual Paths Conference. We have also worked in collaboration with the AFL-CIO Department of Education to modify the model for a series of HIV/AIDS training they conducted in South Africa.

I have included a selective resource list which may help you as you continue and/or begin your journey of ministering in the age of AIDS. May God bless, inspire and keep you in your endeavors.

RESOURCES LIST

Reverend Carol A. Johnson
Founder and Executive Director
Harvard AIDS Ministries
c/o Parker Street
Boston, MA 02138
(617) 427–8840 voice and fax (phone first)
email: cjohnson@div.harvard.edu

The U.S. Department of Public Health
Centers for Disease Control and Prevention
National AIDS Clearinghouse
Religious Resource Data Base
(800) 458–5231

The Balm in Gilead Institute for Minority AIDS Prevention Studies
130 West 42nd Street
Suite 1300
New York, NY 10036

Rollins School of Public Health
Emory University
1518 Clifton Road, N.E.
Atlanta, GA 30322
(404) 727–8742

Kendall Institute
130 Clarendon Street
Boston, MA 02119

The Ark of Refuge
3814 MacArthur Blvd.
Oakland, CA 94619
(415) 788–1240

Catholic Charities USA
1731 King Street
Alexandra, VA 22314
(713) 549–1390

H.E.A.L., Inc.
10155 Merrimack
Richmond, VA 23235
(804) 771–5873

The Lesbian AIDS Project
129 West 20th Street, 2nd Floor
New York, NY 10011
(212) 337–3531

National Red Cross
African American HIV/AIDS Programs
2025 E. Street, NE
Washington, DC
(202) 728–6693

Global NetWork of People Living With AIDS (GNP +)
KEIZERSGRACHT
390–3921016GB
Amsterdam

AFL-CIO Department of Education
816 16th Street, NW
Washington, DC
(202) 637–5331

International Community of Women Living With AIDS
c/o Positively
P.O. Box 11535
Oakland, CA
(510) 658–6930

Coalition of Labor Union Women
1126 16th Street, NW

Washington, DC 20036
(202) 296–1200

Unity Fellowship Church
5149 W. Jefferson Blvd.
Los Angeles, CA 90016
(213) 936–4948

Essence Magazine
1500 Broadway
New York, NY 10036
ESSENCEonline@nyo.com

Black Women's Health Book: Speaking for Ourselves
Seal Press, 1990

Consultants Unlimited
3753 N. 5th Street
Milwaukee, WI 53212
(414) 372–8810

Black Coalition on AIDS
1042 Divisa dero Street
San Francisco, CA 94115
(415) 346–6037

Numerous AIDS, AIDS Ministerial, and AIDS and African-American resources can be found on the World Wide Web (WWW) by searching in WWW, Gopher, and IRC environments. Consult your local computer administrator or contact me at the address, phone/fax, and email address listed above. Light, Love, and Blessing to you all.

16

The Bond Is Called Blackness:
Black Women and AIDS

Sheila Battle

Sheila Battle is a medical social worker with the San Francisco Department of Public Health. Currently she works with HIV-positive African-American families. Ms. Battle's writing has been featured previously in *The Black Women's Health Book,* edited by Evelyn C. White, in the article entitled "Moving Targets: Alcohol, Crack, and Black Women." Ms. Battle has been a social worker for many years working with the elderly, troubled teens, communities, families, and women addicted to crack.

Black women represent the largest growing population infected with AIDS. "In 1993, AIDS and other related HIV infections became the leading cause of death among Black women ages 25 to 44," according to CDC Reports on Morbidity and Mortality, 1993. Unfortunately, this disturbing trend seems fated to continue because of a general lack of concern at the national and local levels of government about Black health issues. If there is to be a change in these statistics, we in the Black community must begin to educate our own, and develop our own programs. And if there is to be a change in the services available to women around HIV issues, we will have to fight that battle as well: At the meeting I recently attended with other HIV service providers in San Francisco to discuss allocation of monies slated for HIV programs, they allocated only 5 percent of these monies for HIV women's programs.

For the past year, I have worked with the Sister Care Project, which was designed by a pediatric medical doctor who felt that Black women should receive prenatal care and antiviral drugs without being committed to clinical trails. Sister Care, which works in collaboration with a program that specializes in providing services to all pregnant and postpartum HIV-positive women and their children, specializes in providing prenatal medical services to pregnant/postpartum African-American HIV positive women. I and several of my colleagues coined the name Sister Care, which means sisters taking care of sisters.

Because so many women I work with have a history of chronic homelessness, use multiple drugs, and have their own communities—the people on the street—we designed Sister Care to let the client choose where she wants to receive prenatal care. In essence, we take our program to the client and provide comprehensive medical/social services. Since most AIDS programs focus on gay men or other populations, Sister Care has been long overdue. I hope that it will open eyes about the tremendous needs for more HIV women's programs.

AIDS has had an unacknowledged affect on Blacks. The attitude that "Blacks don't get AIDS—gays do" has caused much shame, grief, and long-term suffering for those infected with HIV and their loved ones in the African-American community. But this kind of denial cannot dispel national statistics that state that the African-American population is the fastest-growing AIDS-infected population in America in the 1990s and may represent a staggering 50 percent of new reported cases.

Women in Sister Care

The Black women I work with are the hearts and souls of our community. Like all Black women, they are daughters, wives, sisters, lovers, and mothers. Most are between the ages of twenty-five and forty-five. A large percentage of Sister Care clients dropped out of high school in ninth or tenth grade. For many, drugs have been a part of their lives for more than fifteen years. Alcohol, heroin, crack, and amphetamines have numbed their painful life experiences. Most have been involved with the criminal justice system for ten years or more. Then there are the psychological problems: severe depression, organic problems, post-traumatic stress disorder, and anxiety disorders that at times make it difficult to distinguish a mental-health problem from a drug-induced psychological problem.

Most have been arrested for petty theft, drug sales, and prostitution. Along with street life come the uncontrollable forces of beating and rapes. The scars and marks on their body symbolizes their victimization. Thus, they look many years older than their age. Over 80 percent have had five or more children.

Because so many of these women suffer from being abused both mentally and physically by family members, friends, and lovers, abuse is now an intimate part of all their relationships. Domestic violence is a force that controls these women's lives even more than drugs do. They stay in physically abusive relationships because of fear, insecurity, depression, etc. Domestic violence increases when a woman is pregnant. According to information from the March of Dimes, "between seven percent and 20% of women report physical or sexual violence during pregnancy and women who are battered while pregnant are more likely to report alcohol and drug use during pregnancy than non-battered pregnant women." Equally significant is the number of women who stay because the males in their lives are supplying their drugs or using with them.

Incest and domestic violence often intertwine since women who suffer incest learn to accept others' abnormal behavior while suffering in silence. More than 90 percent of women who were molested as children have never sought therapy to deal with the incest. More than 80 percent of survivors of child sexual abuse have had their own children taken away by Child Protective Services (CPS). Women who choose to change are frequently frustrated and give up because CPS requirements are often too stringent; I have met few (CPS) social workers in my professional career who truly have their clients' interests at heart.

In this population, pursuits such as housing, food, and drugs take precedence over medical care, which is sought only during pregnancy. In fact, this is how some of our clients learn they're HIV-positive—because they come in for prenatal services. Their diagnosis means that they must now deal with the triple burden of an AIDS diagnosis, an unplanned pregnancy, and a drug addiction. Because a large percent of these women do not have regular medical checkups and many have long histories of drug use, they present with various medical problems—such as high blood pressure, heart problems, sexually transmitted diseases, and other infections. At times these medical problems pose a risk for the unborn child. And then there is the virus itself: The mother can transmit HIV to her infant during pregnancy, labor, delivery, and breast feeding. The risk of prenatal transmission seems greater at times when there is a high level of HIV reproduction or viral actually in the mother's blood (i.e., during the first one to six months of infection and at later stages of the disease.)

Most newborns fare well healthwise. These infants mainly have problems withdrawing from methadone and other drugs. For infants who test positive "many demonstrate a failure to thrive—they do not gain weight or grow normally. Infected children are often slow to reach important milestones in motor skills and mental development such as crawling, walking and speaking. As the disease progresses, many children with AIDS have neurologic problems such as difficulty walking, poor school performances, seizures, mental retardation and cerebral palsy." In essence, infants who test positive for AIDS develop symptoms related to HIV by their first birthdays. The HIV culture test and/or the polymerase chain reactive test (PCR) are currently used to test newborns or infants. If both of these tests are negative, then the PG24 antigen test is used to be certain antibodies are not present in the infant's blood.

It's unfortunate that very few of our clients seek prenatal care in the second trimester, when the antiviral drugs can be most effective in preventing the risk of HIV transmission from mother to newborn. According to the February 1994 results from the National Institute of Health (NIH) AIDS Clinical Trials 076, zidovudine (ZDV or AZT) can reduce prenatal HIV transmission by as much as two-thirds (1.6), so ZDV has the potential to substantially reduce the rate of perinatal transmission. I am an advocate for AZT during pregnancy, but currently many Blacks practice home folk remedies and others have a lack of trust in the medical system. In addition, many Blacks don't like taking medications for prolonged periods, while others have heard horror stories about AZT—the side effects can be horrendous and can make you terribly sick. Given these obstacles, I think it's vitally important that there be more education in the Black community about AZT and pregnancy—especially since growing numbers of childbearing women are being infected—if the community's resistance to AZT is to be overcome. Such education is a means to provide other options to the belief that "God will take care of it."

Currently, mandatory HIV testing for all pregnant women is being debated nationally and locally. I feel that a pregnant woman should be presented with information about HIV testing, then allowed to make the decision to test or not. There shouldn't be any mandates that says you must do this or that. Such an attitude will definitely keep women from seeking care. Furthermore, I feel that the ultimate purpose of such a mandate would be to convince the entire population that everyone should be HIV-tested—just starting with vulnerable pregnant women first.

Family Relationships

Most women we met through Sister Care have been detached or abandoned from family members, who express anger, shame, fear, resentment, and hurt because of our clients' lifestyles. There are no phone calls or visits. Tensions are not decreased by the fact that family members are often responsible for rearing many of my clients' children. In the Black community it's important to keep children within the family system with their siblings, so these children are cared for by grandparents, uncles, aunts, and cousins. (Although many of my clients have had no contact with their children, they still have that glow that all parents have when talking about their children.) When a parent is absent from a child's life, that child suffers emotionally and spiritually—and children may be confused about their parents' fate. A high percentage of these children were born exposed to drugs before birth and may be experiencing some long-term psychological and physical problems, which most families are not equipped to deal with. Family members' ignorance results from a lack of education about AIDS or denial. Often, in speaking to me, family members have said that my clients (their relatives) "brought it on themselves."

The People in the Street

Because family relationships no longer work, these women have developed other family network systems that comfort, support, and help them. Their new family represents a mixture of drugs, happiness, sorrow, life, death, acceptance, and love—unconditional love. Our society tends to validate only family-system relationships, but it's important to validate and accept input from street family members as well.

I have worked many years with substance-abusing pregnant women who mainly used crack. For some, pregnancy is a time to reflect and make needed positive life changes. It's what finally got their attention: Some sought drug treatment programs, some found permanent housing, and others left abusive relationships. But this is only true of a small percentage: Very few women who are HIV-positive and pregnant stop using drugs. Some of these women don't return to see their babies after delivery because their attention is immediately back to the streets and to their community. I often wonder if their response is denial, shame, or guilt. Maybe it has something to do with the stigma society attaches to a woman who has a baby that could be HIV-positive, who uses drugs, and who has had multiple births. Whatever the reason, positive change is slow.

Racism/Discrimination

For centuries racism, discrimination, and oppression have been a fundamental part of American society's major institutions. Neither the criminal justice system nor medical institutions are any exception. In fact, Blacks may have experienced more institutionalized racism at medical institutions—a notion supported by the Tuskegee syphilis study, among others. Historically Blacks didn't utilize medical institutions because too often services were outside of their communities, waiting time could reach hours, and they didn't want to deal with being disrespected by medical staff for not understanding medical terminology. This still holds true for many in the Black community, where it's common knowledge that word of mouth represents the best way of finding out which medical facilities provide services with respect.

The way in which a medical provider reaches out to a client has a very real impact on the success or failure of the relationship they have with one another. My expertise has been working with a community-based hospital with poor pregnant and postpartum women who mainly are Black. I have worked with medical providers who are respectful to their clients and who take the time to reach out and engage them. In these situations there were many positive outcomes, such as women who came into prenatal care regularly and women who went home with their babies. On the other hand, I have observed medical staff be rude and make derogatory statements about clients: "Why is she having another baby?" "Why don't she have an abortion?" "Who will take care of this baby?" As a Black professional, I have also been mistreated at times by medical staff who have been rude and disrespectful, often disregarding my opinion about clients that I have a bond with—a bond called Blackness. I have also observed medical staff with have a strong internal drive to save and deliver their Black clients—people who essentially give something to the Black community while maintaining a superior attitude over the Black professional staff they work with. When medical staff is disrespectful even to professional staff members, I think it's fair to begin to question their ability to relate to and serve poor clients. It's unfortunate that medical and nursing schools can't seem to shake racist and prejudiced attitudes. Whether verbal or nonverbal, attitude has a tremendous effect on whether a client continues to seek care.

We as people all have our conscious and unconscious beliefs about others, but they must not interfere with our work with people. I believe that all hospitals and medical clinics should have a written protocol regarding treatment for AIDS patients, that information between service providers must be accompanied with a signed release by the client, and that in all situations the client should disclose his or her HIV status.

Social and Economic Issues

In a society where money, status, and finances determine who will participate in the political arena, women's issues and concerns are given little consideration overall. This means that my clients, given their particularly poor financial status and sparse resources, have virtually no voice. They are poor and uneducated, and according to society's rules they don't contribute anything. Historically, Black community leaders advocated for civil rights, jobs, better housing, and education, but AIDS is still not a high enough priority in the contemporary Black community, which already faces a multitude of other problems: drugs, Black-on-Black crime, jobs, teenage pregnancy, and education.

In the early eighties the government declared AIDS in the white gay male community a public health issue, but it has failed to extend that recognition to AIDS and Black women. The gay white male community responded to the AIDS crisis by building an empire of services in their own community with resources, money, and committed people in large numbers. Although many Blacks may feel that this mobilization couldn't happen in the Black community—IT CAN! We have the money in our community to develop our own services. We just need committed Black people in large numbers.

Because the women in Sister Care don't have the advocating power to demand services we, as service providers and community leaders, must be that voice that provides insight about HIV and women's issues to our local and national governments. We must demand money for HIV women's research programs and to develop effective programs in communities with the greatest needs. We need more programs like Sister Care that are willing to go where the client chooses to receive medical services. These programs must include medical services, social services, mental health counseling, and nutritional services, and it is important that service providers work as a group. Working with Sister Care clients, many of whom present with multitudes of problems, we have seen that staff can burn out quickly.

New Ideas

Traditional drug treatment programs do not work for the Sister Care population because these women have lived on the street for such a long time and in chaos. Often the rules and policies of traditional drug treatment programs—no phone calls for sixty days, time limits, and the program's daily scheduled activities—are too difficult for these women to adjust to; consequently, they are discharged prematurely. Well-created and well-administered drug treatment is crucial at this juncture: Accepting the reality of being HIV-positive or having a child that could be HIV-positive adds additional stress to some clients' lives, while other residents fear that they or their children may become infected with AIDS-related problems. In these stressful situations, I have suggested that an AIDS workshop be conducted to ease the fears of staff members and residents. This is only done if the client wants to share her HIV status. Finally, well-planned and well-administered intervention is crucial at this time because this may be the last opportunity for these women to have custody of their children.

My concept of a drug treatment program for Sister Care clients is a treatment program that is less structured around rules, policies, and daily activities, while focussing more on a three-month adjustment phase. This stretch of time is vital in giving women an opportunity to adjust to a new lifestyle and new environment. Four hours a day would be devoted to drug treatment, counseling, parenting skills, and life skills.

Other Black Women with HIV

As a social worker, friend, and volunteer, I have worked with other Black women with HIV. While doing street outreach in the Tenderloin area of San Francisco, I met Black women from all economic backgrounds and ages who were HIV-infected. Most of these women were drug addicts and were receiving no medical or social services. A large percentage of them had full-blown AIDS when they received their AIDS test results, with CD4 counts of less than 200. Many had become infected through prostitution, sharing needles, or heterosexual sex. Thus, my goal became to get them into needed services. I would develop friendships with them on a first-name basis, which broke down any barriers between us. Each week I would take a little more time to talk their language and listen to them. Eventually some did seek medical services, social services, and drug treatment services. It's so important when doing street outreach that you have your resource manual and condoms with you, and that you're nonjudgmental about anything you observe.

I have also worked with Black professional women who are HIV-infected. These women are very hard to work with because they're in the mainstream of the Black community. They are independent and pay their own way. Furthermore, they think this shouldn't be happening to them because they haven't participated in what they think of as truly high-risk behaviors: sharing needles, having sex with bisexual men, or prostitution. Many of these women became infected through heterosexual sex. Their denial and fear are so strong that they often struggle with this disease alone. Some die without telling anyone of their HIV status. Those who do tell family members or friends often regret doing so. "They [my family] are afraid of me now; they don't want to catch it." Their one source of comfort is their doctor.

I have also worked with mothers, aunts, and grandmothers—older Black women who are HIV-positive. These women are immobilized by their fear, shame, denial and guilt, often so much that they won't consider telling anybody that they are HIV-positive—no spouse, children, or other family members. Furthermore, they don't want any health education or AIDS information. Their denial is so strong that it can take two to five years to break. Like their professional sisters, they also experience their doctor as their only source of comfort.

My question becomes, How do we motivate these women to take responsibility for their lives and move on? Changes in the situations that these women face along with other Blacks with AIDS will only happen when Black leaders, Black ministers, and Black doctors begin to address AIDS issues from the pulpit and at community forums. I have seen small changes in some Blacks' attitudes about AIDS, but this increased acceptance of people with AIDS has only come about because so many family members have died of HIV.

In the Black community, the Black church has been one long-standing institution that has provided Blacks with identity and a sense of ownership. It has provided spirituality, comfort, and education. The traditional Black church has changed to meet the diverse needs of today's Blacks. The church of today is involved in youth programs, drug counseling, and services for the elders. It's now time for the Black church to become involved with AIDS.

I have a vision of several Black churches coming together and building a huge AIDS center. This center would serve as a model nationally as well as a model for other Black communities to develop AIDS programs.

In this center these services would be offered:

Spiritual healing
Inpatient drug treatment
Outpatient drug treatment
Health education/outreach program
Medical services
Social services
Groups for AIDS patients
Groups for family members
Counseling
Food program
Research
Prevention materials
Acupuncture
Legal services

At this center, we would love and embrace people with AIDS while learning to deal with our fears, denial, and shame through AIDS education. Professional staff such as social workers, drug counselors, AIDS educators, grant writers, researchers, child care workers, doctors, nurses, lawyers, and outreach workers would be hired from within the community. This center would also be staffed with volunteers from the church. Once trained, mothers, deacons, ministers, and elders would provide the love, nurturing, and acceptance that people with AIDS desperately need.

Blacks have faced many obstacles since slavery, and we have overcome each roadblock successfully by fighting back, standing up for each other, sticking together, and having our own agenda. Never before have we been faced with such a challenge as the one we have before us now: AIDS. In the past we have gotten our strength through leaning on the Lord. It's time to refuel our strength once more and begin to fight AIDS.

17

Coming to Their Own Rescue: Teens Teach Teens about HIV

Nina Brand

Nina Brand, LICSW, coordinates the AIDS Teen Team at the New North Citizens' Council in Springfield, Mass., and is a former volunteer supervisor for YO' Line, a teen-run hotline for youth with HIV/AIDS concerns based at the AIDS Action Committee in Boston. She also presently works as an outpatient therapist for a community counseling center.

"Can you get pregnant through oral sex?" I was asked by a 15 year old on the AIDS Teen Team, a peer education program that is part of the New North Citizens' Council, located in the predominantly Latino North End neighborhood of Springfield, Massachusetts. I had been the AIDS Teen Team coordinator for only a couple of months and was new to the program, the agency, and the community. And I was astonished by the question.

In keeping with our Team policy that no question is a stupid question, I tried to contain my surprise, but that became more difficult as several other Team members looked at me with expressions of "I don't know even though I'm a know-it-all," apparently awaiting the answer to this inquiry. I had thought one of the other teens might jump in, as they most often do, eager to show off their knowledge and verbalize their opinions. Silence. . . .

I guess I had thought that because these teens were choosing to participate in an HIV/AIDS educational program, they would come prepared with accurate information on physiology, biology, and sex. But I was wrong. So together we outlined where we needed to begin. We started with a discussion about where, besides this program, they had learned about subjects such as sex, sexuality, and reproduction. Then they reaffirmed their goal of making such information easily available to other teens. (And that was when I began to recognize my goal: that one day they'd put language to their understanding of the interconnection of access to information and resources and various forms of oppression.)

There were other surprises too, like finding out that several of the members of the AIDS Teen Team who are drawn to the program each year, which runs on an academic calendar, have motives other than an interest in HIV/AIDS for joining. Some speak of wanting the stipend that is awarded to participants while others talk of needing something to do after school because the streets are scary or things at home aren't going well and they need a place to hang out. In my first two years coordinating the program, I've had a hard time rejecting any enthusiastic teen. If, a few weeks into the program, a Team member appears unmotivated, uninterested, or unable to focus during trainings and meetings, we talk about it, but I have not yet needed to ask anyone to leave the program. With a variety of reasons— rather than one common interest—bringing these teens together, the challenge of a group like this developing into a cohesive team can feel enormous.

But the need for the group is clear. First of all, peer education is the most logical way for teens to learn about HIV/AIDS: Teens seem to trust that their peers will level with them more often than adults. I think they project their own desire to be taken seriously onto one another while simultaneously recognizing that some adults don't have their best or realistic interests at heart.

And then there are the risks and challenges of adolescence itself, years marked by specific social, personal, and developmental obstacles laced with cultural norms and values. Some get through it with seemingly little difficulty while others carry their adolescence into their late twenties. Regardless, risk-taking is a normal characteristic of adolescence. Often, teens will participate in risks with immediate consequences, such as drug experimentation. But with HIV, the repercussions of risky behaviors may go unnoticed for years, since it can take that long for someone with HIV to show signs of the virus. And teens, who often don't consider long-term risk, are suffering the consequences.[1] HIV infection and AIDS are presently ranked the sixth leading cause of death for people 15–24 years old, though because of the lengthy time period between exposure to HIV and an AIDS diagnosis, this statistic considerably underestimates the severity of the HIV crisis among teens.[2]

Despite statistics like these, many adolescents still don't believe that they are vulnerable to HIV. Since most of those who contract the virus in their teens either don't know they have it or do not speak publicly about their HIV status, there are few opportunities for youth to hear firsthand accounts from other youth about being seropositive. Peer education programs offer a setting for guest youth speakers to share their experiences with teens who then benefit from both the context of the presentation and the role-modeling of the presenter.

Teen peer education programs ideally encourage healthy interaction and communication, and provide a place of belonging (which in turn reduces feelings of aloneness), both of which are necessary in creating an environment conducive to exploring the range of issues related to HIV/AIDS prevention. One of the roles of the coordinator is that of a guide who helps the group through the tricky terrain, recognizing when to step back and allow the program members to take over. While most teen peer education groups have an adult organizing or facilitating aspects of the program, I recently became familiar with one coordinated by youth themselves, and with the program's creator.

I first heard of Kate Barnhart [another contributor to this volume] through a mutual acquaintance who knew I was interested in talking with other HIV/AIDS peer education coordinators. While Kate's program, the Coalition of Peer Educators (COPE) is based in New York City, she attends college in Amherst, Massachusetts. Now in her senior year, she is already an experienced educator and activist who easily converses about a range of controversial HIV/AIDS-related issues with an eloquent movement between statistical information, theory, and opinion. During our first phone conversation we touched on a wide range of topics, including mandatory HIV testing for foster kids and for pregnant women. Several months later, when we sat down with one another to discuss this piece that I'd be writing about peer education, she mentioned in an offhand manner that she'd been working on peer education for so long that she could write about it in her sleep—then caught herself, looked slightly embarrassed, as though she had insulted me, and apologized lightheartedly. Kate's ease in addressing the subject of peer education bears out her confident remark. She has only recently turned twenty, and in the true spirit of peer education, her age adds to her credentials.

I met with Kate in the Hampshire College AIDS Resource Center where she was awaiting a call from the Centers for Disease Control—searching for data on AIDS-related trials and youth 13–18 years old—to complete her piece for this anthology. Among other services, the AIDS

Resource Center provides peer counseling and information on testing, and is home to the AIDS Action Collective, a group of Hampshire students who promote creative HIV/AIDS learning, with a safer-sex erotica writing contest currently in the works.

Kate commutes to New York City a couple of times a month to continue her work with the Coalition of Peer Educators, which she started in 1993 with teens Elliott Silverman and John Won. Adult consultants John McIlveen and Joe Miller acted as resources for the three. While there are many HIV/AIDS peer education programs throughout New York City, few are created, managed, and facilitated by youth. COPE was founded as a response to the competition between the city's numerous peer education programs for limited resources. In addition to the constant financial obstacles plaguing so many HIV/AIDS programs, ageism—manifested primarily through the stereotyping of teens, their beliefs, and their behaviors—results in institutions discrediting the potential of youth and denying them funding. COPE brings together peer educators from the programs around the city, helping them advocate for their rights while offering support; it functions to empower the city's whole HIV/AIDS youth movement.

COPE created a thirty-hour, four-week HIV/AIDS peer education training curriculum first utilized in August 1994. Collaborating with the Center for Alternative Sentencing and Employment Services (CASES), an alternative sentencing program for young people who have committed felonies, the COPE training offers twenty to thirty youth the opportunity to be trained as HIV/AIDS peer educators. This youth-driven program stands out because it reaches a traditionally underserved population—many of whom are at high risk for being exposed to HIV—within the justice system. Most of the participants have grown up in an environment of poverty and violence. With histories of academic failure, they have minimal skills and reading difficulties. As Kate says, few are "employment-wise."

Those who partake in the COPE training choose to do so; they apply to the program, which allows them to practice job skills such as interviewing. Many participants are aware of their own desire to share AIDS information and become peer educators. Kate reports that soon after the 1994 training's completion, several program graduates started an on-site, ongoing HIV/AIDS peer education group at CASES, while three other program graduates were employed as part-time peer educators at the Teen Outreach Prevention Service (TOPS) of Bellevue/New York University Medical Center, a sponsor of the COPE program.

Like other peer education programs, COPE faces ongoing modification of its HIV/AIDS training curriculum. A positive and crucial challenge for AIDS educators is the continual examination of what material is presented and how it is presented. The scramble for funding adds to the factors leading to changes in a program. COPE's 1995 peer education training functioned with a fraction of the 1994 budget. The search for grant money and private donations is another task that Kate and the other COPE workers are faced with annually.

The creation of a training curriculum takes patience and a willingness to experiment with a range of subjects and activities. The simple, accurate facts about HIV transmission, alone, will not reduce HIV risk for most young people, although this knowledge is important.[3] Ideally, programs such as the AIDS Teen Team and the COPE HIV/AIDS peer education training promote a more positive self-image for the program participants. There are several ways this goal is achieved. Becoming peer leaders—having something positive to offer to the community—increases self-esteem for youth as many teens struggle with the culturally reinforced notion that their ideas hold little weight compared to those of adults.

Additionally, peer education programs provide a group atmosphere in which, over time, it feels increasingly safe to explore difficult material and personal feelings. Working through a range of emotions and learning to resolve conflicts within the group can be an uncomfortable yet empowering process. When young people—or any people—with low self-esteem feel useless in their communities and don't believe they have a voice, there is no reason to expect them to care about the reduction of HIV risk. Peer education programs provide opportunity for youth to feel better about themselves.

The ways in which material is addressed can utilize the natural talents and eagerness of the group members. Experiential learning allows participants' energy and enthusiasm to be channeled into productive training opportunities. Role-plays, games, and activities which involve movement and acting often communicate far stronger messages than simple discussions of a subject. Also, they make room for needed validation of the intensity of feelings that come with topics such as sexual relationships. Normalizing the spectrum of emotions during this time of exploration gives texture to the range of subjects covered in trainings.

With this in mind, an HIV/AIDS peer education curriculum needs to incorporate a host of related topics relevant to the lives of young people (though time and funding often limit what is covered). Initially, a foundation of facts about body parts and their functions along with reproduction may be review for some but much needed by others. This also sets the stage for future discussions on differentiating sex/sexuality from reproduction. Over time, teens become increasingly comfortable talking about these subjects—and it's essential that youth feel free to use their own vocabulary even after becoming familiar with formal terminology. When youth talk with youth about HIV/AIDS, the material is more accessible if it's shared in language that allows them to be themselves, to be real.

"AIDS 101," including basic definitions, modes of transmission, prevention, and testing information is a logical follow-up to initial material on physiology, reproduction, and sexuality. Throughout the curriculum there needs to be the freedom to discuss how the participants feel about all that they are learning; after all, the material is loaded with controversial and emotional content. If this is done from the onset, it becomes a natural part of the group process. Ground rules that address respect and confidentiality may help create some sense of safety as the group members get to know one another.

The following discussion of additional topics is by no means complete, nor does the order signify their importance; the list grows as more young people share with me the complexities of their lives.

Teen pregnancy. Why do some teens want to become parents? What is gained by having/fathering a baby (i.e., status, love, attention?) Do young people feel they have access to information on parenting and birth control? How do thoughts on being sexually active, birth control, and HIV prevention overlap?

Drug and alcohol use. In addition to understanding how HIV is transmitted through sharing needles, how else do drug and alcohol use impact HIV risk? How do various drugs and alcohol make someone feel? How are a person's decision-making skills affected when using drugs or alcohol? What is peer pressure?

Sexually transmitted diseases (STDs). Each year three million young people contract STDs.[4] Which STDs are symptomatic? Where can teens go for confidential STD screenings? What is the connection between HIV transmission and STDs? Have teens learned enough about their bodies to recognize when something doesn't seem right?

Sexual abuse and dating violence. Does anyone ever have the right to expect sex from someone else? What is abuse? What is sexual? What is consent? What is incest? What are power and control? What are the different ways in which physical and sexual abuse happen throughout our society? Who has the right to another person's body and under what circumstances? Is forced sexual activity a form of violence? Are there long-term effects on the self-esteem of someone who's been sexually forced, manipulated or coerced? How is someone's HIV risk affected by abuse?

Domestic violence. Often there are feelings of helplessness and hopelessness that come with witnessing or experiencing violence by family. Where does someone find refuge from family violence? How does violence in a family connect with a person's sense of worth and desire to take care of himself or herself?

Street violence. When homeless teens live on the streets, what risks are associated with trying to find food and shelter? If teens sell sex for money, drugs, or a place to stay, are they at risk for getting HIV? Who is looking out for them, protecting them? When a young person is in a gang, are any of the gang expectations increasing his or her chances of exposure to HIV?

Gender roles. What are the differences in how men and women are "supposed" to behave socially and sexually? How would a teen be perceived by his or her peers for not adhering to such expectation? Where do young people learn gender roles? Is it OK for a man to choose to not have sex? Is it OK for a woman to carry condoms with her?

Gay/lesbian/bisexual (g/l/b) identified teens. What is homophobia? What are the myths and what are the stereotypes about people who partner with people of the same sex? What assumptions do people make about g/l/b youth? Why are the three often clumped together? Is there a difference between identity and behavior? If young people grow up believing negative messages about being g/l/b, how does it affect their self-esteem if they think they're g/l/b? If teens don't feel safe or welcome in their home because of their sexual orientation, preference, or behavior, they may end up living on the streets—does this affect their HIV risk? Are there places for g/l/b youth to get their questions about safer sex answered confidentially?

Classism and poverty. What are the realities of underserved, impoverished youth that may put them at additional risk for HIV? Does prioritizing reduced HIV risk become more difficult when food, clothing, and shelter are difficult to secure? Is HIV a disease that affects one class of people more than others?

Cultural and religious responses to HIV. How might teens with various cultural and religious backgrounds view HIV/AIDS-related subjects such as sexuality, drug and alcohol use, condom use, illness, and death? Can a person feel oppressed by another individual's cultural or religious beliefs? Do all people of a particular cultural or religious background think or act the same?

Disabled youth. Are teens with disabilities sexually active? Are there materials that address the needs of disabled youth and HIV education? Are peer education groups and safety-net parties wheelchair accessible? In what ways do people make assumptions about young people with disabilities that limit their ability to obtain resources, consequently increasing their risk for getting HIV?

Education and literacy. How much does someone's educational achievement contribute to an overall sense of accomplishment (vs. failure)? How do youth who have had a hard time in school feel about themselves? How does a person's inability to read limit the amount of HIV information he or she can access? Who is at risk for illiteracy?

Legal rights. What legal rights do young people have within the justice and social service systems? Under what circumstances—if any—is it fair for teens to be tested for HIV without their consent? Where can young people go for affordable legal assistance?

Body piercing, branding, and tattooing. Often IV drug use is seen as the primary way in which the use of dirty needles spreads HIV but with increasing numbers of young people choosing to pierce, brand, and tattoo their bodies, how can teens assess the safety of these procedures?

Tolerating difference. Who benefits from intolerance? How does being judgmental constrict the potential of HIV education? How is the success of a peer education program measured? On written questionnaires, most AIDS Teen Team members demonstrate a solid understanding of AIDS-related information. They can correctly roll a condom onto a cucumber in a flash.

And they can convert a condom into a rectangular barrier (for mouth-to-anus or mouth-to-vagina contact) just as fast. At area high school health fairs, they attract far more attentive students than other represented organizations because often they're the only teen-run table. The participants in the COPE program pre- and post-test for knowledge and post-test for presentation skills. Does this mean that program members and the teens they reach are changing their behaviors? What is a reasonable expectation?

Last year two AIDS Teen Team members told me they were pregnant while a third fathered a baby girl, obviously demonstrating that three of the thirty program participants—at least—had unsafe sex. They each shared with me that they weren't using a condom or any other means of birth control. I am not fully aware of the numerous related, important factors that were particular to these three teen pregnancies (i.e., how much choice they had in having sex, how interested or supportive their sex-partners were in considering condom use). But I did notice that while both pregnant teens told me they weren't really trying to get pregnant, each was looking forward to giving their mother a first grandchild because both their moms were sick with AIDS.

It seems as though the impact this virus has already had on the lives of some teens plays a significant role in their ability and desire to recognize and reduce their own HIV risk. Without ongoing support addressing the difficult and overwhelming circumstances facing many teens, peer education may only make a small dent—if that—in the statistics. But the significance of peer education programs is as much in the process as it is in the outcome. I'm reminded of this when AIDS Teen Team members moan if a meeting is canceled; when a young person who shows up to school 50 percent of the time makes it to every training; and when Team members drag a sibling, cousin, or friend into a meeting saying, "This is the group, this is the one I told you about."

NOTES

1. Andy Humm and Frances Kunreuther, "The Invisible Epidemic: Teenagers and AIDS," *Social Policy* 21, no. 4 (spring 1991): 40–46.

2. Centers for Disease Control and Prevention, U.S. Department of Health and

Human Services, *Pregnancy, Sexually Transmitted Diseases and Related Risk Behaviors* (Atlanta: Centers for Disease Control and Prevention, 1994).

3. Clark Robenstine, "HIV Education at the Secondary Level: An Urgent Necessity," *NASSP-Bulletin* 77, no. 557 (December 1993): 9–16.

4. Center for Population Options, *Peer to Peer: Youth Preventing HIV Infection Together* (Washington, D.C.: Center for Population Options, 1993).

18

Haitian Teens Confront Aids: A Partners in Health Program on Social Justice and AIDS Prevention

Loune Viaud
with Paul Farmer and Guitèle Nicoleau

Loune Viaud is the former Program Director of HTCA and has been involved in the program for over four years. She is currently the Associate Director of Partners in Health. *Paul Farmer*, M.D., Ph.D., author of *AIDS and Accusation* and *The Uses of Haiti*, is an Assistant Professor in the Department of Social Medicine at the Harvard Medical School and an infectious disease specialist at Boston's Brigham and Women's Hospital. He is the former Executive Director of Partners In Health and has been active in the development of all HTCA materials. *Guitele Nicoleau* is the former Director of HTCA and has been involved in the development of all HTCA materials. She is currently writing her thesis for her Ed.D. at the Harvard Graduate School of Education.

What Is Partners in Health?

Partners in Health (PIH), established in 1987, is a nonprofit organization governed by a team of North American and Haitian community activists, including physicians and anthropologists. PIH works in partnership with community-based organizations to improve health in poor communities and to redress inequities in access to health care. Over the past eight years, PIH has been involved in over forty projects, many of them related to AIDS prevention. For example, we have helped to design and operate a community-based AIDS prevention program in rural Haiti; we have helped a Boston-based community group find funding for a day-treatment program for persons with AIDS/ARC; we have published booklets and other materials to assist Haitian community health workers in their AIDS prevention efforts; we have helped to find funding for an AIDS prevention program for a low-literacy area of Western Africa; we have provided in-service education regarding AIDS and AIDS-related discrimination to hospitals in the Boston area; we have published reports and original research in the scholarly literature devoted to AIDS and AIDS prevention.

Our largest project dealing with AIDS, however, is HTCA, the first peer-outreach AIDS prevention project for Haitian adolescents living in New England.

The Accusation: Was It Accurate?

Perceptions of Haitians and of the role they were alleged to have played in the AIDS pandemic are remarkable for their misunderstanding and misinformation. When AIDS was first recognized in the U.S., the Centers for Disease Control (CDC) characterized four groups as being at high risk for contracting and transmitting the new disease: homosexuals, hemophiliacs, heroin abusers, and Haitians. The CDC included Haitians as a separate risk group, because Haitians did not seem to meet the same diagnostic criteria for AIDS as the other identified groups. It was claimed that, when interviewed, Haitians with AIDS and living in the United States reported that they had not engaged in same-sex sexual relations. Most had never had a blood transfusion and all denied intravenous drug use. Because most other cases of the syndrome known at the time implicated one or more of these risk factors, researchers concluded that AIDS among Haitians was "a complete mystery." Later evidence revealed sloppy interview protocols. The cultural biases of the researchers contributed to the production of erroneous data about Haitians in the United States. A refusal to acknowledge the findings of Haitian researchers in Haiti also contributed to the scientific community's misclassification of Haitians as a risk group.

So was born the famous "Four-H Club." Because these classifications all depended on assessment of group identity, rather than on behavior, all gays, all Haitians, all hemophiliacs, and all IVDU were assumed to be at risk of AIDS. In classifying Haitians as a risk group, regardless of their relative participation in the acts that put them at risk for infection, scientists also drew upon the "foreignness" and "otherness" of Haitians and Haitian-Americans—they are poor, Black, speak another language, and supposedly engage in voodoo cult practices. Furthermore, according to these scientists, there was strong evidence that linked Haitians to the origin of the U.S.

AIDS epidemic: three cases of transfusion-related transmission (only one of which, at an unspecified date, took place in Haiti), and the case of a former nun whose sole sexual contact was said to have been in Haiti, where she worked for thirty years. She died in Canada in 1981 "of a disease that her doctors retrospectively recognized as AIDS" (Farmer 1992, 2).

Social scientists joined in and speculated that the origin of AIDS was to be found in "voodoo practices." One hypothesis suggested that the sacrificial offerings in voodoo ceremonies are "infested with one of the Type C oncogenic retroviruses, which is closely related to HTLV . . . and this blood is directly ingested by the priests and their assistants." (Farmer 1992, 3). These social scientists further speculated that many of the voodoo priests are homosexual men who are in a position to satisfy their sexual desires, especially in urban areas.

Contrary to these speculations, more careful and responsible analysis reveals that AIDS in Haiti was not as "mysterious" as had been claimed. It was far more likely, in examining the data, that AIDS made its appearance in Haiti, the U.S., and other Caribbean countries at about the same time. In the Caribbean, Haiti had the largest number of actual AIDS cases, but when these numbers were calculated in proportion to the total population, the AIDS "attack rate" in Haiti was lower than that in Barbados, Jamaica, Martinique, Guadeloupe, French Guiana, the U.S. Virgin Islands, and Grenada.

That the CDC and the World Health Organization should choose to highlight the actual numbers of cases to determine risk groups in the case of Haitians was a significant scientific flaw. Finger-pointing at Haitians living in the U.S. was based on yet another critical error on the part of the scientific community. In 1981, to calculate the prevalence of AIDS in Haitians living in the U.S., the Centers for Disease Control (CDC) compared the sixty known Haitian AIDS cases to a total population of 100,000 Haitian immigrants—a number which is considerably lower than the estimated 500,000 Haitians living in the U.S. (Farmer 1992). By using such a low population figure, the CDC inflated AIDS prevalence among Haitians living in the U.S.

This inflation of the severity of the epidemic among Haitians in the U.S. and the use of actual numbers of AIDS cases as opposed to the proper epidemiological calculations based on percentages clouded rather than illuminated the nature of the AIDS epidemic in Haiti. The "mystery" of AIDS in Haitians is not a mystery at all. Haiti and the other countries of the

Caribbean are historically connected to each other and to the U.S. by a political economy that links rather than isolates them. Most of them are relatively poor, Haiti being the poorest among them. Most of these countries rely on tourism and trade with the U.S and Europe to generate income and foreign aid to support their weak economies. With few skills to offer a global technological market, men and women in these countries sometimes must offer their bodies in the sex industry. As in most areas of the world, prostitution is an industry that walks hand in hand with underdevelopment and poverty.

The Accusation: Its Effects

The classification of Haitians as a risk group had significant consequences for the large Haitian communities in East-Coast cities like New York, Boston, and Miami. There were reports of parents who would not permit their children to attend schools with Haitian-American students; of Haitian cab drivers who had learned to say that they were from Martinique or Guadeloupe for fear of not finding passengers; of families evicted from rented housing for having "black skin and French names"; of sudden firings and quests for jobs for which Haitian-born applicants were "just not right." In Brooklyn, the walls of a predominantly Caribbean neighborhood were sprayed with "Haitians = Niggers with AIDS." In New York, it was reported that Haitian children had been beaten up (and in at least one case, shot) in school; Haitian store owners were going bankrupt as their businesses failed. In Boston, a Haitian high school student was told by one of her teachers that Haitians contracted the virus because they have sex with monkeys. In South Florida, a social service organization received hate mail that conveyed such slogans as "Hire a Haitian—Help Spread AIDS," and "There were [sic] no AIDS in the USA until the illegal criminal Haitian dogs came."

This harsh attack on Haitians sparked a fiery response from the Haitian community. Haitian community leaders in Miami, New York, and Boston formed coalitions to counter what they took to be racist, anti-Haitian attitudes. Haitian doctors and activists lobbied public health officials; they conducted seminars to prove that the labeling of Haitians was a discriminatory act with no scientific basis. Under the considerable pressure they exerted, the New York City Department of Health removed Haitians from its official list of risk groups in the summer of 1983.

In spite of these actions, the official labeling of Haitians as a "risk group" persisted. In 1983, the U.S. Public Health Service, supported by the CDC listing, recommended that Haitian-Americans not donate blood. In defense of their position, the CDC insisted that their literature expressly stated that each risk group contained large numbers of persons not at risk. They further affirmed that they had not meant to imply that persons were at risk of AIDS through mere casual contact with members of the risk group.

But the apology of the CDC meant little in the face of the severe damage inflicted upon the Haitian community by the stigmatization and discrimination that resulted from the labeling. The disagreement between members of the Haitian community and the CDC continued until April 1985, when the term "Haitian" was quietly removed from CDC listing.

But, the "Haitian = AIDS" perception remained in the public imagination, and so did the ban on Haitian blood. In a memorandum issued in 1984 by the federal Food and Drug Administration (FDA), it was stipulated that Haitians who had reached the U.S. after 1977 were prohibited from donating blood. On February 5, 1990, the FDA went one step further: It issued another memorandum that extended the ban to all Haitians, regardless of when they came to the U.S. Considering the information on HIV disease among Haitians that was widely available at the time, the conclusion most Haitians were forced to draw was that these policies were based on racism. Their reaction to the FDA was quick and furious. Massive demonstrations ensued in New York, where over a hundred thousand Haitians crossed the Brooklyn bridge, and in Miami, where more than five thousand Haitians marched outside FDA offices. In Boston, another five thousand Haitians took over the plaza in front of City Hall and demanded that the FDA lift the ban on Haitian blood.

While these demonstrations were going on, Haitian doctors and researchers gathered in New York and Washington to go over the data. Their conclusions are nicely summarized in April 5, 1990, by the *Boston Globe's* Derrick Jackson: If the FDA was honest about geographical bans, it would have halted blood donations by all San Franciscans. In that city, the new-case rate last year, according to the federal Centers for Disease Control, was ten times that of Haiti, 114.5 per 100,000. The FDA would also have banned natives of San Juan and New York City, where respective rates were 86.8 and 69.4. Most of you readers would have been banned. The city said its new case rate last year was 58.1 per 100,000. The CDC's rate for greater Boston is 16.0, still higher than Haiti's. Haitian community leaders held a preliminary meeting with the FDA Commissioner, who subsequently recommended a full hearing before the Advisory Board that advises the FDA on public health policies. The hearing was held on April 20, 1990, with the FDA, the CDC, and the National Institutes of Health (NIH) on one side and the Haitian community, represented by the doctors and researchers of the Haitian-American Health Coalition, on the other.

The FDA's Advisory Board agreed that the Haitian arguments were compelling and recommended that the FDA lift the ban on Haitian blood. The FDA, however, did not follow its own board's recommendation until eight months later, after the increasing political pressure of large demonstrations held in Washington, D.C., and the boycotting of Red Cross blood banks by communities of color in support of Haitians.

Like the CDC's removal of Haitians from its high-risk list, the FDA's removal of the ban on Haitian blood was done without comment and without any admission of having erred in the scientific methods that enabled them to label a whole population as a risk group. This silent withdrawal of the Haitian name in the official literature has perhaps reinforced the "Haitian = AIDS" equation in the public imagination. Today, fifteen years into the pandemic, Haitians are still viewed suspiciously by many as AIDS carriers, and Haiti as a place that is infested with AIDS.

A Community-Based Response

The "Haitian = AIDS carrier" status has affected the Haitian community in numerous ways. It has fostered discrimination against Haitians in schools, in hospitals, in the workplace, and anywhere else people come into contact with Haitians. Put in a defensive posture by the accusation, Haitians spent more time in the early years of the pandemic defending their name and less time working to slow its spread in the Haitian-American community and in Haiti. As was true for other groups, AIDS also carried feelings of blame, guilt, and shame. In these early years of the epidemic, to admit in public that AIDS was present in the Haitian community felt like a defeat of the spirit of Haitian pride and self-assertion that the anti-FDA demonstrations symbolized. Consequently, individuals and families remained guarded and in denial about incidents of AIDS. Within the community, little was known about the disease, and the information that was being provided by the U.S. medical establishment and the media was suspect, given the role of these institutions in creating discrimination and disseminating accusation. Even among those involved in AIDS prevention, there was often more energy for countering the effects of AIDS-related discrimination. Darline, one of our peer educators said: "I think that, when they find out they were wrong, it won't affect them. They'll just say, 'Hey, to err is human.' I feel that they don't know how they've hurt the Haitian people. They don't know how they've wounded us."

Meanwhile, although Haitians were not universally at risk for AIDS, it remained a significant and growing problem in our community. Like other communities of color in the United States and abroad, the Haitian community was experiencing increased rates of heterosexually transmitted HIV infection. Haitian professionals in hospitals and community-based service organizations were seeing more and more patients and clients with signs of HIV infection. The virus showed no preference for men, women, or children: all were affected. Families, already stretched to the limit in their attempt to make good on their dreams of securing a better life for themselves in the United States, suddenly had one more life-threatening, stigmatizing element to add to their burdens. Take, for example, our experience here in New England. It is estimated that more than 80,000 Haitians make their home in Greater Boston. As of January 1, 1995, 447 Haitians in Massachusetts had been diagnosed with AIDS, according to the Massachusetts Department of Public Health. Of these, 259 are from Boston, 53 are from Cambridge, 33 are from Brockton and 28 are from Somerville. A significant number of infected people are young adults: 25 percent are between the ages of 20 and 29; 56 percent are between the ages of 30 and 39. Because the virus has such a long incubation period, this evidence suggests that these adults engaged in high-risk behaviors (particularly unprotected sex, and to a lesser extent, intravenous drug use) as teens and young adults.

Cultural Considerations

Although cultural factors have not conclusively been shown to increase rates of HIV transmission, Haitians do have distinctive ways of understanding and responding to serious illness. These culturally-unique factors must be taken into consideration in attempting to create effective prevention programs. The following list enumerates six considerations we have found relevant to any effort to create AIDS-prevention programs for the Haitian community in Boston or elsewhere in North America:

1. *Prevention as low priority.* Among many Haitians, preventive efforts against sickness often take a distant second place to more pressing concerns: lack of employment, lack of housing, financial obligations to family members in Haiti, poor access to services, and discrimination. As a result, illness prevention often takes a back seat to the resolution of more immediate social and economic problems.

2. *Linguistic factors.* All Haitians speak Haitian Creole; fewer than 10 percent speak French. These linguistic considerations make Creole an obvious first choice when attempting to create effective preventive tools and programs, but low rates of literacy make even Creole a problematic language for health education: because so many have been denied access to schooling in Haiti, many Haitians who are currently in the United States are unable to read or write. Those few who are literate are often literate in French, until quite recently the "official" language of Haiti. Many of the teens that HTCA serves are literate in English only, even though they speak Creole far more fluently than English.

3. *Sexual and social mores.* Given the nature of HIV transmission among Haitians, it is imperative that heterosexual behavior in our community be adequately understood. And yet Haitian sexual and social mores have not been the subject of significant scientific inquiry, nor have they often been the topic of open forums in the Haitian community. In order to develop culturally appropriate preventive programs, these questions must be investigated.

4. *Fighting the stigma.* An atmosphere of mistrust has enveloped AIDS-prevention programs in the Haitian community. This mistrust, which has legitimate foundations, is the result of the inaccurate labeling of Haitians as intrinsically at risk for AIDS. Any attempt to address AIDS in the Haitian community must come to terms with the resentment born of anti-Haitian discrimination resulting from this stigmatization.

5. *Social institutions.* In the Haitian-American community, churches, community organizations, and Creole radio and television programs serve as the

chief forums for addressing community issues. Among these institutions, there are varying levels of commitment to public discussion of AIDS as a sexually transmitted disease. Some community organizations are attempting to address AIDS by providing services to persons with HIV disease. Some of the churches have been less enthusiastic in raising other AIDS-related issues such as the nature of HIV transmission. Developing community awareness and disseminating information about HIV depends upon our ability to develop a shared agenda and language for AIDS programs in the Haitian community.

6. *Gender inequality.* The ability of young women to protect themselves from HIV infection becomes a direct function of power relations between men and women. Sexism has thus weakened women's ability to negotiate safe sexual encounters. Data from preliminary work on HIV transmission in Haiti revealed that men (both those with AIDS and seronegative controls) had substantially greater numbers of partners than did women enrolled in these studies. We can say that the face of AIDS in the Haitian community is a feminine face. Because HIV is more efficiently transmitted from males to females, the increased sexual activity of men amplifies the possibility of transmission to women (and, through them, to children). The social forces such as poverty, sexism, and other forms of discrimination become translated into risk for women, especially poor women and women of color, due to their subordinate status as women. The experiences of poor women with AIDS, whether in rich or in poor countries, call into question the dominant understandings of AIDS, which have not included an appreciation of the mechanisms by which poverty and sexism put poor women at risk of HIV infection. Dominant readings are likely to foster images of women with AIDS in the Haitian community as promiscuous or as prostitutes, but very unlikely to reveal how political structural violence come to be important in the AIDS pandemic today. The factors that sap women's ability to control sexual encounters must continue to be addressed in order to help women organize themselves not just against AIDS, but against the forces that rob them of control over their bodies and their lives. "In societies where the female has a weaker hand," note Desvarieux and Pape (1991, 277), "effective methods of prevention have a better chance of working if the woman does not have to rely on either the consent or the willingness of her partner."

Haitian Teens Confront AIDS: A Social-Justice Model

The founding of Haitian Teens Confront AIDS, in 1989, marked the first initiative to address the twin epidemics of AIDS and discrimination as faced by Haitian teenagers in the greater Boston area. As noted, epidemiological studies indicate that 25–30 percent of AIDS cases in the Boston-area Haitian community were registered in people between the ages of twenty and thirty-five. Given the five- to ten-year incubation period of the virus, it was safe to assume that, for many people, infection occurred during adolescence. Other data suggested increased rates of infection among the adolescent population statewide.

Prior to the founding of HTCA, no educational efforts had been undertaken that targeted and involved Haitian youth. HTCA was initiated in order to respond to the need for AIDS preventive education among Haitian youth and provide them with the tools to confront the discrimination they were facing in their daily lives. The project was divided into several phases, which are outlined below.

Phases I and II

Production of a Teen Video

Experts in health education have been unequivocal in the need for age-specific and culturally appropriate prevention programs. We chose the medium of video because of its popularity among teens, and also because of the high rate of illiteracy among precisely those teens most at risk for exposure to HIV. PIH's underlying philosophy was that the "target audience"—in this case, Haitian teens—should be directly involved in the production of the video. PIH, therefore, worked with Haitian performing artists and Arts in Progress to recruit and train Haitian high school students from Boston and Cambridge. The video—which the teens wrote, acted in, and directed—is the first ever to be targeted specifically to Haitian-speaking adolescents. Presented in Haitian Creole with English subtitles, Pitimi San Gad confronts AIDS in its complexity as a sociomedical problem. In "soap-opera" format, the video introduces the teenage members of a Haitian family as they face dilemmas of sexuality, cultural identity, gender inequality, and the threat of a new disease. The tape includes a brief presentation of how the teens worked together to produce the video.

Clerna, a 19-year-old who had recently arrived from Haiti, introduces the narrative with the following comments:

> The video is one of the tools we created to confront AIDS. It was written, directed, acted in, and produced by us, the teens of Haitian Teens Confront AIDS. The video is an expression of our desire to inform other teens about HIV transmission. It is equally an expression of our experience as young Haitians in the United States, where we are faced with issues of cultural identity, racism, and the role of AIDS as one more factor complicating the quality of our lives here. But our message must be one of courage. We are not about to bow down before either AIDS or discrimination.

In its distribution to educational, community and youth organizations in North America and Haiti, the video has received a very enthusiastic reception. Six years after its production, its remains, as far as we know, the only such tool available. Its success, and that of other tools created during the first year of HTCA, led the team of youth and adult educators in HTCA, naturally to the complementary activities of the early phases of the project.

Peer Education and Leadership Training

As mentioned above, seventeen students were recruited and trained in the epidemiology and transmission of HIV, in group education and discussion, and in dealing with issues of discrimination. Skills in acting and other performing arts were also polished. When coupled with their experience as Haitian teens, these new skills and the new information they received about AIDS resulted in the formation of a talented and committed group of teens. The teens saw themselves—and were perceived by other members of the teen and adult, Haitian, and non-Haitian communities—as a significant community resource.

In recent years, the teens have conducted peer and community education activities in a variety of settings. Each activity has brought the project closer to an awareness of the impact of the role the teens can play in developing greater understanding between the U.S. and Haitian communities. To illustrate, take the example of one particularly busy weekend for the HTCA teens. At a conference at the Harvard Graduate School of Education in May 1990, four teens engaged teachers, administrators and students in a discussion about issues of racism, discrimination, AIDS, and Haitians. The same day, at the Graham Parks Elementary School, the teens directed an AIDS session with the participation of Haitian and non-Haitian students. Also on that day, at the Cambridge Hospital's Haitian Health Fair, four other teens engaged a Haitian audience in a discussion of AIDS, how it is transmitted, and how it can be prevented. These points were discussed in tandem with a consideration of the impact of religious beliefs and social mores on efforts to prevent AIDS. This audience, comprised primarily of adults, was very forthcoming with its concerns and its ideas. This discussion was one of our first indications of the powerful role that HTCA could play in breaking down generational barriers and providing opportunities for parents and their children to engage in fruitful dialogue about sexuality, gender inequality, religious beliefs, and other potentially taboo issues that are rarely discussed across generations. These experiences represented, for us, true examples of the possibilities of building cultural and generational bridges through the cultural work and leadership skills of the teens. Increasing compassion for those living with AIDS was always a central concern of those involved in planning and running the project.

Clébert Jean-Baptiste was one of the first Haitians diagnosed in the United States with HIV. He served as a Person With AIDS/Adult Educator for HTCA until he became very ill and was unable to continue in his role. Clébert died in the winter of 1993.

Phase III

During the summer of 1990, artists and educators worked with the teens to further develop peer-education and leadership skills, and to enable them to undertake a significant schedule of educational sessions and performances over the coming year. During July and August 1990, for twenty hours per week, the teens participated in workshops that were planned by them and the artist/educators. During the academic year, the teens worked for twenty hours per month. Their activities included Saturday workshops and weekly meetings spent planning and conducting educational presentations and discussions. The workshops were led by HTCA artists, educators, and physicians, as well as by other educators and physicians from community-based organizations active in HIV/AIDS education in the Greater Boston area. The goals of the workshops held in this period and the focus of our activities were as follows:

1. HIV/AIDS education. To continue to increase the teens' knowledge of HIV and AIDS as it affects the lives of adolescents and young adults; to address the issues surrounding the primary modes of transmission in the Haitian and non-Haitian communities; to discuss sexual and drug-abuse practices that put teens at risk for contracting HIV; to identify culturally relevant and specific preventive measures; to conduct personal risk assessments; to articulate nonstigmatizing social responses to the disease; and to identify the ways in which the community can respond with compassion to people with AIDS.

The group has produced other materials that are available to the public— *Lavi Nouvo,* "New Life," a musical play about existing risk practices and alternative relationships based on trust and respect, and *Silabè SIDA: Sa ou konnen pa ka fè ou pè,* "ABC's of AIDS: what you know can't hurt you." The latter is a collection of fictional short case studies based on real instances of HIV infection in the Haitian community. Physicians and case workers from Haitian community-based organizations were invited to relate their experiences with the management of cases of HIV infection. Using these cases and their own experiences, the HTCA teens and educators developed the case studies, and determined the kind of factual and culturally relevant information which was to be included in a manual that could serve as a tool for teaching, discussion, and self-education. Cases from the manual were field-tested in church- and school-based sessions with encouraging responses from the audience.

2. Peer education and facilitating. To enable the teens to develop their skills as discussion facilitators and educators using the video, *Pitimi San Gadò,* the musical play, *Lavi Nouvo,* and the handbook of short case studies, *Silabè Sida,* which were developed during Phase I and II of HTCA.

3. Community outreach. To plan outreach sessions targeting Haitian and non-Haitian teens and adults, using the skills of HTCA teens as bilingual and bicultural "culture brokers." These efforts led directly to a series of peer-outreach activities in area schools and churches.

Since the inception of the project, the teens have traveled to New York to make presentations to a gathering of community-based educational programs; they have lent their voices to the Bridges Program of the Boston-based AIDS Action Committee (a commemorative event for PWAs who have passed away). *Pitimi San Gadò* has been widely screeened; the teens have performed *Lavi Nouvo* before youth and adult audiences numbering between 250 and 800. They have used *Silabè SIDA* in its embryonic stages with recalcitrant church audiences who preferred not to see the video because it spoke of condoms. They have participated in school health fairs, ranging from junior high to high schools. When Magic Johnson disclosed his HIV status to the world, the teens were sought out to offer their response as peer educators to the local papers; and their work has been featured on special television and radio programs on the Haitian community and AIDS education initiatives in Boston. The activities undertaken by the teens and staff of HTCA and PIH in Phase III far surpassed all expectations, both in number and impact.

Phase IV

In 1991 we began experimenting with a mechanism, proposed and designed by the teens, to recruit new peer educators. We held a six-week summer seminar on HIV/AIDS for youth in the community. The seminar included presentations by the teens and the use of the HTCA material to generate discussions among the participants. The process had a dual purpose: (1) to identify and select potential teen educators and facilitators, and (2) to implement a peer training and mentoring process for the new recruits. In addition, we have begun the process of determining which aspects of the project we will integrate into a long-term youth-development and community-education program of Partners In Health.

Seven peer educators were recruited from the summer seminar to serve as peer educators. They ranged in age from thirteen to twenty and lived in Cambridge, Dorchester, Mattapan, Somerville and Waltham. Partners In Health awarded each of them a stipend, presented as a "scholarship" for their work in the course of the year, and they received payment in monthly disbursements. They were responsible for planning and conducting all the activities of HTCA. These seven teens chose to participate in order to follow in the footsteps of the first seventeen teens who left their mark on the Haitian community as vocal members actively participating in the effort to curb the spread of HIV in the Haitian community. Since 1991, we have conducted these seminars yearly as a form of outreach and recruitment of new peer educators. Scores of teens have participated in this year-long program.

Expanding Community Outreach and Strengthening Organizing

While we have been successful in implementing our AIDS prevention activities and programs, we saw a persistent need for more coordination and collaboration between community organizations in order to create greater awareness among a much larger youth audience. In 1992 HTCA, along with two other Haitians organizations working with adolescents, submitted a successful collaborative proposal to the Massachusetts Department of Public Health. The collaborative experience has allowed the adolescents within several programs to develop a common language for speaking with their peers and adults about the issues surrounding AIDS prevention. *The Annual Congress for Mobilizing Haitian Youth for AIDS Prevention* is the most significant fruit of the collaboration between the three peer HIV/AIDS-education programs for Haitians adolescents. This event brings together between five hundred and eight hundred Haitian adolescents from the Greater Boston area for a day-long series of activities. The Congress is designed to create greater awareness about HIV/AIDS among Haitian youth and to mobilize them to protect themselves and each other from HIV infection. The students come together to perform original skits, poetry, and dances; compare prevention slogans; attend workshops on HIV/AIDS, relationships, sex and sexuality, and other related subjects, including gender inequality; and hear presentations by Haitians living with HIV/AIDS, speakers from the Department of Public Health, the AIDS Action Committee, the Multicultural AIDS Coalition and Haitian community leaders.

Phase V

In the summer of 1994, we expanded our work by initiating a second, complementary cohort, whose work focuses more exclusively on outreach activities. This group meets twice a week. The first group devotes most of its time to organizing the Parent-Youth Forums and the Youth Congress, while the second group devotes its activities primarily to wide outreach in the Cambridge area, using the HTCA materials, "safety net" parties and other strategies and venues. Both groups have participated in the other's activities (i.e., the Forum, the Congress, and "safety net" parties) and it is clear to us that further focusing the activities of each group has strengthened the overall impact of HTCA.

The primary focus of the first six months is to prepare the teens to conduct a series of activities throughout the school year as peer educators. In addition to intensive tutoring in the facts of HIV/AIDS, they receive training in facilitation skills, condom use demonstration, substance abuse prevention and violence prevention. In every aspect of the training program, we have worked to develop overall leadership skills and an understanding of cultural identity. During the Saturday meetings, we reserve time to discuss Haiti's political situation and to have general discussions about parent/youth communication or youth/youth communication.

We talk about the differences between Haitian adolescents in the U.S. and Haitian youth in Haiti. We trigger these discussions with *Chache lavi, Detwi lavi,* a half-hour video produced by Zanmi Lasante, the sister organization of Partners In Health, that tells the story of a young rural Haitian woman who dies of AIDS. The young woman, whose family loses their land and becomes impoverished, responds to the overtures of a truck driver, hoping he will help her family out of poverty. After she gives birth to his child, she finds herself alone and penniless, and seeks work in the city as her only hope of surviving and procuring a brighter future for her daughter. What happens in the city is emblematic of the lot of poor women in Haiti and elsewhere.

This videotaped story brings up many discussions about the differences between Haitian adolescents in the U.S. and Haitian youth in rural Haiti, the plight of women, and the ways in which the lives of women, in particular, are framed by economic and gender inequalities. In these discussions, the youth, both male and female, shift from blaming the woman for her naiveté in falling for a duplicitous man to compassion for her, her family, and her daughter. The shift occurs as the adult educators in the program help the youth explore the social and personal complexities of the character's situation. The girls, in particular, begin to recognize the ways in which they, too, can find themselves victims of often unnamed and disempowering social forces. In their empathy for the character, they engage the boys and each other in impassioned discussions about the role of men in creating and sustaining economic and gender inequalities— extrapolations that also take them to the larger global forces that shape these inequalities. The peer educators take the insights gained from these discussions and frame them to generate community dialogue in their outreach efforts with youth and adults. In so doing, they help members of the community articulate the intersection between AIDS, gender and economic inequalities, and the social realities of Haitians living in Haiti and the U.S.

Working with other community organizations, HTCA has recently made information about AIDS in Creole more accessible to Haitian youth in Massachusetts. The project was created in conjunction with a "youth only" AIDS telephone hotline, a project of the AIDS Action Committee. Every Wednesday night from 6 to 9 p.m., HTCA peer educators respond confidentially to Haitian youth who call in with questions and concerns about HIV/AIDS. This anonymous hotline is proving to be yet another important HIV education resource to Haitian adolescents and adults in the community.

Incorporating Social Justice Concepts into AIDS Prevention

We started HTCA with a clear understanding that AIDS is deeply related to social inequality. The texture of the discussions that generated the HTCA educational materials and the dialogues with the larger community have permitted us to appreciate the important intersection between HIV prevention and social justice. With each new cohort of 12–18-year-old girls and boys that enters HTCA, we see a persistent tendency to ascribe blame to the victims in the educational materials that serve as the basis of discussion. Using these tools—*Pitimi San Gadò, Silabé Sida, Lavi Nouvo, Chache lavi, Detwi lavi,* and other materials produced for non-Haitians, the youth are able to enter into discussion that problematize the social world they and the characters in the stories inhabit. Through these discussions, the youth test their own emerging concepts of who they are as young Haitians growing up in this country and often caught between Haitian and U.S. systems of values. They enter with each other and the adults and young adult educators of the programs into deep discussions about the differential treatment that girls and boys receive from their parents in matters of relationships between boys and girls, schooling, and family responsibilities. In no uncertain terms, the girls bemoan the societal pressures to adhere to the social constructions of a "good girl"—one who, among other attributes, is silent yet strong and who upholds the moral values of the community even at the expense of herself. In the heat of discussion, they are often heard to forcefully defend their right to the opportunities for exploring who they are in relationships without fear of being stigmatized as "bad girls." They decry the feelings of being "boxed in" by the societal expectations of underachievement ascribed to black youth, in general, and girls in particular. The educational tools provide a safe context to articulate and explore the conflicting feelings they hold about how to define themselves culturally, how to understand and make personal sense of the Haitian and religious values attached to maintaining virginity and of the explicit expectations of sexual activity they pick up around them in schools, the media, and in observing the social world of U.S. adolescents. The internal group discussions and community dialogues also serve as the arena in which many of the girls take the boys to task when they over-identify, for example, with the macho image of Mario *Lavi Nouvo* and when they find themselves feeling unsupported by both boys and girls as they defend the alternative character in the musical. Through these discussions, the youth also begin to articulate the variety of ways in which they can constructively challenge gender roles, racist constructions of their identity, and the economic barriers to the health of their communities.

The opportunities to engage the peer educators and other youth in the community have clearly opened a window into the peculiar and evolving needs of Haitian adolescents. They have provided an important context for adults to hear the social issues that frame the world of Haitian adolescents, and to help shape the voices in which youth can personally and socially respond to inequalities that would make them victims of rather than actors in their own realities. Our evolving appreciation for the importance of HTCA's dialogical processes as a socializing construct has made us aware of the necessity to sustain, over a long term, an educational program that links social justice to prevention. Such a commitment is further underscored by our heightened collective awareness of the complex relationship between power, powerlessness, and sexuality as they are revealed in the increased rates of infection among poor women and women of color. That AIDS is the leading cause of death among young women of color in U.S. cities forces all of us to recognize the importance of attacking the myths that would have us believe that women are in complete control of their bodies and lives. As the peer educators of HTCA become increasingly aware of these facts and as they construct personal and social meaning around HIV prevention and social justice, they express their resolve to create links between their work in AIDS prevention with broader campaigns to make the world a more just place to live. They want to address poverty, racism, and sexism as powerful social forces that put women, especially, at risk for HIV infection.

In the next few years, HTCA plans to reinforce and broaden the scope of its program by strengthening its current activities and continually responding to the emerging HIV/AIDS educational demands of the Haitian community both in the U.S. and in Haiti. For example, given our strong links to Zanmi Lasante, our sister organization in Haiti, PIH will further support its efforts to bridge the gap between North America and Haiti by involving some of the HTCA teens in a major AIDS prevention program in rural Haiti. The goal of broadening and strengthening will also be realized in the compilation of a comprehensive AIDS prevention package in the effort to share HTCA's experiences, teaching tools, and methods proven effective in the Haitian-American community in addressing AIDS and discrimination.[1]

Conclusions

HTCA has reached thousands of Haitians of all ages and has created the opportunities for Haitian youth to develop their individual and collective voices in many debates around AIDS and other problems facing Haitian and non-Haitian communities. HTCA's presence as a culturally responsive AIDS-prevention program has helped to develop an emerging new language of prevention in the Haitian community—one that is built on hope, cultural pride, political activism, and compassion. With each new cohort of HTCA teens, we witness the development of politically and socially active teens who are not afraid to take on the challenges of engaging each other and members of the community in the difficult discussions surrounding human sexuality, gender inequalities, homophobia, and social injustice. Their new-found language for understanding and negotiating social meaning around AIDS and social justice enables many of the HTCA teens to say, "Once you are a peer educator, you remain so for the rest of your life." Their voices, combined with those of each new cohort of HTCA, can continue to bring into relief the complex dynamics undergirding HIV transmission among members of the Haitian community, and can also play a significant role in rectifying errors of perception concerning Haitians and AIDS.

Realizing that long-term HIV prevention requires a constant presence of an HIV/AIDS discourse, our goal is to provide a stable context for articulating the concerns of Haitian youth around gender inequality, social justice, and HIV/AIDS in the community. We will continue to follow the example offered by the theology of liberation by breaking the complicity of silence on social injustices, creating an "option for the poor," and struggling with the poor against their repression.

ACKNOWLEDGMENTS

We want to thank all the teens of HTCA (1989–1995). We would like also to thank Joyce Bendremer, Ophelia Dahl, Denny Stein, Janie Simmons, and most of all Tom White. Partners In Health is grateful for the support of the Thomas J. White Foundation, the World AIDS Foundation, the AIDS Action Committee of Massachusetts, the Department of Public Health/AIDS Bureau, the Massachusetts Prevention Center and the Cambridge Hospital. Requests for reprints should be sent to Partners in Health, 113 River Street, Cambridge, MA 02139.

NOTES

1. In disseminating this package, we hope to help other groups generate discussions and to promote dialogue about a disease that will be in our midst for the foreseeable future. PIH has already begun to make good on its goal of global linkages by initiating with Socios En Salud in Carabayllo, Peru, a Peruvian version of Zanmi Lasante's health surveillance project, Proje Veye Sante. By training thirteen young adults from Carabayllo to undertake a community wide health assessment, the project enjoins the insights learned from rural Haitian women's vigilant participation in naming their health needs, and the youth-engaged processes of HTCA. We view each of these linkages as further elaborations of our goal to create and sustain a discourse of health and social justice in social action.

REFERENCES

Abbott, E. (1988). *Haiti: The Duvaliers and their legacy.* New York: McGraw-Hill.

Albert, E. (1986). "Illness and deviance: The response of the press to AIDS." In D. Feldman and T. Johnson (eds.), *The social dimensions of AIDS: Method and theory.* New York: Praeger.

Casper, V. (1986). "AIDS: A psychological perspective." In D. Feldman and T. Johnson (eds.), *The social dimensions of AIDS: Method and theory.* New York: Praeger.

Centers for Disease Control (1982). "Opportunistic infections and Karposi's sarcoma among Haitians in the United States." *Morbidity and Mortality Weekly Report* 31: 353–54, 360–61.

Collaborative Study Group of AIDS in Haitian-Americans (1987). "Risk factors for AIDS among Haitians residing in the United States: Evidence of heterosexual transmission." *Journal of American Medical Association* 257(5): 635–639.

Desvarieux, M., and J.W. Pape (1991). "HIV and AIDS in Haiti: Recent developments." *AIDS Care* 3(3): 271–79.

Farmer, P. (1988). "Blood, sweat, and baseballs: Haiti in the West Atlantic system." *Dialectical Anthropology* 13: 83–99.

Farmer, P. (1990). "The exotic and mundane: Human Immunodeficiency Virus in Haiti." *Human Nature* 1(4): 415–46.

Farmer, P. (1992). *AIDS and Accusation: Haiti and the Geography of Blame.* Berkeley and Los Angeles: University of California Press.

Farmer, P. (1995). *Culture, poverty, and the dynamics of HIV transmission in rural Haiti.* New York: Gordon and Breach.

Farmer, P., and K. Jim. (1991) "Anthropology, accountability, and the prevention of AIDS." *Journal of Sex Research,* 203–21.

Farmer, P., and A. Kleinman. (1989). "AIDS as human suffering." *Daedalus* 118(2): 135–60.

Laguerre, M. (1984). *American odyssey: Haitians living in New York.* Ithaca, N.Y.: Cornell University Press.

Moore, A., and R. Lebaron. (1986). "The case for a Haitian origin of the AIDS epidemic." In D. Feldman and T. Johnson (eds.), *The social dimensions of AIDS: Method and theory.* New York: Praeger.

Nachman, S., and G. Dreyfuss. (1986). "Haitians and AIDS in South Florida." *Medical Anthropology Quarterly* 17(2): 32–33.

Pitchenik, A., M. Fischl, G. Dickerson, D. Becker, A. Fournier, M. O'Connell, R. Colton, and T. Spira. (1983). "Opportunistic infections and Karposi's sarcoma among Haitians: Evidence of a new acquired immunodeficiency state." *Annals of Internal Medicine* 98(3): 277–84.

Reid, Elizabeth (1993). *The HIV Epidemic and Development: The Unfolding of the Epidemic.* New York: United Nations Development Programme.

Remafedi, G. (1988). "Preventing the sexual transmission of AIDS during adolescence." *Journal of Adolescent Health Care* 9: 139–43.

Siegal, F.P., and M. Siegal. (1983). *AIDS: The medical mystery.* New York: St. Martin's Press.

Smith, H. (Dec. 1983). *AIDS: The Haitian connection.* MD, 46–52.

Sontag, S. (1988). *AIDS as metaphor.* New York: Farrar, Straus, Giroux.

Valdeserri, R. (1989). *Preventing AIDS: The design of effective programs.* New Brunswick, N.J.: Rutgers University Press.

Viera, J. (1985). "The Haitian link." In V. Gong (ed.), *Understanding AIDS: A comprehensive guide.* New Brunswick, N.J.: Rutgers University Press.

Viera, J., E. Frank, T. Spira, and S. Landerman (1983). "Acquired immune deficiency in Haitians: Opportunistic infections in previously healthy Haitian immigrants." *New England Journal of Medicine* 308: 125–29.

19

HIV Does Not Erase Desire: Addressing the Sexual and Reproductive Concerns of Women with HIV/AIDS

Risa Denenberg

Risa Denenberg is a family nurse practitioner, teacher, and writer with a background in the feminist women's health movement. As a provider of health care to individuals and families with HIV/AIDS since 1988, she was in a front-line position to recognize the impact of gender on survival in women with HIV infection. In an effort to improve primary care services for women with HIV/AIDS, Denenberg authored *OB/GYN Care for HIV-Positive Women*.

Janine is a 26-year-old HIV-positive woman who is the mother of one child, four-year-old Jeannette, who has tested HIV negative. When Janine came to the clinic for her gynecological exam, I asked her my usual questions, including,

"Do you plan to have more children?"
"But I can't," she responded.
"What do you mean?" I inquired.
"When the doctor gave me my diagnosis, he told me I couldn't have any more children."

This authority had convinced Janine that his negative value judgment about her worthiness to bear a child was a medical certainty. In fact, Janine had not disclosed her HIV status to her current boyfriend, because he desperately wanted her to have his baby. She was afraid he might leave her if he found out she was "sterile." *And* she was having unprotected sex with him because she couldn't ask him to use a condom.

Professionals working with women living with HIV/AIDS often admit to feelings of profound discomfort when confronted with clients who have unsafe sex, want children, or become pregnant. This bias appears to cross disciplines and is evidenced in doctors, psychologists, and social workers, as well as in peer counselors and community outreach workers. Yetthe insertion of value judgements in such situations causes tension and failure in the client-worker bond. These failures inevitably affect the achievement of medical and psychosocial goals for the client, and invariably the client is blamed for such failures. This article addresses some of the important sexual and reproductive issues facing HIV-positive women and their families.

The framework for presenting these issues is within the context of harm reduction. Harm reduction is a philosophy and practice wherein the worker sets aside all judgments in order to meet clients "where they are at" regarding a problem or crisis. In doing so, the worker also commits to assist the client with technical information toward achieving the client's goal, while reducing the potential harm that may occur due to the client's behavior. This model assumes that all individuals have good and logical reasons for their desired goals, and do not desire to harm themselves or others, but simply do not know how to avoid doing so.[1] The worker is reminded that setting aside personal values for the purpose of engaging a client is not the same as abandoning one's values. Harm reduction has been recognized as a valuable theory for working with problems related to addiction; however, it is equally effective in the arena of sexual and repro-ductive counseling.

Issues of Sex and Safety for Women

For many women, sex has never been safe, and is often only conditionally pleasurable. For all women, sex is fraught with risk—the risk of pregnancy, risk of censure, risk of sexually transmitted diseases, risk of rejection, risk of violence, risk of tainted reputation. These real risks are juxtaposed with the stereotype of female attractiveness and sensuality that the media bom-bards us with. Women feel, on the one hand, inadequate to achieve pleasure, and on the other, afraid of its consequences. In effect, the barriers to pleasure and the promise of pleasure create a tension that must be addressed in discussions of female sexuality. It's this very tension that re-quires acknowledgement in teaching endeavors regarding achieving a healthy female sexuality, and in learning the skills necessary to reduce risk and harm from its expression.

Unfortunately, by adulthood, most women have already experienced varying degrees of harm from sexual expression. Still, sexual drive, and the promise or hope of sexual pleasure and bonding, is a powerful force in women's lives, one that must be reckoned with when considering strategies for reducing harm.

It is helpful to emphasize that taking risks is not the problem. Despite the rhetoric of "risk reduction" in issues of sexuality, it is more useful to recognize sexual risk-taking as a normal part of human development. Adolescents and young adults must take risks to achieve goals appropriate to their developmental growth such as asserting a sexual identity, choosing partners, becoming independent from the family of origin, creating a chosen family, and bearing and raising children. Taking such risks amounts to "trying on" different outfits to see not only what looks good, but also what is most comfortable. This process can allow for healthy individuation and potential to form healthy bonds with others.

However, for many young women, the above scenario does not occur. Early sexual abuse, incest, peer pressure, unplanned pregnancy, or serious medical complications from adolescent pregnancy or sexually transmitted infections may intervene to permanently damage a woman's health and self-image. For women at highest risk of heterosexual transmission of HIV, these problems are intertwined with rampant poverty and drug abuse in their communities. The consequence of these events in women's lives is a tragic waste of potential, creativity, and productivity. The problem is not that women experiment with sex and sexuality, it is that they are forced to do so in an inherently unsafe environment.

Issues of Gender and Inequality

This unsafe environment is also one that sustains gender inequality. In every culture, beginning at birth, gender specifies roles, expectations, and the entire spectrum of an individual's future. This is a fluid reality in which the magnitude of gender difference can change over time or appear unequally among individuals living in the same era. However, neither the biologic fact of female gender, nor its effect on women's lives can be entirely erased. Female gender places girls at greater risk than boys of childhood sexual abuse. Females are far more often the victims of domestic violence, domestic sexual abuse, acquaintance rape, and sexual assault. Women persistently have less earning power than men, creating greater dependency. The consequences of sexual intercourse frequently includes pregnancy for females, a fact that many women directly consider to obstruct sexual pleasure. Conceiving, menstruating, carrying a pregnancy to term, aborting a pregnancy, miscarrying, laboring to deliver a baby, and breastfeeding all take their physical toll on a woman's well-being throughout her lifespan.

Biologic differences between men and women result in social inequality in many spheres. In the medical setting, women have been subject to sexist standards of health care. For example, women's subjective symptoms or medical complaints are often relegated to "stress," "neurosis," "hysteria," or "hypochondria." This happens far less frequently when men offer the same symptoms such as headache, fatigue, palpitations, chest pain, itching, rashes, night sweats, loss of appetite, trouble swallowing, insomnia, or trouble concentrating. Thus, women often learn not to trust the signals of imbalance or ill health that their bodies offer. Furthermore, symptoms of serious illness often go overlooked by medical practitioners, and women are often sicker than are men when they receive treatment for similar medical conditions.[2]

Gender inequality is under public scrutiny and changes are occurring in many areas. However, women still experience a marked disadvantage relative to men in areas such as in the home, in employment, in accumulation of wealth and resources, and in responsibility for raising children. Women cope in various ways with the inequality that they experience in their lives. The extra work that women perform both biologically and socially for their communities takes its toll on the ability to achieve personal health and fulfillment. And for women currently at highest risk for HIV infection, sexism is compounded by the impact of racism and poverty in their neighborhoods. In working with HIV-positive women, it is critical to understand this background. For many HIV-positive women, HIV infection is not their most urgent problem.

Sexual Function in HIV-Positive Women

Commonly, a woman's response to discovery of HIV infection is to shun sexual relations for some period of time. This often is a symptom of depression and altered self-esteem. It may also be accompanied by poor appetite and sleep disturbance. HIV-positive clients need support and encouragement to continue expression of healthy and safe relationships where affection and sexuality are experienced. It is important to recognize that sexual dysfunction is a normal initial response to the crisis of learning that one is HIV infected. Women may need to go through the established stages of grieving—both in anticipation of their own death, and for loss of their previous self-image as healthy and whole. The actual current staging of HIV illness must be taken into account in order to assist clients in working through this successfully. It may help to counsel the client individually and with her partner. The message that sexual dysfunction (like poor sleep and appetite) is most likely temporary, and that sexual interest will resume, is the most realistic and hopeful message. This also sets the stage for working on issues related to safety and sexuality, whereas these issues are often overlooked when the woman reports that there is no current sexual partner, or no current sexual behavior with an intimate partner.

It is important to keep in mind that for women clients, intimate and sexual relationships may take place with men, women, or both. Lesbian clients need to have their partners and families included in care planning, and clinicians need to know safe-sex guidelines for woman who have sex with women. Further, women often need support and assistance in learning how to disclose their HIV status to sexual partners, how to incorporate the use of barriers into sexual relationships, and how to experience pleasure during sex.

Childbearing Concerns

Until recently, the Centers for Disease Control recommended that HIV-positive women be discouraged from bearing children.[3] This is not the first time that primarily poor woman have received the message not to procreate. Nor is it the first time that these women have responded to such a message with the belief that the government and medical providers are insensitive to their communities or have genocidal goals in mind. It is not an unrealistic concern, considering the intergenerational effect HIV is having in poor communities in the United States. The public response to a pregnant, HIV-positive woman amplifies the medical and governmental message. In general, HIV-positive men and women are bombarded with messages not to engage in activities which have previously been considered normal. The slogan "living" with AIDS becomes a cruel joke to persons living under such proscriptions. Women are especially prone to denying their normal interest in sexual activities and childbearing, and are often unable to locate any support for reasserting a healthy sexual and reproductive response under the constraints of HIV illness. Affirming that all individuals have a right to our own hopes and dreams regarding our future is the best starting place for beginning to understand the dilemmas confronting an HIV-positive woman. Supporting the sexual and childbearing goals of all HIV-positive people is not only ethically imperative, but it is the most practical way of offering hopeful messages and helpful interventions.

Women with HIV infection who are not overwhelmed by illness generally have the same attitudes and emotions regarding childbearing as they had prior to their diagnosis. Efforts to interfere in this type of personal and family decision making is not only an invasion of the woman's privacy, but tends to impose distance between the professional and the HIV-positive woman. When providers are seen as supportive of women's rights and abilities to make informed personal decisions, the provider/client relationship is generally preserved.

Several researchers have shown that HIV-positive women do not differ significantly from similar HIV-negative women in making personal decisions regarding carrying or aborting a pregnancy.[4,5,6] Women at risk of HIV infection are also likely to experience the profound effect of the epidemic on their families, extended families, neighbors, friends, and community. Often there is extreme disruption of norms in family formation and child-rearing due to intergenerational death from AIDS. Ethnic, religious, and cultural background greatly influence women's response to this devastation.

Implications of Current Research in Counseling Pregnant Women

HIV-positive women have confronted barriers to accessing promising drug trials due to concern regarding their "reproductive potential" (i.e., the fear regarding possible damaging effects of experimental medication on a fetus). Some drug trials have required women to undergo permanent sterilization in order to enroll; others require proof of contraception or periodic pregnancy testing. Research centers may mandate the use of the intrauterine device (IUD) for birth control in females who wish to enroll despite the consensus that this method may pose risk of infection and thus is contraindicated in HIV infection.[7] Due to the low enrollment of women in drug trials, we really know very little about the efficacy, dosing, and reproductive side effects of AIDS drugs in women's bodies.

On the other hand, the scientific community has been very interested in researching transmission of HIV from mother to child during pregnancy and labor. Many women view this lack of interest in women, coupled with this enhanced interest in their children, as oppressive. At the same time, HIV-positive women are very concerned about issues of HIV transmission during pregnancy.

HIV-positive women who are asymptomatic do as well as other similar (but HIV-negative) women during their pregnancies, and do not appear to have higher rates of complications such as prematurity or low-birth-weight babies. The mother's HIV antibodies are always passed on to the fetus, but the virus is only transmitted about 20–30 percent of the time.[8] Therefore, the pregnant woman has a good chance of having an uninfected baby. However, even these babies need to be followed carefully, and the diagnosis of "positive" or "negative" may not be certain for many months.

A trial was conducted by the AIDS Clinical Trial Groups (ACTG #076) in which the drug Retrovir (AZT) was given to pregnant women and their newborns to observe the effects of the drug on perinatal transmission of HIV. The trial was ended in 1994, when it was determined that Retrovir reduced HIV transmission significantly in the women enrolled in the study.[9] While this is very hopeful information, there are still many unanswered questions. We don't yet know if all women will experience the same benefit as those enrolled in the trial, and we don't know the long-term effects on the children who were exposed to AZT during fetal development. One very important concern about the trial results is that there will be more public pressure to require HIV antibody testing of all pregnant women. It is very important that advocates of HIV-positive women understand that forcing pregnant women to be tested for HIV, or to take AZT during pregnancy, represents a grave violation of their civil rights. It is only by protecting women's reproductive rights, and being sensitive to their dilemmas and problems, that we can hope to impact positively on their decision making.

Harm Reduction in Sexual Counseling

To use a harm reduction model in sexual counseling, all judgments must be put aside to support a client's goals and provide technical information. In initiating discussions regarding sexual behavior, it is helpful to start by acknowledging that individuals don't always know what we want or what we might do in a given sexual situation. For the following complicated reasons, sexual goals are difficult to put into words:

- Our sexual fantasies are private, but sometimes difficult to separate from our desired sexual actions.
- Our sexual relationships are shared, and therefore not entirely subject to individual planning.
- Many of us have unresolved issues concerning our own sexuality which may inhibit our ideal sexual responses.
- Drugs and alcohol often affect our sexual behaviors.

Taking a comprehensive sexual history is the critical underlying task. It is essential to ask clients if they have experienced sexual abuse, incest, or rape. Many HIV-positive women report a history of childhood sexual abuse. Studies show that a history of unresolved sexual abuse often leaves women vulnerable in sexual situations, rendering them more likely to experience adolescent pregnancy, substance abuse, domestic violence, and HIV infection.[10] Advising these women to "negotiate" with their partners may be ineffective because they may feel powerless in all sexual situations. Other more thoughtful interventions, geared toward bolstering the client's self-esteem, and supportive counseling to resolve or lessen the symptoms of sexual trauma will be more helpful than slogans to "use condoms." Of course professionals must be prepared to respond appropriately whenever abuse is disclosed. Clients should always be reassured that the abuse was not their fault and that healing (or resolution) is usually possible with the proper support. Furthermore, it is likely that such women or their children are at current risk for sexual or physical abuse, because women who were abused as children may choose abusive partners as adults. Any such disclosure will require appropriate crisis intervention to secure safety for the woman and children at risk.

All clients should be asked if they have had sexual relations with men, women, or both; if they have exchanged sex for money, drugs, or shelter (survival sex); if they have any current sexual partner(s); and how they feel about their current semicolon sexual situation. A current sexual situation can be explored by assessing specific sexual acts, sexual satisfaction, discomforts associated with specific sex acts, use of contraceptives, and use of barriers for protection from STDs. The current trend to ask the (useless) question, "How many sexual partners have you had over your lifetime?" is easily discarded if the questioner imagines being asked this question herself.

Once a history is obtained, certain tentative "goals" can be formulated with the client. This presents an opportunity for the client to "try on" various ideas presented by the counselor. The client is guided to articulate what fits her best. Again, the underlying assumption is that individuals have good and logical reasons for their behaviors but will be able to modify behaviors to increase personal safety if basic goals are not obstructed. Naming behaviors allows the client to compare a description of what she is doing with what she believes she might want to be doing. After taking a history, the counselor may say something like this: "So, you and your partner both want to have unprotected intercourse, but for different reasons. He doesn't believe than a man can be infected through sex with a woman, *and* he wants to have a baby with you. You want to have unprotected sex with him, because you are afraid that if you tell him that you have the virus, you will lose him. But now you understand that unprotected sex may lead to a pregnancy and to infection for your partner. You are not sure right now how you would feel about a pregnancy. Is that right?" If the client finds this to be an acceptable assessment of her goals and desires, two interventions could be offered immediately: the use of temporary non-barrier contraception (such as birth control pills) to prevent a pregnancy until more resolution is reached, and the use of a vaginal spermicide (contraceptive spermicides come in the form of suppositories, creams, or films—which can be used discretely) to decrease his risk of infection until disclosure is possible. Both of these interventions will buy time for the client, and incorporate the knowledge that most behavior change is incremental, not monumental.

In another situation, after obtaining a history, the counselor might say: "So, you want to hold on to your boyfriend, and you're afraid to tell him you're HIV-positive because he may become very upset or even leave you. You try to avoid sex with him as much as possible, but you still want to have sex with your female partner occasionally. Your boyfriend doesn't want to use condoms because he wants you to have his baby, even though he knows you do not want another child. Is that right?" One obvious intervention is to assist the client to use barriers with any liaison outside of the primary relationship. This reduces the risk of STDs and HIV transmission to all concerned. The more difficult intervention is to guide the client through a discussion of the inevitable disclosure to her partner and their conflict over childbearing. It is reasonable to ask her directly how she would feel if her partner contracted HIV from her, or if she became pregnant in the next few months.

Of course the client may not agree that the counselor has correctly described her goals and plans. This, too, offers an opportunity to fine-tune the discussion in order to look closely at what is really going on. The woman in the second example may say, "I don't want to tell him, but not because he would leave me. I just don't want to tell him everything I have done in the past or everything I do, for that matter. And he has done things too. He could already have the virus, for all I know." She may be more willing to disclose her HIV status than the fact that she has other sexual partners at the present time. In this case, the client may agree to couples counseling so that she can disclose her serostatus in a supportive situation. Then the couple can be assisted in defining sexual and reproductive goals as a couple. The client could be assured that her confidences regarding other sexual partners would be respected.

There are many possible situations that may be encountered in sexual counseling of individuals and couples. Individuals may be gay, lesbian, bisexual, or heterosexual. Couples may be concordant or discordant in their HIV status, or the status of one or both partners may be unknown. Clients may need technical information about potential transmission of HIV for specific sexual acts. Some clients practice unsafe sex consensually; others may practice unprotected sex without discussing the consequences with their sexual partners. Many individuals, regardless of HIV status, practice a variety of sexual acts, in which some would be considered safe and others unsafe. In most situations, however, by using the sexual history and techniques which clarify sexual goals, interventions can be planned with clients that reduce risks without interfering with sexual autonomy.

The most difficult part of this work is learning to set aside personal judgment about sexual goals and behaviors, while holding on to values that protect others from harm. Most professionals tend to agree that a child at risk of sexual abuse by an adult requires investigation and protection. However, consensus may be more difficult regarding partner notification of

HIV for consenting adults. It is important to spend adequate time discussing these difficult concerns with colleagues in a supportive atmosphere.

Harm Reduction in Reproductive Counseling

General admonitions regarding safer sex may not take into consideration that couples may engage in unprotected intercourse for the purpose of procreation. This may be an individual or mutual goal within a couple. Single heterosexual women and lesbians also may engage in unprotected sexual intercourse in order to get pregnant.

Again, the first step is to take a comprehensive history. Once this is initiated, a portrait of individual and family goals can be painted, and interventions that will be specific and useful can be introduced. It matters how questions are posed to clients. Taking an appropriate and comprehensive sexual and reproductive history allows the provider many opportunities to educate, support, and intervene. If a trusting relationship has been built, and the client expects the counselor to support her goals, difficult questions can be raised and not perceived as obstructing the client's intent. On the other hand, it becomes a crisis between the woman and her counselor if a pregnancy occurs before the topic has been broached and thoroughly discussed, so that goals are understood and supported.

The HIV-positive woman or couple who wish to have children have a great need for accurate and up-to-date information. The risk to the pregnant woman who is HIV-positive but asymptomatic is considered to be similar to the obstetrical risks of an HIV-negative woman who is matched for parity, socioeconomic status, drug use, etc.[11,12] For the symptomatic woman with little immune reserve, the risks to the mother are much greater. Risk of viral transmission to the fetus during pregnancy and delivery may be reduced by good prenatal nutrition and good prenatal care, as well as by use of AZT, where desired.[13,14] Sperm washing techniques are not currently available, but may be in the future, in order to render semen from an HIV-positive donor safe for insemination.[15] Breast feeding may transmit HIV from mother to baby.[16]

The focus of the discussion will be to address the areas of uncertainty. In some situations, there will be the risk of HIV transmission to an uninfected partner. Is the couple willing to assume such a risk? How much risk is acceptable? What are the parents' strengths and weaknesses at parenting? Will the parents be able to accept if the child is HIV-infected, becomes ill, or dies? Can the parents imagine how they might feel during the first few months after the child is born when there is no way to know for sure if the child has the virus? How will they feel about the possibility that the HIV-positive parent (or both parents) might not live long enough to raise the child? What are the family support systems and extended family network that will be able to help in the event of illness or death of a parent?

Many women want a child to replace children they have lost either through their own inability to provide a stable environment or through a death from AIDS or other causes. Some couples want to parent a child together, even though one or both already have had children with a prior partner. This is rocky but important terrain to cover. Identification of the skills and resources needed to become successful at parenting may assist clients to attain their goals or to modify them. For example, if a woman receives support and counseling for her desire to regain custody of a child in foster care, she may find renewed energy to work on that goal, and her desire to achieve a new pregnancy may diminish.

Conclusion

Let's go back to Janine, whom I introduced at the beginning of this article. In working with her, my first goal was to correct the misinformation she had received, and to listen carefully to her emotional response (anger and curiosity) to the correction. I gradually provided additional information regarding HIV infection and pregnancy. I broached the topic of HIV transmission and disclosure to her partner, Rick. When she was ready, I offered to be present during the disclosure. Finally, over time I counseled the couple, who were able to initiate the use of condoms as a temporary measure "until things become clearer." Thankfully, Rick tested HIV-negative. Some months later, after the couple worked through many feelings and issues, they decided they wanted to have a child together. At this point, they articulated the shared value to the family of reducing the risk of transmission to Rick. (Janine said, "At least our baby could have one healthy parent.") With instruction and guidance, they were able to successfully learn to detect Janine's fertile days, and they learned to inseminate

Rick's semen at home, without risking transmission. Janine is now pregnant, and she and Rick are still together as a couple.

NOTES

1. Edith Springer, "Effective AIDS prevention with active drug users: the harm
reduction model," *Counseling Chemically Dependent People with HIV Illness,* ed. Michael
Shernoff (New York: Haworth Press, 1991): 141–58.

2. American Medical Association, Council on Ethical and Judicial Affairs, "Gender
disparities in clinical decision making." *Journal of the American Medical Association* 266
(1991): 559–62.

3. Centers for Disease Control, "Recommendations for assisting in the prevention
of perinatal transmission of human T-lymphocyte virus type III/lymphadenopathy-
associated virus and acquired immunodeficiency syndrome," *Morbidity and Mortality
Weekly Report* 34 (1985): 721–26.

4. F. D. Johnstone et al., "Women's knowledge of their HIV antibody state: Its effect
on their decision whether to continue the pregnancy," *British Medical Journal* 300 (1990):
23–24.

5. P. A. Selwyn et al., "Knowledge of HIV antibody status and decisions to continue
or terminate pregnancy among intravenous drug users," *Journal of the American Medical
Association* 261 (1989): 3567–71.

6. A. Sunderland et al., "The impact of influence of human immunodeficiency
virus serostatus on reproductive decisions of women." *Obstetrics and Gynecology* 7, no. 6
(1992): 1027–31.

7. Ann Kurth and Howard L. Minkoff, "Pregnancy and reproductive concerns of
women with HIV infection," in *Primary Care of Women and Children with HIV Infection,*
eds. P. Kelly, S. Holman, R. Rothenberg, and S. P. Holzemer (Boston: Jones and
Bartlett, 1995), 59–88.

8. European Collaborative Study, "Risk factors for mother to child transmission of
HIV-1," *Lancet* 339 (1992): 1007–12.

9. Centers for Disease Control, "Zidovudine for the prevention of HIV transmission
from mother to infant," *Morbidity and Mortality Weekly Report* 43 (1994): 285–7.

10. James Cassese, "The invisible bridge: Child sexual abuse and the risk of HIV
infection in adulthood." *SEICUS Report* 21.4 (1993): 1–7.

11. F. D. Johnstone, "Pregnancy outcome and pregnancy management in HIV-
infected women," in *HIV Infection in Women,* eds. M. A. Johnson and F. D. Johnstone
(London: Churchill Livingston, 1993), 187–98.

12. H. L. Minkoff et al., "Pregnancy outcomes among women infected with HIV
and matched controls," *American Journal of Obstetrics and Gynecology* 163 (1990): 1598–
1603.

13. R. D. Semba et al., "Maternal vitamin A deficiency and mother-to-child
transmission of HIV-1," *Lancet* 343 (1994): 1595–97.

14. Centers for Disease Control, "U.S. Public Health Service recommendations for human immunodeficiency virus counseling and voluntary testing for pregnant women," *Morbidity and Mortality Weekly Report* 44, RR-7 (1995).

15. A. E. Semprini et al., "Insemination of HIV-negative women with processed semen of HIV-positive partners," *Lancet* 340 (1992): 1317–19.

16. WHO/UNICEF, Consultation on HIV Transmission and Breastfeeding, *Consensus Statement and Press Release* (Geneva: World Health Organization, May 1992).

20

Native Women Living beyond HIV/AIDS Infection

Linda Burhansstipanov, Carole laFavor,
Shirley Hoskins, Gloria Bellymule,
and Ron Rowell

Each of the authors is an advocate for culturally competent quality of care for Native peoples infected with or affected by HIV/AIDS. All are involved in the HRSA Special Initiatives to gain access to quality care and to implement culturally relevant case management programs for HIV/AIDS-infected Native American women. *Linda Burhansstipanov,* MSPH, DrPH, CHES (Western Cherokee) is the director of the AMC Native American Cancer Research Program (Denver, Colo.), director of research at the American Indian Clinic (Bellflower, Calif.), and a consultant to the National Native American AIDS Prevention Center (Oakland, Calif.). *Carole Lafavor* (Ojibwa) is the editor of *Positively Native,* a quarterly newsletter created to develop confidentially as well as an unobtrusive support mechanism for Native Americans who are HIV-positive or who have AIDS. Carole is a national advocate for access to state-of-the-art treatment and quality of care for Native peoples, as well as integration of traditional healing within the treatment paradigm. *Shirley Hoskins* (Kickapoo/Potawatomie) is the director of the Native American HIV/AIDS Coalition of the greater Kansas City area and is responsible for implementing a protocol to accurately identify Native Americans within her state database. She also developed culturally relevant case management support services for Native Peoples within Kansas and Missouri. *Gloria Bellymule,* RN (Cheyenne) is a case manager for the Ahalaya Project in Oklahoma and is responsible for developing and implementing the most comprehensive, culturally competent case management model for Native Americans on the continent. She has advocated for services which, prior to her involvement, were denied to Native Americans infected with HIV (e.g., medications for dual-diagnosed clients). RON ROWELL, MPH (Choctaw) is the Executive Director of the National Native American AIDS Prevention Center and is responsible for organizing both local and national initiatives to better meet the needs of Native peoples. He has taken a leadership role in raising the awareness of HIV as a problem within Native communities since 1987 and regularly works with Congress and federal agencies on HIV/AIDS quality-of-care issues.

Overview

The Health Resources Service Administration (HRSA) funded the Special Initiatives Project of the National Native American AIDS Prevention Center (NNAAPC) in 1993 to develop services around the country for American Indians, Alaska Natives, and Native Hawaiians who were HIV-infected. As a result of this two-year project, nine Native American organizations were funded in October 1993 and three additional projects were funded in late January 1994. The projects represented geographically diverse sections of the country (e.g., Alaska, Hawaii, southwestern, central, northeastern states) and included Native Americans who lived in the urban and rural areas, as well as on reservations. As a result of these projects, NNAAPC developed a national database of AIDS-infected American Indians, Alaska Natives, and Native Hawaiians. As of October 1995, this database includes 269 Native American clients, of whom 91 have asymptomatic HIV, 76 have symptomatic HIV, and 102 have AIDS. In addition to collecting accurate data about HIV among Native Americans, these projects also initiated culturally relevant and/or competent case management programs, implemented a national network of Native Americans who were living with HIV/AIDS, and spread awareness throughout Indian Country that HIV was finally being raised as a health priority within Native communities.

According to the NNAAPC national AIDS database (February 1995), Native women are overrepresented among the Native AIDS cases (18 percent) when compared with nonminority populations. This overrepresentation of women is consistent with other minority populations. Women are the fastest-growing population at risk for contracting HIV. Approximately 52 percent of the women are asymptomatic with HIV, 16 percent are symptomatic with HIV, and 32 percent have been diagnosed with AIDS. The primary mode of transmission among Native female clients was through heterosexual contact (52 percent). Other specified common modes of transmission included IV drug use (32 percent), blood transfusion (7 percent), unknown (6 percent), and maternal (3 percent). The mean age of adult women clients is thirty-six years. The CD-4 counts for adult women clients range from 5 to 952, with a mean of 342. There were no statistically significant differences between male and female clients on the basis of demographics or health status.

As a result of these NNAAPC-supported projects, culturally competent HIV/AIDS programs were initiated in geographically and culturally diverse Native American communities. Of striking significance was the overwhelming impact of these programs, as was evidenced by the participation of Native American HIV/AIDS clients in case management service programs. Based upon documentation from Ryan White and other-supported HIV/AIDS case management programs throughout the U.S., Native American HIV/AIDS clients visit non-Native facilities/service organizations once and typically do not return until the final stages of the disease are manifest. However, through the provision of HIV/AIDS programs developed by and for Natives, according to project staff, client participation and retention within the NNAAPC SPNS case management programs was approximately 90 percent.

Western Medicine in Comparison with Traditional Indian Medicine Access to Care Issues Affecting Native American Women and HIV/AIDS

Western Medical Physician	Traditional Medical Healer
"What are your symptoms?" asks the Western medical doctor.	The traditional Native healer waits patiently for you to tell him/her whatever you want to, in whatever order you choose.
A physician says, "You can pray if you want, but here's a prescription for AZT. Don't forget to take it."	After praying as he or she gathers and prepares herbal medicines for you, the Native healer gives it to you to take, then counsels you about the importance of your state of mind when you take the medicine, and the importance of a prayerful life.
When you make an appointment with your physician, the receptionist asks about the kind of insurance you carry, and may ask, "Do you think this is a twenty-minute visit, or will you need a half an hour?"	When you go to your Native healer, you bring tobacco, corn pollen, or some other offering of respect and honor (depending on your tribe's tradition), and you stay as long as you need to (e.g., in one meeting one of the coauthors stayed four hours).

These are just a few examples of the discernible differences between Western medicine and the healing practices of Native Americans. It is not as simple, though, as saying allopathic doctors treat symptoms and Native healers treat people, because the implications of that statement are enormous. To follow through on the promise to treat the whole person requires a tremendous commitment—some would say a spiritual commitment. According to a respected Dakota healer, "To be a healer, you have to be ready anytime day or night. If someone calls and needs your help, you go. If someone comes by and gives you tobacco, asking for your help, you give it, without question. Creator says you must be ready at a moment's notice. I am a pipe carrier. I go whenever I'm asked. Native women know our healers take their commitment seriously. This gives us confidence in them, and in their concern for us. Confidence in one's healer is strongly believed by HIV-infected Native women to be an important factor in their longevity with HIV.

To follow through on the promise to treat the whole person also requires a host of skills that may be more culturally inherent than learned. One of those skills is looking to other living things for advice. When asked how people with HIV should evaluate all the treatments being recommended, Ojibwa elder Lillian Rice replied, "I believe that somewhere there's a medicine for HIV. Mother Earth provides all we need. Animals know what to eat to help themselves. Out walking once we saw where a bear had been eating ginger roots. Well, why were they eating that? They needed it for some reason. The HIV virus came from an animal. That animal must know what to take for it, how to live with it. Or look at your dog, for example. Have you seen him outside eating grass? He does that when he doesn't feel good. That's how Indian people did it hundreds of years ago, we watched and learned from animals. We should watch the animals where HIV came from. What do they do?" Women who have this belief feel that Native healers use all avenues to help us heal from, and live with, our illness. It is a secure feeling to know we are being assisted by so many levels—by more than just Western medicine.

Another Native healer once said, "Listening is probably the most important thing I do. Listening as a child to my grandfather, he taught me about plants and their uses. Now, it's important that I listen to people who come to me for help, listen to the mood of the community, and listen to the spirits. If you're not a good listener, you won't be a good healer." When you sit with a healer with that attitude, you feel listened to, which breeds trust, and a sense that your life is important to them. This feeling of security and confidence in your healer is an important factor in the quality and quantity of life for people living with HIV.

Often in HIV circles you hear of people closely monitoring their blood work, especially T-cell counts to determine their state of wellness. Many Native women with HIV do not keep track of T-cell counts, or only want to know what it is if they have to make a decision about a Western medical treatment. That is because we believe it's more important to pay attention to how we feel rather than what our blood level is. We know blood tests are a very small part of watching our health. We are much more than T-cell counts. Too many times we've heard people say they felt good, even great, until they heard their T-cell count had dropped, and then they began to feel terrible—their quality of life changed in a flash because they gave too much weight to lab tests, and not enough to how they really felt. Native healers teach us to pay attention to all aspects of ourselves—to our physical symptoms, to our emotional state, and to our spiritual well-being.

That brings us to another teaching from Native healers—that our journey does not end when we die; we are transformed and go on to the spirit world. Thus: (1) it's important to pay attention to our spiritual, as well as our physical and emotional journey, and (2) death is not a failure, it is only another step along the Red Road. We're a praying people, and spiritual health is the most important kind of health for which Native people strive. As long as we are spiritually healthy, physical health, regardless of what it is, can be accepted.

People in this country were done a grave disservice at the beginning of the 1900s when other kinds of therapies were pushed aside by modern medical schools at the onset of high-tech scientific medicine. Treatments that had been used for hundreds of years, which had been brought to North America in the trunks and minds of people from all over Europe and Africa, were outlawed or declared folk medicine by the more (so-called) sophisticated scientific circles. One has to wonder if part of the prejudice then came from the fact that in many circles women were the primary healers, and almost 100 percent of the allopathic medicine was implemented by men. After being labeled witchcraft on the one hand, many medicines still found their way into the U.S. Pharmacopeia as treatments for one malady or another. For example, aspirin was originally an Ojibwa medicine scraped from the inside of the bark of the aspen tree, but until it was crushed and formed into tiny white pills and a price was put on it by a pharmaceutical company, it was considered medicine-man voodoo by allopathic doctors.

It has taken many people more than ninety years to get out from under that blanket oppressing their choices. While Native healing ceremonies were outlawed and derided, we didn't lose them because there were many brave and spiritual people in the tribes that refused to bend to the "great white father's" orders and went underground with the ceremonies, preserving them for their descendants. These are the traditions and treatments that we now rely on as we live with HIV. And we thank our ancestors every day for their courage in life-threatening situations to preserve traditions that are now saving our lives.

Many Native women choose the guidance we receive from our grannies and other tribal elders over that of scientific America. A Seminole elder stated, "Good medicine is for healing. To do it, a lot of it is belief in it. If you don't believe in something, if your hearts not in it, it'll be hard to heal." What could any scientist add to that? The CDC is not our leader, or whom we turn to for advice. Our elders and healers are our leaders. They are because they show us over and over they care about us as people, not as a group of symptoms. They are because, over and over, we get better under their care; we learn to live full, spiritual lives under their care. Mourning Dove, a Salish woman, gave us hopeful words to live by when she instructed us, "everything on earth has a purpose, every disease and herb to cure it, and every person a mission. This is the Indian theory of existence." It is a theory that has kept the Native circle surviving and thriving for centuries despite plagues, massacres, reservations, poverty, starvation, drugs and alcoholism, and now HIV/AIDS.

Needs Identified by HIV/AIDS-Infected Native Women

Issues and concerns described in this next section are compiled from interviews with Native American women who are HIV positive or have AIDS, or from Native women case managers. The women come from a variety of tribal affiliations and geographic areas and all are involved with the NNAAPC SPNS projects.

The Need for Gender-Specific HIV/AIDS Services

The National Native American AIDS Prevention Center (NNAAPC) received HRSA SPNS support to sponsor HIV/AIDS planning and service projects in diverse regions of Indian Country. During the 1995 summary of the funded projects, common unmet needs were identified and among those was the need to provide gender-specific and sexual orientation-specific HIV/AIDS support programs. Likewise, there is a need to have female Native American case managers and direct outreach services for Native American HIV-positive women. The perception among American Indian women infected with HIV or AIDS was that services were gender-specific for males and did not meet their needs, were unavailable to them, or were so difficult to access that they were unable to utilize them.

The Need for Culturally Competent Services

There is a dearth of culturally relevant and competent support services for Native Americans of both sexes. The majority of support services are designed for homosexual males or IVDU, and consequently the model for successful support groups has been developed by and for homosexual men. For example, one component of these successful models is identification and implementation of a buddy system. However, this model has not been implemented for families, teens, and mothers, and their needs for buddy systems which are geared toward the family structure.

There is great need to have services where men and women of color can feel comfortable. Native women who have HIV or AIDS have identified some factors that increase one's comfort in a support group. Among the most frequently mentioned factors is having someone who looks like you or is a member of another Indian nation in the group. This eliminates the need to constantly explain your Native culture and to justify or rationalize why specific factors are of greater or differing priority within Native communities than in non–Native cultures.

Although being HIV-positive creates an immediate commonality and bond among infected individuals, there are so many subtleties within the culture that are difficult, or inappropriate to share. For example, Native women who are infected with HIV frequently participate in different healing ceremonies, which require many weeks of preparation (physically, mentally, and spiritually). These preparations are difficult for those outside of the culture to understand and vary among the tribes, and the intensity of such ceremonies is frequently misunderstood. Those outside the culture frequently react inappropriately to the significance and depth of a cere-mony. For example, during an HIV support group with multicultural women, a Native woman who is HIV-positive briefly described her participation within a Sundance during the last summer. She recounted that the ceremony included cutting and giving up part of the body. The members of the HIV support group who listened to this became shocked by this portion of the ceremony and focused on it alone and missed the entire significance of both this component of the ceremony as well as of the entire ceremony. In comparison, when a woman says that she participated in a Sundance to another Native woman, the phenomenal impact and power of that type of healing on both the woman and her community is immediately understood and respected.

Another common problem in not having access to culturally specific support programs is that non-Natives frequently request specific information regarding Indian healing ceremonies. When such information has been provided, many non-Natives have attempted to "take" certain components of the ceremonies that are appealing to them and incorporate those facets within their own, personally developed healing protocols. This bastardizing of ceremonies is greatly resented by the Indian community and considered insulting because it diminishes the potential impact and sacredness of the Indian ceremony. This is among the reasons why it is inappropriate for Indian people to ever describe in detail specifics of ceremonies. This bastardizing has become rampant among followers of "New Age" practices.

Examples of culturally competent services would be the inclusion of traditional forms of counseling, spiritual healing, and community support, such as through the Talking Circle for American Indian women or Talk Story for Native Hawaiian women. Likewise, many indigenous peoples who are infected with HIV and AIDS have found great support through participation in the Native American Church. Culturally competent services also include access to sweats, traditional healers, and herbalists.

NNAAPC has identified a total of five support programs specifically designed for American Indian women. These programs have been located in the following states: Kansas/Missouri, Minnesota, New York, Oklahoma, Washington. An example of a model program is in Minnesota. A Native American women's support group meets once a week. Transportation is provided to women without cars, child care is provided, and lunch is often included to give the women, especially the mothers, a break in cooking for large families. The women smudge and pray, and sometimes have Talking Circles. At other times they do Indian crafts while discussing how HIV infection impacts their lives and the lives of their families.

The Need to Develop, Implement, and Assess Culturally Competent HIV/ AIDS Gender-Specific Counseling Services

Native women felt that the counseling models currently being implemented were based on non-Native belief structures and needed to be modified to be culturally acceptable to HIV-positive Native women. For example, many counseling paradigms implement very directive and restrictive protocols. But Native people appear to respond more positively to nondirective models that provide for alternative choices (e.g., including options to incorporate traditional healing within one's treatment program).

The Need to Collect Information on Relatives Who Have Family Members Infected with HIV/AIDS

There is a dearth of information about families affected with HIV, especially Native American families. Due to the initial populations significantly infected with HIV, the services which evolved were targeted to meet the needs of gay men and IVDU. These services are based on single males and have received positive client satisfaction ratings. However, as the pattern of infection shifts, service agencies are confronted with the demand to implement protocols which meet the growing needs for family-structured services, and they lack access to accurate information about the family structures to develop or implement such services. For example, successful retreats for HIV-positive clients have primarily been focused on the individual. There is a need to also provide retreats which address the needs of whole families affected by HIV (e.g., those with one or both parents and/ or children affected). An example of such a program is the Minnesota American Indian AIDS Task Force, which has been a leader in providing culturally specific retreats for whole families with day care available for children of clients. Another is the Indian Health Council, Inc. (San Diego, Calif.) and their retreat, the Native Traditional Family, Youth and Elder Retreat and Healing Ceremonies. The goals of the retreats were to (1) provide Native American HIV infected and affected individuals with social support; (2) educate participants of the healing potential to body, mind, emotion, and spirit through participation in ceremonies and healing activities; (3) improve the quality of life of the HIV infected and affected Native American by helping the participant work toward obtaining balance in one's life in the traditional manner; and (4) increase self-esteem and empowerment by "remembering" the power and healing inherent in Indian culture. Retreat highlights included morning sweats, HIV-positive "Talking Circles" (one for men, one for women, another for gays and lesbians), youth activities, sessions on learning traditional songs, and puberty ceremonies for the youth.

The Need to Provide Family-Oriented Nutritional Services

Many services that initially appear to be universal, regardless of one's sex, sexual orientation, or culture, are found to have unique characteristics as data become available. For example, nutritional programs were created to meet the needs of infected individuals, who initially were primarily homosexual males or IVDU. These nutritional programs (where available) have been very well accepted and successful among these populations. However, there appear to be either limited or no food programs that address the nutritional needs of women who have children. For example, an American Indian woman from the central states attempted to collect sustenance through the AIDS food pantry. She has six children and was provided food for herself alone. How many women (of any color!) would eat in front of their hungry children or husband? Nutritional and vitamin therapy counseling also is usually geared to men's nutritional needs and not to women's nutritional requirements (e.g., an elevated intake of calcium, iron, and so on).

The Need for Confidentiality within Small, Sparsely Populated Communities

A nagging issue within the overall Native community is confidentiality. Indian Country is very small and almost everyone knows everyone else. Of the Native American projects funded through NNAAPC, there was a consensus that a high-priority need was to develop a protocol to maintain confidentiality within sparsely populated, rural, tightly knit communities (e.g., neighbors see an HIV case manager drive toward an individual's home and it is assumed that someone who lives there must have AIDS). Efforts also need to go toward making confidentiality less necessary by removing the stigma surrounding this illness (e.g., through the implementation of culturally relevant HIV/AIDS education programs targeted to the entire Native community).

Most women who either are, or suspect that they are HIV-positive greatly fear the loss of confidentiality. At the client's request, the extended family members may not be informed of the diagnosis. Cultural support and family support may be available, but by the choice of the client, the women are not accessing their support. Native women typically won't even take brochures, fliers, or any HIV-specific information for fear someone from the community might see the printed information and "guess" about their HIV status. In addition, Native women appear to go to great extremes to keep knowledge of the HIV infection from their children. Obviously, if they have children who can read, this need to keep the disease hidden interferes with them receiving printed HIV/AIDS information. This driving need to keep the diagnosis private increases the feelings of isolation experienced by women who are HIV-positive or who have AIDS. Even when opportunities exist to bring HIV-infected women together to a fun activity, such as a picnic or an Indian craft workshop, those women whose families are unaware of their diagnosis do not participate and remain isolated. They also miss out on the healing benefits of a loving, supportive family and community. For those Native women who have chosen to share their diagnosis with family, they report a significant level of understanding and support, and urge others to do the same.

The Need for Family-Structured Transportation Services

Transportation services are available for individuals who are eligible for HIV/AIDS services and have been identified on client satisfaction assessments to be an essential form of support for individuals to access HIV/AIDS services. These services need to be expanded to allow women and their children or extended family members to travel with them. These noninfected companions are frequently prohibited from accessing the free or low-cost transportation. This is particularly pertinent in Indian Country, where transportation to and from providers' clinics may be three hundred miles one way. The infected women do not want to travel that distance alone.

The Need for Services for Clients Who Are HIV-Positive as Well as for Those Who Have AIDS

At the present time in communities such as Kansas City, emergency assistance services are available for people who have AIDS. These services include access to conventional care networks such as Salvation Army or Metropolitan Lutheran Ministries. Access to these types of services is also needed for clients who are HIV-positive. However, due to severe federal and state budgetary cuts, services are being limited to people who have AIDS. Those who are HIV-positive are unable to access prophylactic forms of treatment.

The Need for Respite Care

Another form of support which is greatly lacking is respite care for families and caregivers. For example, in one Native family where the mother is HIV-positive, the caregiver is a teen-age son. There are no support services for him. This is particularly obvious when vacations or summer begins and he is unable to participate in other youthful interactions because someone needs to care for the mother and he is the most responsible family member. His caregiving duties increase during vacations because he is also helping to care for younger siblings.

The women who are HIV-positive and the primary caregivers to their families have periods of time when they are unable to provide homemaking services for their families and need some assistance with those tasks. They also need items such as diapers, plastic liners, blankets, and sheets provided to the home during those periods when the woman is too weak or ill to go out and obtain household products.

An example of a positive model in the preimplementation phase is in Minnesota. The Minnesota American Indian AIDS Task Force is planning to develop housing for Native people with HIV. It will include single rooms and two- and three-bedroom units for families, as well as a guest apartment for families who come to visit from their reservations or homes located in other cities. Support for family members will be provided in both contemporary and traditional (e.g., Talking Circle) ways.

The Need for Products Which Positively Influence Self-Esteem

Self-esteem is important to maintain a quality life. Many of the women who have AIDS have lost weight and live on welfare incomes. The women do not purchase nice things for themselves, but rather buy items for their children and husbands. There needs to be a clothing bank for women so that they can dress in clothes that fit. Another approach would be to have care packages available which focus on the woman's appearance (and self-esteem). These packages may include items such as cologne, nice powders, scarves, cosmetics, or free haircuts. They may also include tribe-specific items (e.g., sage or cedar to smudge, or specific herbs or pollens for prayer ceremonies).

The Need for Increased Funding and Revised Program Priorities

Almost all HIV/AIDS service agencies have experienced severe budget cuts. These cuts have affected quality of care provided to all peoples affected with HIV and AIDS. However, among the frustrating perceptions is that the agencies appear to cut services to women and families before cutting monies that go into the service agency administration (e.g., purchasing computers or hiring administrative staff).

The Need for HIV/AIDS Education within Native Communities

Several of the female clients being served through the NNAAPC-funded projects expressed concern over the community's reactions to their HIV/AIDS status. The immediate societal judgment was that these were "bad" women and they deserved what they got. (This is the same societal perception and judgment of infected homosexual men.) However, there appears to be very successful gay men's support networks and few or no female support resources.

Case Management Issues

Little to no information is available that is appropriate for Native American women, children, or women with families. HIV/AIDS services were designed to treat infected males. This creates some cultural issues for Native women since the majority of Indian tribes have very strong female modesty issues and it is difficult to wait for personal care in waiting rooms filled with men, especially men who typically are not Native. Culturally, this is very inappropriate, and women will go without care rather than be surrounded by men from other cultures. This dramatically demonstrates the need for Native case manager projects which address the modesty issue (e.g., private waiting room for Native American women and their children).

The majority of services which are targeted to males who are affected with HIV/AIDS do not provide any form of child care. Contrary to non-Natives, who frequently utilizes babysitters to care for their young while they work or do errands, in general Native American children participate and accompany their mothers for most activities. Lack of child care at the HIV/AIDS treatment facilities creates an additional challenge to obtaining services.

Case managers need access to training that increases their ability to address family issues, including ways to assist families who have two people who are HIV-positive. Typically one of the two infected family members is a caretaker and has additional needs for providing for the entire family as well as her own health needs. Case managers need access to both training and resources to provide appropriate support services to these caregivers.

There is a dearth of case management services available for women who have multiple problems. The majority of Native female clients have dual and triple diagnoses (e.g., HIV-positive, alcohol and substance abuse, and/ or mental problems), as well as living in poverty and being unemployed. Multiply diagnosed clients are very high-maintenance case loads, and there are few Native female case managers to oversee the growing number of women and families affected by HIV and AIDS. Case managers who supervise multiply diagnosed clients need to implement aggressive follow-up. Due to budgetary limitations that require the case manager to carry too many clients and particularly with Native clients, to travel long distances to meet with these women and their families, this follow-up may not be feasible.

Support services for children who are not infected, such as support groups, could go a long way in relieving some of the stress on the woman. Native case managers believe that Indian women tend to not live as long or have as high a quality of life as do others affected by HIV and AIDS. Among the primary explanations for this perception of poorer survival is that Native women with HIV/AIDS place the needs of their children and family above their own health needs. Case management which was designed for families could address their priorities and provides overall family support which would ease the woman's additional stress related to coping with caretaking for the family while feeling sick, or failing to take care of herself because her needs come after her family's needs are met.

Provider Issues

Providers need to be knowledgeable of other systems of care to assure that Native HIV-positive women are cared for. Many of the providers who serve in Indian Country have limited access to knowledge of other HIV/AIDS support programs and therefore are unable to refer the woman to appropriate services. Many Native women are interested in traditional Native healing. Care givers unfamiliar with Native traditions cannot facilitate this need.

Health care providers have little accurate information about people of First Nations other than what has been misrepresented via Hollywood and similar forms of media. There is a dearth of data on Native American women who are infected with HIV or have AIDS. This paucity of information extends to informational pamphlets, fliers, and brochures which are culturally or gender-specific to women, lesbians, prostitutes and so on. Obviously, this means that the providers are unable to do a literature search or data run and obtain accurate information on HIV/AIDS within Native American women. This creates a great disadvantage for providers who are devoted to providing appropriate care or treatment in a culturally competent manner. As a result of providers receiving insufficient information, they tend to not treat American Indian women as aggressively as they do men. Basically, they do not know how to treat women who are very modest and traditional. They are unable to discuss personal issues with these women in a culturally acceptable manner. This lack of effective communication affects the providers' ability to discuss care issues such as Pap smears, vaginal thrush, cervical cancer, estrogen replacement, birth control, hormones, and so on.

Title I, II, and Ryan White Limitations

Ryan White–established systems have been too focused on individuals and are too inflexible to meet the needs of HIV-infected women. Individuals who work within Ryan White–supported programs have difficulty deviating from the stringent mandates to appropriately meet the needs of Native women and/or families infected with HIV. The majority of the systems are unable to provide assistance with family emergencies which involve children, such as when the mother needs to be hospitalized and her children require care and supervision. A major fear for women is that if they are hospitalized, their children will be taken from them and put in foster care.

Child care issues are greatly affected by the Indian Child Welfare Protection Act which specifies that the placements of Indian children follow certain priorities: (1) with other family members; (2) with members of the same tribal affiliation; and (3) with members of another tribal affiliation. The intent of the Act and subsequent law is to prohibit the adoption of Indian children into non-Native homes, which results in loss of access to culturally appropriate rearing. This becomes an issue if there are no responsible family members or that the woman's home tribal community is unaware of her HIV status and confidentiality would be violated if they were told.

Since the initial HIV and AIDS cases were homosexual males and IVDU, the Ryan White system has been geared toward single individuals. According to case managers who provide services to Native peoples, there are only two times a year when Ryan White–funded agency staffs ask women for participation. Typically this is for some type of retreat. It is felt that these agencies have funds for women-specific programs, yet it isn't allocated for women's issues with children.

Interviews with American Indian women infected with HIV or AIDS repeatedly introduced a great deal of resentment and anger towards Title I and II, Ryan White–funded agencies. Among the common areas of resentment was the feeling of "tokenism." For example, women from the Kansas and Missouri areas stated that the only time agencies look for women or children is when they want sad, pitiful, sympathetic story-lines. Once the women and children showed up and had their photos taken, there were no attempts to provide any follow-up care for those Indian families. An example of a program which has found a way to overcome the initially perceived Ryan White "barriers" to providing services to Native women and children infected with HIV are the Seattle programs which provide child care, prenatal care, and a variety of support services to HIV-infected women of all colors.

Case Study: Nan (As Told by a Native American Female Case Manager)

On April 1, 1995, I received a phone call from a crying woman. I couldn't understand what she was saying because she was very upset. She started to speak, but then there were sounds of someone entering the room in which she sat. She immediately said, "I can't talk. I'll call you later." Within the hour, the woman called back after getting her crying under control. She told me that she had been reading a pamphlet about the Ahalaya Project, then she paused. I told her that I could help her. I was not in my office at the time, but returned there.

The woman told me she was calling from her hospital room and apologized for hanging up the phone so abruptly during her previous call. She said that a nurse had walked into her room, causing her to panic because she didn't want anyone to know that she had AIDS. I asked her whether she was sure that she had AIDS or whether she was HIV-positive. She said, "I have an infection in my brain called *histoplasmosis*." She had been hospitalized in February 1994 at the local Indian hospital. The hospital had run numerous tests on her, and eventually referred her to a non-Indian hospital. The doctors at the non-Indian hospital, after running more tests on the woman, asked her if she lived around birds or chickens. At the time, she thought, "This doesn't make sense. I'm sick, and they're asking if I live around chickens." The doctor then asked her if she had ever been tested for HIV, and she said she had not. Subsequently, the woman tested HIV-positive.

The doctors told her that the infection she had was called *histoplasmosis* and was an infection usually found in the lungs of an individual who had inhaled dust containing spores that cause the disease. She said, "You might know I'd be the only person to have this disease in my head. I guess I just don't follow the normal process even with my diseases," and she laughed. I knew at this point that she was more relaxed. I explained the Ahalaya Project's case management services to the woman. She wanted to know if she could become a client of the project, and I told her that I would go to visit her and initiate the intake process. She gave me detailed directions to her rural home, and we set up a meeting on Monday, April 4, 1994, to do the intake.

Nan is a 46-year-old Shawnee/Delaware female who became infected with the human immunodeficiency virus (HIV) through heterosexual contact. She has seven children, two of whom are grown and married. The other five children live with Nan, and range in age from seven to fourteen years old. She is a very strong-willed Native female who believes in traditional healing. She expressed that her family subscribes to the practices of the Native American Church.

When I met with Nan, we spoke about ways to inform her family of her HIV status. She said that she wasn't ready to do that, but that she would let them know in time. Nan later found a way to talk with her mother and tells her that she is HIV-positive. The family had a Native American Church gathering for Mothers' Day. During this gathering, one of her family members was praying and let it be known that Nan is HIV-positive. Nan's uncle told her other family members to help her inform the rest of the family members of Nan's HIV status. Nan said that she didn't know at that point in time how to react, but she felt that from that point on, it was easier to talk with her family. She said she had a good feeling, one of relief.

Nan has become a great voice in the Native community and is making a difference at the local and national levels. She has been a speaker on numerous panels regarding issues affecting females throughout Indian Country.

Nan has been an advocate to Native people at the Indian Health Service (IHS) on a variety of topics, including, but not limited to: (1) standing up for the rights of Native Americans to have a better quality of care; (2) requesting that AIDS medications be added to the IHS formulary; and (3) asking her physicians if they would like for her to speak with their staff on issues pertaining to HIV and Native women.

Nan has also participated in a video produced by the American Red Cross titled "Care and Compassion for People Living with AIDS." She also went to Washington, D.C., and spoke with congressmen and representatives in regards to the Ryan White CARE Act. She presented a resolution to the National Congress of American Indian's conference committee on "Health Care in HIV/AIDS."

I asked Nan what she does to cope with HIV and what she feels her needs are. "Speaking about HIV," she said, laughing. She said, "My needs are making my bills meet at the end of each month and making sure my children are taken care of. Living with HIV has given me a new outlook on life and has enriched by spiritual belief and my belief that the Creator gave us things to use and to use in a good way, and this is what I believe in. I'm now celebrating my new lease on life, but I'm dealing with bills and illnesses, blues, colds, and my children. But I'm doing what I need to do, and I'm not as irritable as I used to be. I've found a calmness, but I need to work hard on keeping it this way."

I asked Nan what she considers the most imperative needs of Native American women living with HIV/AIDS. She responded,

More compassion and care. It's hard for Indian women to live with and talk about AIDS. I had a good support system. Women just don't want anybody to know, not even their families. Somehow it is important to let them know they can share a lot of the hurtful things with someone. It's better to release the burden. They also feel like their kids are more important than anything else and that if people know of their HIV [status], they may be ostracized. Women need spiritual and psychological help to deal with the feelings of being scared to let anyone know. Indian women can hide their feelings well, so people think they're okay, but they may be holding all the hurt feelings inside which also brings their health down.

We need someone to talk about this disease too. I've had someone to talk with, and believe me, it helped. I had to find my own strength, and I feel strong with all the good things happening to me because of love, care, compassion, and people truly caring about me. Indian women need someone to make them care for themselves, so they will think of themselves as an important person because if you can't take care of yourself, who's going to take care of your kids? We need to heal self, mind, body, and especially spirit.

It's hard for women to go and get health care because of confidentiality issues. There is also a fear of everybody finding out by just going to the hospital. As they say in Indian Country, "Everybody knows everybody." When I first went to the hospital, I wanted to steal my chart because I saw a red sticker stating HIV positive, and I said, "Don't they know that's why Indian women won't come for health care?" We've got to do something to make the health care system keep [the patient's] confidentiality.

Education is my big deal. It is the only way I have to fight this disease — not just how to get it, but also how to treat others [who have it] and when to get care and treatment. People don't want to find out because it's perceived that if you get tested and find out you're positive, they automatically label you as a bad person. It makes you want to curl up and hide and hope daylight doesn't find you again. We need to do something, and I'm trying to help in my own way.

As the primary case managers for Nan, we are proud of her efforts to care for herself and to reach out to the Native community to help others. We will continue to support her and her family and to help advocate for her health, social, mental, and spiritual needs.

REFERENCES

This chapter's references are from on-going service and case management projects funded by HRSA SPNS through NNAAPC projects. These projects include:

Planning grants
Service grants

Outreach
AZ: Indian Community Health Service
HI: Papa Ola L kahi
KS: Native American HIV/AIDS Coalition
NC: Tuscarora Tribe of North Carolina
AK: Chugachumuit
AZ: Navajo Nation AIDS Network
MN: Minnesota American Indian AIDS Task Force
NY: American Indian Community House
WA: Seattle Indian Health Board
WI: Milwaukee Indian Health Board
CA: Indian Health Council
MN: Positively Native

21

Can Needle Exchange Better
Serve Women?

Kaveh Khoshnood and P. Clay Stephens

Kaveh Khoshnood was born in Iran and immigrated to the U.S. in the early 1980's. He is now an epidemiologist with the Yale AIDS Program, where he is involved with a project that provides medical services to needle-exchange clients. He is currently a member of the New Haven Mayor's Task Force on AIDS and the Connecticut HIV Community Planning Group. *P. Clay Stephens* has worked at grassroots social service and women's health care delivery at free and community clinics. Her involvement in the Women's Health Movement led her to the world of commercial sex workers and injection drug-using women which, in turn, led to her early commitment to HIV/AIDS efforts. In Boston she participated in clinical HIV research at Fenway Community Health Center, served as Director of HIV/AIDS Services for the AIDS Office of the Public Health Department, Commonwealth of Massachusetts, and as Clinical Manager for Community Medical Alliance, now a nationwide model of managed care for persons with HIV. She is now Research Scientist with the Bureau of HIV/AIDS Epidemiology at the State of New York Department of Health in Albany, New York.

A growing proportion of the Acquired Immunodeficiency Syndrome (AIDS) cases in the United States is made up of injecting drug users. The major factor in the transmission of Human Immunodeficiency Virus (HIV), the etiologic cause of AIDS among drug injectors, is the sharing of contaminated drug paraphernalia, particularly syringes. Among women, over 50 percent of AIDS cases can be attributed to intravenous drug injection either by the woman herself or indirectly through sexual exposure to an injection drug user.

Needle Exchange Programs

Needle exchange programs (NEPs) have been suggested as a means to increase the availability of sterile needles and syringes and to decrease the reuse of injection equipment by IDUs (injection drug users). These programs provide new sterile syringes to IDUs in exchange for their used ones. In addition, most programs also provide some or all of the following: bleach for disinfecting injection equipment, cotton, cooker, clean water, alcohol wipes (for disinfecting skin to prevent skin infections and abscesses), condoms, and educational materials.[1] Similar to their "bleach and teach" predecessors, many NEPs hire former drug injectors for their staff to better communicate their risk reduction messages to IDUs. Moreover, other public health services are offered to this hard-to-reach population in the context of NEPs. These services, some of which are offered on site and others through referrals, include HIV counseling and testing, screening for tuberculosis and sexually transmitted diseases (STDs), and assistance with drug treatment and primary medical care.[1]

History

The first known NEP came into existence in the summer of 1984 in Amsterdam as a response to the growing epidemic of hepatitis B virus among IDUs.[2] "Jonkibonden" (Junkie Union), an advocacy organization of IDUs, contacted the health officials in Amsterdam and demanded increased access to syringes to prevent the further transmission of hepatitis B virus among its constituency. Although over-the-counter (OTC) sale of syringes in Amsterdam is permitted, members of the Junkie Union were concerned about some pharmacists' refusal to sell syringes to IDUs and the potential for a hepatitis B outbreak.

In the United States, many researchers and public health officials found the argument for such programs convincing, but did not believe that the political climate and the legal obstacles to syringe possession and distribution would allow the establishment of these programs here at home. Moreover, opponents of NEPs raised a number of issues regarding potential negative effects of these programs including an increase in drug injections among their clients and in the community in which they operate, a reduction in number of IDUs seeking drug treatment, and an increase in the number of discarded syringes in the community. African-American and Hispanic community leaders expressed their concerns in national forums that NEPs contribute to the devastating drug problem in their communities, and would shift funds away from needed drug treatment programs.

Nevertheless, small NEPs began operation in the United States within a few years of the first program in Amsterdam. The early programs were established by activist groups or individuals and were often operated illegally and with personal funds. Modifications in the law began to allow some of these programs to operate legally. This was also the case in New Haven, where an underground NEP existed prior to the establishment of the legally sanctioned program operated by the New Haven Health Department.[3] By September 1, 1993, at least thirty-seven NEPs existed in the United States.[1] About half of these programs operated legally, but with unstable funding. It must be noted, however, that at the time of this writing, *federal* dollars are still not available for syringe exchange services. Several legislative restrictions ban the use of federal funds for NEPs.[1,4] This ban cannot be lifted unless "the Surgeon General of the United States [determines] that such programs are effective in preventing the spread of HIV and do not encourage the use of illegal drugs."[4] Paradoxically, until recently, federal funds were also not available to conduct evaluation research of these programs. The first federally funded research of a NEP was the New Haven needle exchange evaluation project funded by the National Infectious Disease Association (NIDA).

New Haven Needle Exchange Program

New Haven's needle exchange was the first program of its kind in the state of Connecticut and began operation in November of 1990. Much of the early history and the operation of this program has been described previously[3,5,6] Briefly, in 1989, the New Haven Mayor's Task Force on AIDS recommended access to sterile syringes as an important HIV prevention strategy. This recommendation stemmed from the knowledge and the experience gained by New Haven Health Department outreach team in their effort to reduce HIV transmission among IDUs in New Haven. The city of New Haven was the first city in Connecticut to initiate street outreach to IDUs in 1987. The multicultural, indigenous outreach workers delivered AIDS information, and "safety kits" (filled with bleach bottles, water bottles, and condoms) to IDUs in various neighborhoods in the city. To better understand the reason for high rates of syringe sharing, a sample of active IDUs in New Haven were surveyed by health department outreach workers. The survey conducted in 1987 showed that fear of arrest, scarcity of sterile syringes, and the high cost of syringes in street black markets were the top three reasons for syringe sharing among this group of active IDUs.

To increase IDUs' access to sterile syringes, members of the New Haven Mayor's Task Force on AIDS testified before the Connecticut State legislature asking for the removal of legal barriers to sterile syringe access. This could be achieved by altering legislation that prohibit the sale and possession of syringes in Connecticut, by authorizing establishment of NEPs, or both. The response from the Public Health Committee was not favorable. The next year, a bill was introduced by representatives William Dyson from New Haven and Joseph Grabarz from Bridgeport requesting decriminalization of syringe sale and possession as well as funding for three demonstration NEPs in Connecticut cities with a high prevalence of HIV and drug use. In March 1990, the Public Health Committee had a second hearing focusing on the decriminalization of the sale and possession of syringes without a prescription. After much debate, a compromise bill was prepared authorizing funding for one demonstration NEP. In May of 1990, the Connecticut House passed Public Act No. 90–214, *An Act Concerning a Demonstration Needle and Syringe Exchange Program,* by a vote of 99 to 36. This was followed by a favorable vote of 26 to 10 in the Senate. Governor O'Neill then signed the bill into law effective July 1, 1990. The law altered the state statues pertaining to the sale and possession of syringes (and needles) without a prescription and the "drug paraphernalia" law by adding the demonstration NEP to the list of exceptions to the General Statutes and exempting those who administer or participate in the NEP from penalty for the delivery, use, or possession of drug paraphernalia. This Public Act also appropriated $25,000 for essential costs of the demonstration project in fiscal year 1990–1991, authorized the Connecticut Department of Health Services to oversee the program, and mandated that the program be evaluated.

The New Haven NEP operates out of a mobile van six hours a day, four days a week. The van visits several sites during the course of each day. These sites were chosen based on their proximity to areas with a high prevalence of drug use. The original staff of NEP were all outreach workers involved in the bleach distribution program in the city prior to their involvement with the NEP. In addition to sterile syringes, needle exchange clients receive bleach and water bottles, condoms, and easily understood literature about HIV transmission risk. Moreover, NEP staff provide all clients with information regarding drug treatment services and assist those requesting drug treatment. As part of the enrollment process, clients are asked to choose a pseudonym and to complete a brief survey used for program evaluation. Program pseudonyms are non-identifying, client-specific codes used to link client visits. Upon enrollment, clients are offered a single sterile syringe if they do not have a used syringe to exchange. All future exchanges, however, are made on a one-to-one basis to a maximum of five (this number was mandated by law; however, with the change in legislation in Connecticut decriminalizing sale and possession of up to ten syringes in July 1992, the maximum number of syringes exchanged per visit was increased to ten).

Results

The client-based research component of the New Haven needle exchange program demonstrated the following:

1. The research showed lack of evidence for a "client-shift" hypothesis to explain the observed drop in HIV prevalence in tested syringes over time.

2. Minority drug injectors and those with ten or more years duration of drug injection are the clients with the longest participation interval in the program.

3. While regular clients of the program have substantially reduced their levels of drug injection associated risk behavior, they have not significantly reduced their sex-related risk behaviors.

4. The research demonstrated marked decreases in both enrollment and participation in the program, along with increases in syringe sales in New Haven pharmacies, immediately following the decriminalization of syringe sale and possession in Connecticut.

5. Although a gender-specific analysis was not done as part of this work, several differences are noteworthy:

    a. No gender differences were found for NEP clients who had a single visit versus those who were more regular.

    b. In comparison to men, women reported increased sex-related risk behavior, including having multiple partners and exchanging sex for money and drugs.

    c. Women were less likely to enroll in the New Haven NEP following decriminalization of syringe sales in Connecticut.

TABLE I

Comparison of New Haven needle exchange clients who made one visit versus others,
November 1990–June 1992

Variables[1]	Clients with one visit N = 466	Clients with two or more visits N = 922	P*
	N (%)	N (%)	
Sex			.858
Men	342 (73)	710 (77)	
Women	93 (20)	198 (21)	
Missing	31 (7)	14 (2)	
Age			.034
< 35 yrs	257 (55)	439 (48)	
> 35 yrs	173 (37)	447 (48)	
Missing	36 (8)	36 (4)	
Race			.152
White	170 (36)	407 (44)	
Nonwhite	260 (56)	494 (54)	
Missing	36 (8)	21 (2)	
New Haven residency[2]			.270
Yes	128 (27)	183 (20)	
No	29 (6)	55 (6)	
Missing	309 (66)	684 (74)	
Duration of injection			.235
< 10 yrs	207 (44)	396 (43)	
> 10 yrs	206 (44)	455 (49)	
Missing	53 (11)	71 (8)	
Frequency of injection			.483
< 1 per day	102 (22)	178 (19)	
> 1 per day	299 (64)	666 (72)	
Missing	65 (14)	78 (8)	
Cocaine use			.877
Yes	300 (64)	617 (67)	
No	110 (24)	231 (25)	
Missing	56 (12)	74 (8)	

1. All variable categories are not shown
2. Question added in the second year of the program.
*Based on chi-square analysis; all variable categories were considered in the analysis.

Why Might Needle Exchange Be Important to Women?

Two aspects of needle exchange may differentially affect women as compared to men: length of HIV survival in used injection syringes and access to new, sterile syringes.

HIV-1 Survival in Used Injection Equipment

HIV survival modeling[7,8,9] based on data from the New Haven NEP has indicated that provision of needle exchange decreases the circulation time of used syringes and in turn, decreases the likelihood that an individual user will encounter a syringe containing viable HIV.

Survival of HIV-1 for greater than one week has been documented in fluids such as water, blood, and culture medium (for review see Sattar, 1991). The duration of survival and quantitative load of HIV-type 1 in injection syringes has been of interest not only as a key to understanding transmission[10,11,12] but also as a scientific basis for needle exchange programs.[8,13,14] The lack of ready access to large numbers of actual-use syringes and the absence of appropriate technology has, to date, hampered this work. Needle exchange programs have provided syringes for inspection and testing[15,16] but current PBMC (peripheral blood mononuclear cell) quantitative culture techniques require an amount of whole blood in excess

TABLE 2

Comparisons of needle exchange clients who participated in the follow-up study with those who did not

	Follow-up done?		
Variables[1]	Yes (N = 197)	No (N = 873)	P★
	N (%)	N (%)	
Sex			.163
Men	147 (75)	691 (79)	
Women	50 (25)	182 (21)	
Age			.093
< 35 yrs	91 (46)	433 (50)	
> 35 yrs	102 (52)	421 (48)	
Missing	4 (2)	19 (2)	
Race			.015
White	70 (36)	391 (45)	
Nonwhite	126 (64)	473 (54)	
Missing	1 (<1)	9 (1)	
Duration of injection			.005
< 10 yrs	75 (38)	392 (45)	
> 10 yrs	122 (62)	410 (47)	
Missing	0	71 (8)	
Frequency of injection			.832
< 1 per day	158 (77)	631 (72)	
> 1 per day	39 (13)	162 (19)	
Missing	0	80 (9)	
Syringes sharing (% of time)			.768
Some sharing	70 (36)	289 (33)	
No sharing	125 (63)	488 (56)	
Missing	2 (1)	96 (11)	
Cocaine use			.136
Yes	150 (76)	569 (59)	
No	46 (23)	230 (33)	
Missing	1 (<1)	74 (8)	

1. All variable categories are not shown.

★P values are based on chi-square methods. For ordered categorical variables, i.e., age, duration of injection, fraction of time injecting with shared syringes, we employed chi-square approximations using Kruskal-Wallis test.

TABLE 3

Comparisons of injection risk behavior of New Haven needle exchange clients at baseline and at follow-up interviews

Baseline	Follow-up			N	p
Frequency of injection (per day)				193	.6021
	> 4 times	1–3 times	< 1 time		
> 4 times	30	23	11		
1–3 times	35	42	14		
< 1 time	7	16	15		
Syringe sharing (% of time)				192	.0001
	Always	Sometimes	Never		
Always (100%)	0	1	5		
Sometimes (1–99%)	2	18	44		
Never (0%)	0	1	106		
Syringe cleaning (% of time)				17	.1953
	Always	Sometimes	Never		
Always (100%)	9	4	1		
Sometimes (1–99%)	1	1	0		
Never (0%)	1	0	0		
"Shooting gallery" use (% of time)				192	.0081
	Always	Sometimes	Never		
Always (100%)	1	1	7		
Sometimes (1–99%)	2	6	29		
Never (0%)	1	15	130		
"Risky injection"				187	.0061
	Yes	No			
Yes	16	41			
No	20	110			
Cocaine use				192	.7503
	Yes	No			
Yes	126	20			
No	18	28			
Ever applied for drug treatment?				188	.8752
	Yes	No			
Yes	130	20			
No	19	19			

of that typically found in used equipment.[17–21] While extensive ethnographic and epidemiologic attention has illuminated the handling and use of syringes,[22–25] specific information on duration and level of infectiousness is desirable. Survival of more than seven days and viral load information would also provide support the use of harm-reduction techniques such as nonsharing and bleaching/cleaning of injection equipment.

In a recent study, two HIV-1 wild-type strains were loaded into multiple syringes in simulation of 'street' use. Viable HIV-1 was recovered from syringes after storage for as long as twenty-eight days.[26,27] Viral loads during that survival period appear to be sufficient to effect transmission. This survival time in the barrel of a syringe far exceeds previous estimates and

TABLE 4

Comparisons of number of syringe-sharing partners of New Haven needle exchange clients at baseline and at follow-up interviews

Baseline	Follow-up			N	p*
Different sharing partners[1]				188	.0020
	0	*1*	*> 2*		
0 partner	109	6	8		
1 partner	15	5	4		
> 2 partners	29	5	7		
New sharing partners[1]				182	.0001
	0	*1*	*> 2*		
0 partner	147	1	3		
1 partner	13	0	0		
> 2 partners	16	1	1		

1. Past three months.
*Paired Wilcoxon signed-rank median test.

TABLE 5

Comparison of sex-related risk variables of New Haven needle exchange clients, by sex, at baseline, and at follow-up interviews

Sex-related variables	Men (N = 147)			Women (N = 50)		
Baseline	Follow-up		p*	Follow-up		p*
Live with sex partner			.13			1.00
	Yes	*No*		*Yes*	*No*	
Yes	34	22		14	10	
No	13	77		9	17	
Sex for drugs (ever)[1]			N/A			.02
	Yes	*No*		*Yes*	*No*	
Yes	N/A	N/A		3	0	
No	N/A	N/A		7	0	
Sex for money (ever)[2]			.69			.25
	Yes	*No*		*Yes*	*No*	
Yes	2	2		7	0	
No	4	32		3	8	
Condom use[3]			.03			.73
	1	*2*	*3*	*1*	*2*	*3*
1	23	6	2	10	0	3
2	20	4	1	1	2	1
3	11	4	26	4	2	6

1. At baseline, this question was not asked from men. Many "no" responses were left blank.
2. Many "no" responses were left blank.
3. Past one month; only those who reported having a sex partner were included. 1 = Always (100% of time), 2 = Sometimes (0–99% of time), 3 = Never (0% of time); all variable categories are not shown.
*Paired Wilcoxon signed-rank median test. All variable categories were included in analysis.

TABLE 6

Comparisons of clients enrolled in the New Haven Needle Exchange Program
three months before and after decriminalization of syringe sale and
possession in Connecticut

Variables [1]	Pre-Decrim [2] N = 164	Post-Decrim [2] N = 80	
	N (%)	N (%)	p*
Sex			.04
Men	120 (73)	68 (85)	
Women	44 (27)	12 (15)	
Age			.02
< 35 Yrs	95 (58)	37 (48)	
> 35 Yrs	66 (41)	40 (52)	
Missing	3 (2)	3 (4)	
Race			.01
White	94 (57)	31 (39)	
Nonwhite	68 (41)	45 (56)	
Missing	2 (1)	4 (5)	
Duration of injection			.35
< 10 Yrs	70 (43)	39 (49)	
> 10 Yrs	82 (50)	35 (44)	
Missing	12 (7)	6 (8)	
Frequency of injection			.11
< 1 per day	21 (13)	6 (8)	
> 1 per day	126 (77)	67 (84)	
Missing	17 (10)	7 (9)	
Syringe sharing			.61
No sharing	91 (51)	39 (49)	
Some sharing	44 (27)	15 (19)	
Missing	29 (18)	26 (33)	
Cocaine use			.96
Yes	97 (59)	47 (59)	
No	53 (32)	26 (33)	
Missing	14 (9)	7 (9)	

1. All variable categories are not shown.
2. Decrim = decriminalization.
*P values are based on chi-square methods. For ordered categorical variables, i.e., age, duration of injection, frequency of injection, we employed chi-square approximations using Kruskal-Wallis tests.

provides a scientific basis for both needle exchange and the mathematical modeling used in the evaluation of such schemes.

The longer the survival time, the more likely those with no or diminished access to sterile, unused syringes are to become infected. It is particularly important as in simulation only a single bolus, or dose, of infected blood was studied. In street use, actual HIV survival duration would extend well beyond the last contribution of fresh, infected blood, thus resulting in survival totals in excess of the basic survival time. In fact, if an "infected" syringe was used by an uninfected individual, that uninfected bolus might also serve to extend the "infectivity" of a syringe by providing a fresh supply of uninfected lymphocytes.

Women are more likely to than men to use or borrow previously used equipment, to inject later in mixed gender groups, and to be at risk of HIV transmission via both needle use and sexual transmission. The longer the survival of HIV in injection equipment, the more likely women, as compared to men, are to become infected in the absence of needle exchange or access to new equipment.

Access

Prior to HIV, women accounted for between 20 and 25 percent of all injecting drug users.[28,29,30] That percentage has remained relatively steady over time, varying only slightly by region and type of injectable drug. In New Haven, prior to the legalization of possession of injection equipment, the percentage of women using the NEP was consistent with these national estimates, i.e. 27 percent of NEP clients were women.[31] After legalization, the gender ratio shifted as the percentage of women participating dropped to 15 percent.[31]

Why the Decrease in Utilization by Women?

Why might these women have ceased to use NEP and, if still injecting, how might they have obtained the necessary equipment?

The women who ceased to use injecting drugs may have entered drug treatment, may have ceased to use on their own without organized treatment, or may have ceased to use involuntarily due to hospitalization, incarceration, or entry into other restrictive settings. It is difficult to see how the moment of legalization of possession of injection equipment would affect any of these situations directly. Women who continued to inject but who no longer utilized NEP might include those who moved from the area, who found NEP inconvenient (or perhaps to otherwise not meet their needs), who arranged for others to exchange their needles for them without alerting the NEP staff to that activity, and of course, those women who choose to purchase their syringes at pharmacies directly or through an intermediary. There is recognition of secondary exchange, i.e., having another individual exchange one's syringes, either openly — as available in San Francisco's Prevention Point NEP, where women outnumber men as secondary exchangers[32] and in the Netherlands — or discreetly in schemes which do not formally permit such secondary exchange. Again, however, there is little to support the notion that the moment of legalization would cause women to increase their rate of secondary exchange.

Remaining is the possibility that although NEP served as a safe and no-cost source of injection equipment during the prelegalization period, 1986 to 1992, after legalization other sources of equipment, in this case legal purchase, better served women.

In needle exchange schemes, as in virtually all other public health interventions, men and women regard access to and benefit from the intervention according to their individual and social roles and expectations. NEP was, in the Netherlands and many of the programs in the U.S., designed to fit into and make use of the neighborhood society in areas where injecting drug users congregated. Prevention Point was particularly adept at using routes and methods of communication and distribution already in place in the drug injecting populations of specific neighborhoods to announce the presence of, and complete the actual exchange of, syringes.[33] As the majority of injecting users were, and remain, male, and the street corner society has also remained primarily a male society, it is logical to assume that those programs most closely resembling the street culture, by design if not intent, best served male clients and those able and willing to operate in that culture.

Legalization in New Haven opened up a new alternative to that street culture setting. Purchase of injection equipment at a pharmacy, while adding the burden of cost of the syringes, does have several advantages: it allows for more discreet purchase, the hours and days of availability are greatly expanded, one cannot be as readily identified by the location of the purchase as an injector, and the burden of any time spent in completing forms or other registration/research activities is removed. Unfortunately, also removed is the regular or semiregular contact with the staff and services provided by NEP. In New Haven these range from HIV-risk reduction counseling, harm-reduction instruction, medical care, and referrals to community services including drug dependency treatment.

Designing Programs and Policy for Women

While enlarging the choices available to an individual which will allow that individual to reduce their own and others risk of HIV is laudable, might there be other messages available in the movement of women away from

NEP upon legalization? Are there ways in which NEP can be organized that might address the particular culture, social roles, and norms of women injectors?

It is also vitally important to recognize, at the point of service design for injecting women, that for those women with children, loss of custody of and access to her children has often been the price of seeking service or care for herself. The threat of such loss has been used by the legal and social service bureaucracies to leverage the individual woman into certain behaviors, programs, and situations. Further, as many women with HIV/AIDS have made clear, to be identified as an injector or as HIV-infected is to identify not only yourself but often your children as well.

Again, Prevention Point has led the way by allowing and supporting secondary exchange.[32] This better meets the needs of those who cannot attend an NEP due to disability or illness, community status, profile, or role, or due to the need to provide care for other family members such as children or elders.

Hours can be modified to assure that some exchange is available when children might be expected to be in school and when day work hours are over. Weekend exchange might be explored for many of the same reasons. Staffing might be adjusted to include one or more exchange periods staffed exclusively by women and offering collateral education, instruction, and services specifically for women. If the access needs of women differ greatly from those of the men served, programs could consider women-only stops or could dedicate an entire van to women and women and their children. Similar to other outreach to women, child care remains an issue. Given the types of vans in use, or in the case of the two van approach in New Haven (one is NEP; the other is medical care and referral) and their preset routes through the community, programs might be able to set up a situation wherein a woman could bring her children to a nearby site for very short-term child care. This would allow her to complete her exchange without having her children at the actual exchange site. The site chosen for a van stop and the provision of service and referral to all that come, rather than restricting such access only to those registered or enrolled NEP clients, also serve to lift the stigma of being seen at or near such sites. Attention must also be paid to the language and cultural determinants such that these aspects of service design support NEP access and use by women. Further, prevention/intervention policy must be extended and/or modified to meet the access and usage patterns of all injection drug users. This can be accomplished by the legalization of sale, possession, and the exclusion from evidentiary use of injection equipment and drug paraphernalia[34] and the distribution of a full range of sterile—and exchangeable—injection equipment.[35] As injection represents only one of the risk routes of HIV infection, needle exchange programs' distribution protocols should also include safer sex technique instruction, supplies, and materials.

Summary

As the dual concepts of one-stop-shopping and harm reduction gain support, the nonjudgmental, nonpunitive, and user-friendly nature of needle exchange makes such programs an ideal locus for a broad range of risk and harm-reduction and health-enhancing activities. These include primary and targeted health care (contraception, HIV, pediatric) and a wide range of social service intake and referral activities (housing, food, addiction services). The recent positive evaluation of needle-exchange schemes by the National Academy of Science provides further support for the expansion of NEP nationally. This expansion, in turn, can provide the ideal moment for direct attention to services specifically designed to address the needs of women.

NOTES

1. Centers for Disease Control and Prevention and the University of California, San Francisco and Berkeley, *The Public Health Impact of Needle Exchange Programs in the United States and Abroad,* September 1993.

2. E.C. Buning, "Effects of Amsterdam Needle and Syringe Exchange." *International Journal of Addictions* 26 (1991).

3. E. O'Keefe E, "Altering Public Policy on Needle Exchange: The Connecticut Experience." *AIDS & Public Policy Journal* 6 (1991).

4. Office of National Drug Control Policy, "Needle Exchange Programs: Are They Effective?" *Bulletin No. 7* (Washington, D.C., July 1992).

5. E. O'Keefe, E.H. Kaplan, and K. Khoshnood, *Preliminary Report: City of New Haven Needle Exchange Program* (New Haven, Conn.: New Haven Health Department, AIDS Division, 1991).

6. E.H. Kaplan and E. O'Keefe, "Let the Needles Do the Talking! Evaluating the New Haven Needle Exchange," *Interfaces* 23 (1993).

7. E.H. Kaplan, "Modeling HIV Infectivity: Must Sex Acts Be Counted?" *Journal of Acquired Immune Deficiency Syndrome* 3 (1990).

8. E.H. Kaplan and R. Heimer, "A Model-Based Estimate of HIV Infectivity via Needle Sharing," *Journal of Acquired Immune Deficiency Syndrome* 7 (1992).

9. E.H. Kaplan and R. Heimer, "HIV Incidence among Needle Exchange Participants: Estimates from Syringe Tracking and Testing Data." *Journal of Acquired Immune Deficiency Syndrome* 7 (1994).

10. I. Raineri, H. Senn, C. Schneideggar, R. Hornung, R. Luthy, and M. Vogt, "Detection of HIV-1 from Needles Discarded by I.V. Drug Users in Zurich and Basel Using Polymerase Chain Reaction: Assessment of In Vitro Infectivity (ThAP 111)," in *Final Program and Abstracts of the Fifth International Conference on AIDS,* Montreal, 1989.

11. E.H. Kaplan, "Needles that Kill: Modeling Human Immunodeficiency Virus Transmission via Shared Drug Injection Equipment in Shooting Galleries," *Reviews of Infectious Diseases* 11 (1989).

12. A. Wodak, K. Dolan, A.A. Imrie et al., "Antibodies to the Human Immunodeficiency Virus in Needles and Syringes Used by Intravenous Drug Abusers," *Medical Journal of Australia* 147 (1987).

13. E.H. Kaplan and R. Heimer, "A Circulation Theory of Needle Exchange," *AIDS* 8 (1994).

14. E.H. Kaplan, "Evaluating Needle-Exchange Programs via Syringe Tracking and Testing (STT)," *AIDS and Public Policy Journal* 6 (1991).

15. J. Guydish, G. Clark, D. Garcia, M. Downing, P. Case, and J.L. Sorensen, "Evaluating Needle Exchange: Do Distributed Needles Come Back?" *American Journal of Public Health* 81 (1991).

16. D.D. Chitwood, C.B. McCoy, J.A. Inciardi, D.C. McBride, M. Comerford, E. Trapido, V. McCoy, J.B. Page, J. Griffin, M.A. Fletcher, and M.A. Ashman, "HIV Seropositivity of Needles from Shooting Galleries in South Florida," *American Journal of Public Health* 80, no. 2 (1990).

17. G.J. Bayliss, W.J. Jesson, B.A. Evans, and K. McLean, "Isolation of HIV-1 from Small Volumes of Heparinized Whole Blood," *AIDS* 3 (1989).

18. G.J. Bayliss, W.J. Jesson, P.P. Mortimer, K.A. McLean, and B.A. Evans, "Cultivation of Human Immunodeficiency Virus from Whole Blood: Effect of Anticoagulant and Inoculum Size on Viral Growth," *Journal of Medical Virology* 31 (1990).

19. B.A. Castro, C.D. Weiss, L.D. Wiviott, and J.A. Levy, "Optimal Conditions for Recovery of the Human Immunodeficiency Virus from Peripheral Blood Mononuclear Cells," *Journal of Clinical Microbiology* 26, no. 11 (November 1988).

20. B. Chesebro and K. Wehrly, "Development of a Sensitive Quantitative Focal Assay for Human Immunodeficiency Virus Infection," *Journal of Virology* 62, no. 10 (1988).

21. J.B. Jackson, R.W. Coombs, K. Sannerud, F.R. Rhame, and H.H. Balfour, Jr., "Rapid and Sensitive Viral Culture Method for Human Immunodeficiency Virus Type 1," *Journal of Clinical Microbiology* 26, no. 7 (July 1988).

22. S. Koester, R. Booth, and W. Wiebel, "The Risk of HIV Transmission from

Sharing Water, Drug Mixing Containers and Cotton Filters among Intravenous Drug Users," *International Journal of Drug Policy* 1 (1990).

23. J.P.C. Grund, C.D. Kaplan, N.F.B. Adrianns et al., "Drug Sharing and HIV Transmission Risk: The Practice of Frontloading in the Dutch Injecting-Drug-Users Population," *Journal of Psychoactive Drugs* 23 (1991).

24. B. Jose, S.R. Friedman, A. Neaigus et al., "Syringe-Mediated Drug-Sharing (Backloading): A New Risk Factor for HIV among Injecting Drug Users," *AIDS* 7 (1993).

25. H.W. Feldman and P. Biernacki, "The Ethnography of Needle Sharing among Intravenous Drug Users and Implications for Drug Policies and Interventions Strategies," in R.J. Battjes and R.W. Pickens, *Needle Sharing among Intravenous Drug Users: National and International Perspectives* (National Institute on Drug Abuse Research Monograph 80, Rockville, Md., 1988), 28–39.

26. P.C. Stephens, R. Heimer, B. Griffith, B. Jariwala Freeman, and E. Kaplan, "HIV-Type 1 Survival and Load in Injection Equipment: Policy and Prevention Implications for Women," NIH/CDC HIV Infection in Women Conference, Washington, D.C., 1995.

27. P.C. Stephens, R. Heimer, B. Jariwala Freeman, D. Negioanu, and B. Griffith, "Survival of Human Immunodeficiency Virus (Type 1) in Injection Equipment" (submitted for publication, 1996).

28. D. Glaser et al., "Opiate Addicted and Non-Addicted Siblings in a Slum Area," *Social Problems* 18, no. 4 (1971).

29. M. Hilton, "Abstention in the General Population of the USA," *British Journal of Addiction* 81 (1986).

30. K. Marsh and D.D. Simpson, "Sex Differences in Opioid Addiction Careers," *American Journal of Drug and Alcohol Abuse* 12, no. 4 (1986).

31. K. Khoshnood, "Client-Based Evaluation of New Haven's Needle Exchange Program," Ph.D. dissertation, Yale University, 1995.

32. L.D. Wenger and S. Murphy, "They Are Not Just Giving Out Needles: The Impact of Needle Exchange on the San Francisco Drug Injecting Community (Session 4000)," 122nd American Public Health Association National Meeting, Washington, D.C., 1994.

33. P. Case, personal communication, 1988.

34. L. Stern and J. Grund, "Harm Reduction among Injection Drug Users," Presentation to Yale AIDS Program, Internal Medicine Department, Yale–New Haven Hospital, New Haven, Conn., April 1995.

35. D. Des Jarlais, S. Friedman, and T. Ward, "Harm Reduction: A Public Health Response to the AIDS Epidemic among Injecting Drug Users," *Annual Review of Public Health* 14 (1993).

22

Leather, Lace, and Latex: Safer Sex for Women

Denise J. Ribble

Denise J. Ribble, RN, BSN, MPA, is Director of Nursing and Director of The Treatment Mall at the Middletown Psychiatric Center, Middletown, New York. She is also a member of the Orange County AIDS Council and Cochair of the Orange County Sexual Abuse Task Force. Ms. Ribble has been an AIDS activist since 1981 and is particularly concerned with women's health safety and empowerment.

In some ways, talking to women about safer sex in a workshop format is both easy and simple: keep body fluids that contain HIV out of your body. On the other hand, talking to women about safer sex is incredibly complex. One must take into account societal, gender, and cultural contexts. Values, beliefs, and taboos are also important, particularly considering that AIDS raises the taboos of sex, drug addiction, homosexuality, and death. Also take into account that some of the women in the room are HIV-positive, and that most of the women will have had many and varied experiences with medical and mental health systems. Add to that women's sexuality and sexual behavior, conditioning, upbringing, religion, language, and roles. And don't forget denial, embarrassment, self-esteem, and the capacity to learn (or unlearn). Each group of people and each individual in the group will have different reasons for being present based on their own experiences. It is vital to respect that.

For a presenter, there are the above expectations. There is also the aspect of creating a comfortable and safe environment for this intimate discussion. It is important to be positive and at the same time value-neutral. I do a lot of question-and-answer, tell me what you know, role-playing and experiential interactions to create participation. I use drama to get attention and movement to keep it. I use self-revelation and the true stories of others' experiences to connect.

In order to create value in a safer sex discussion, I believe it is important to explain the Buddhist concepts of "shiki shin funi" and "esho funi." "Shiki shin" refers to the mind and the body and "esho" refers to the body and environment which exists in the spiritual relationship of "funi–two but not two." This is likened to the head and tail of a nickel, each separate, but integral to the identity of the nickel.

It is in this state of "two but not two" that helps people reconcile paradoxes like spontaneity and self-responsibility, how we move on and let go while keeping the dear and precious in our lives. I am reminded of a short parable my life partner tells. She says, "You are taking out the garbage, and you have two armloads full. Meanwhile, a friend comes to your door bringing you a beautiful gift which requires both hands to receive it. You have to decide whether to cling to the garbage or accept the beautiful gift, for you cannot accept the gift if both your arms are holding garbage."

Talking about safer sex is often like this parable. Like most people, I have been both a gift *and* a garbage bearer. I think it is apropos that the Chinese character for crisis (or risk) contains the symbols for both danger and opportunity. It is important to examine safer sex and carry on a dialogue (in the tradition of story-telling in a community) about what is our greater purpose in coming here. In the age of AIDS there is both danger and opportunity. In my experience, women's lives are at stake.

In this article, I will be using a mixed format of the text from one of my talks and, in italics, my commentary. My commentary includes my perspective, things I have learned, points I try to make, and tips for doing this kind of presentation. I hope by using this format, that anyone reading it will be entertained and possibly learn something they can use in their own life.

It's a Friday night somewhere. My topic is safer sex—Leather, Lace, and Latex. Two weeks ago I talked about abstinence and saying no with a group of about twenty women. Two months ago, safer sex with 275 mostly male (but not totally) Marines. Next week I'll be talking to a mixed crowd of gay, straight, bi-, lesbian and transsexual/gender men and/or women. Next month I'll be presenting a three-week curriculum developed by Jennifer Tiffany at Cornell Cooperative Extension called, "Chatting with your kids about AIDS" to the PTA in the town that I live in. I've spoken to seniors, people with hemophilia and their partners, women in safe homes, women in jail. Sometimes I do a single evening presentation. Other times I might present safer sex with assertiveness training or a behavioral change model. That might take multiple meetings, but it seems to have a more lasting effect that a one-

night-stand. Tonight, I'll be talking to a mixed group of about seventy-five lesbian, bisexual, and heterosexual women.

I began talking about safer sex with women for a number of reasons. First was my experience working in a primary care clinic which treated HIV disease (GRID and CRID at that time). We had two hundred women enrolled at our clinic—half of them lesbians—at a time when the rest of the world seemed to be in an acute state of denial about bidirectional transmission, different symptoms in women, treatment exclusion, and woman-to-woman transmission. Women who were infected or affected needed a safe space to become empowered about AIDS. Second, I have worked in women's health for my entire adult, professional life. And finally (this is by no means an exhaustive list), I like talking about sex. So . . .

"Good Evening!! My name is Denise Ribble and tonight I'm going to talk with you about safer sex. This discussion will be frank and explicit. It will cover a variety of consensual sexual activities between adults. *(I can also talk for three hours about abstinence but that is not what I'm here for tonight!)* If anybody needs to leave at any time, please feel free to do so. If you need to talk with someone before you go, please see ———— or ———— who are just outside the door." *(Cover any housekeeping details here.)*

"Why am I talking with you about safer sex? I'm talking with you about safer sex because safer sex is one of the best ways you can avoid sexually contracting the virus, HIV, that is thought to cause AIDS. It is important to learn about safer sex so that you can decide about protecting yourself. If you are already HIV-positive, safer sex may help you protect yourself from getting more HIV or other germs, and from transmitting the virus. As I talk about things tonight, each one of you will need to decide for yourself how much you enjoy any particular sexual activity, how risky it is, how you can make it safer and . . . will you? I will NOT be giving you any lists of safer or unsafe behaviors. *Adult women learn by making choices and applying their experiences to a new situation. Choices are causes whose effects can be evaluated if one is not afraid to examine the nuances of consequences. This type of decision making is very personal and adaptable to a variety of situations. This is the context within which I talk to women about safer sex and risk reduction, since this allows individual women to craft decisions that meet their circumstances, values, and contexts. This is why I do not present lists. Lists, I believe, give and impose a false sense of security particularly to women. After all, I recall a time when vaginal secretions and oral sex [woman to man, woman to woman, man to woman] were not on any "lists." It is also a normal denial response to ascribe safety to any desired and desirable activity that doesn't appear "on the list." Give a woman a list and you may help her be safe for a day. Teach a woman about risk and she can reduce harm to herself for a lifetime.* Safer sex is a conscious party where you engage your mind AND your genitals. I believe that sex can be both safe and erotic.

"Before we get started, I would like to find out what you already know. And, if you're willing, I would like you to tell me what you would like to learn about tonight. *Many of the women attendees are there because they are interested in talking about or listening to others talk about sex. In my experience, many people intellectualize at this point. It is important to establish a zone of comfort and safety first. It is important to break through denial and embarrassment. But gently, ever so gently. On the other hand if you don't keep it moving you might find yourself answering many intellectual questions and having no time left to talk about safer sex.*

"What does A-I-D-S stand for?"

"What is HIV?"

"How can HIV be transmitted?"

"Who can get HIV?" *(Correct any misconceptions.)*

"Does anybody have any questions?" *(Usually questions about HIV antibody testing come up here.)*

"The virus that causes AIDS is found in some body fluids. Which ones?" *This is a good time to talk about the concentration of virus in different body fluids and to differentiate between blood (including menstrual blood), semen, vaginal secretions, and other body fluids that pose less risk of transmission. I like to use household measures when discussing concentration of HIV in body fluids since it is easier for most people to understand than nanograms per decaliter.*

"The important thing is to keep body fluids that contain HIV out of your body.

"Does anybody have any questions?

"Now, I would like you to all stand up. I'm going to ask you a series of questions. First, I want you to think back fifteen years. Where were you? Who were you? What were you doing? These questions will cover the last fifteen years. Next, if you answer yes to any of these questions, I want you to sit down. However, I want you to wait to sit down until the last question is asked. Otherwise, this room full of strangers will know YOUR risk factors and that might not feel safe or comfortable for everyone. Lastly, if you do NOT answer yes to any of these questions, please remain standing. Are you ready?

"First question: Have you ever used drugs or alcohol as an addiction, as a recreation, or to the point of impaired judgment? By addiction I mean to have a disease of physiological dependence on a substance like alcohol, heroin, cocaine, or pot. By recreation, I mean . . . you know . . . just a few lines of coke now and then, just a six pack on the weekends. And by impaired judgment I mean that you don't remember exactly what you did, with whom, even once in the last fifteen years.

"Don't sit yet. If you answered "YES" to this question, you'll sit in a few minutes.

"Second question: Have you had unprotected sex with a man or a woman anytime in the last fifteen years? By unprotected I mean without the use of a latex, vinyl, or plastic barrier to prevent someone else's blood, semen, or vaginal secretions (body fluids) from getting inside your body. By sex I mean oral, anal, vaginal, or digital intercourse between a man and a man, a man and a woman, or a woman and a woman. This includes sex by consent, sex for the purpose of getting pregnant, sex by force *(If he or she hurts you or forces you, we aren't talking about safer sex anymore, but violence and abuse. I might also discuss a partner's unwillingness to practice safely as abusive)*, and sex for the purpose of making a living. Man or a woman? Do I have to explain that?

"Third question: Have you been exposed to blood or blood products, like a blood transfusion, a needle-stick injury or a lab accident in the last fifteen years?

"Fourth question: Have you ever been so in love (or so infatuated) that you'd do anything or almost anything? *Lust and love are sometimes the greatest of risk behaviors, particularly for women. Our society supports the use of both sexual desire and love to control women. To give yourself up to either is, therefore, a risk, a disowning of self-responsibility, which undermines self-protection.*

At this point you can add questions that are more specific to your audience.

"If you answered YES to any of the questions, please sit down now. If you did not answer YES *PLEASE* remain standing." *At this point most of the audience will sit. It is important to really encourage anyone who answered NO to all the questions to remain standing.*

"So, how does it feel to be the one *(or two or three)* people left standing out of 100?

"You said embarrassed—awkward?

"But the only people who are not at risk for HIV are you who are still standing right now.

"What does that mean for the rest of us who sat down?

"We're at risk!!!!"

If time permits, I might discuss here how the audience is advised to protect themselves; examples like "just say no", negotiate safer sex (negotiations can only take place between two people who are relatively equal in power) and "talk to your partner." I particularly like "talk to your partner," where I encourage the audience to ask me questions about my own risk status to which I respond with some accurate and some inaccurate answers, thus making the point that people rarely tell the truth about their risky behaviors.

"Does anybody have any other questions, because I'd like to move out of the intellectual part of this discussion and start talking about safer sex.

"What's 100 percent safer sex?" *(Abstinence is the most common answer to this question.)* "Abstinence is 100 percent safe. But is it sex? Let's try again. What's 100 percent safer sex?" *(Now will come a few other suggestions: lifetime monogamous sexual relations between two HIV negative people, masturbation, massage, etc. Be prepared for silence or to correct any misperceptions.)*

"How about masturbation or massage? Dry kissing? If my lover is squeezing my nipples, sucking on my earlobes, fucking my armpit or between my breasts is that 100% safe? If she or he *(remember your audience is lesbian, bi-, and straight women)* is nibbling on my neck (and they're not Dracula) is that safe? How about phone or video sex? If they're riding my thigh or ass, or I'm riding theirs, is that safe? What about touching or caressing breasts or testicles (balls)? Are these things safe? What do we call these things after we learn about the 'big event.' Foreplay. But remember, the beauty of foreplay is its capacity to arouse us. Are these things sexual— at least more sexual than abstinence—and are they safe?

"Why are these things safe? Because no body fluids are getting into our bodies. Now I want to bring up a 'what if . . . '. Let's take the example of somebody riding my thigh. What if I just had quadriceps surgery and had staples in my thigh. Rubbing on my thigh might pose a risk, right? However, if I just had quadriceps surgery and I had staples in my thigh, it is likely I'm going to let someone ride it? NOT!!!! Let's use common sense. *(This always reminds me of the question about getting an STD from a toilet seat. There are some STDs you might be able to get from a toilet seat. However, it is not likely. When most of us use a public toilet, we look at the seat and decide whether or not we're going to sit down. Common sense.)*

"I want to go back for a minute to squeezing my nipples and rubbing my breasts. How many of you know how to do a breast self-examination?

How many of you do it every month? Ok. Somebody tell me; walk me through a breast self-exam verbally. You can all follow along if you want to." *(Be prepared to do this without audience participation.)*

If talking to a mixed male and female audience, I would also talk about testicular self-examination, PAP smears, and gyn exams. Caring enough about yourself to self-examine and get a check-up underlie the ability to protect yourself. With lesbian audiences, breast exams and PAPs are very important to stress. I give out the toll free number for breast cancer information—which is 1–800–935–0434—and other toll free numbers.

"What about kissing? Is kissing safe? It takes approximately two quarts of saliva *per kiss* to put you at risk. *(Hold up two quart containers or a half gallon container.)* Imagine two quarts of saliva per kiss. Seems more like drowning perhaps than kissing to me. The important thing about kissing is not necessarily the saliva, but . . . what?" *Here I discuss bleeding gums and cold sores, columnar epithelium (which can "absorb" HIV. This is why vodka, mouthwash, and douching aren't good risk reduction strategies), brushing your teeth, checking yourself and checking your potential kissing partner. The basic points here are to check yourself for "openness" and check the other person for what they may give you. I find it helpful to get a volunteer to role-play an encounter with you where you're checking them out by getting them to talk to you about safer sex, laugh and smile so you can assess lips, tongue, teeth, and mouth.*

Vignette—Lips, Teeth, Tongue, Mouth

She(he) was the kind of woman(man) who threw her(his) head back when she(he) laughed, a full laugh, with her(his) mouth open, her(his) teeth gleaming. Her(his) teeth, not perfectly white, not perfectly even, were clean and her(his) breath was sweet. She(he) had a beguiling gap between her(his) front teeth and I could imagine her(him) taking my breast in her(his) mouth with my nipple sliding through that gap. Her(his) laugh was throaty, not harsh, her(his) voice melodious, not hoarse. Looking at her(his) soft, full lips, I could imagine her(him) kissing me. And tonguing me through a veil of plastic, while I straddled her(his) face and she(he) fucked me with her(his) mouth.

"Now I'd like to talk about oral sex. First, I want to talk about a man or a woman having oral sex with a woman. *(I say "man or woman" to help the audience get past the seemingly automatic reaction of denial which is "this doesn't apply to me" and "with a woman" to help focus on the receivership aspects of oral sex.)* It takes about a quart of *normal* vaginal secretions to put you at risk during oral sex. *(Hold up a quart-sized container.)* In my dreams, I make that much, but in reality most women do not. However, the operative word here is "normal." What does a *normal* vaginal secretion look like? *(I am always amazed that in a room FULL of women, this question is greeted with absolute silence. Be prepared.)* A normal vaginal secretion can be clear or slightly cloudy, like mucus. If it's curdy and white/yellowish or smells like bread is that normal? *(No—probably a yeast infection.)* If it's chalky white, is that normal? *(No—possibly chlamydia. Here I also talk about chlamydia—its prevalent occurrence and it's relationship to Pelvic Inflammatory Disease and infertility. I also discuss that it is generally tested for ONLY on a woman's request and not routinely during a GYN exam.)* If you see what looks like blisters or "popped" blisters on the labia (lips) or vaginal opening, is that normal? *(No—possibly herpes.)* If the vaginal secretion is green and fishy or foul smelling, is that normal? *(No—possibly Trichimoias. I also discuss in our culture how we are conditioned to believe that ANY smell is abnormal even though we all have a normal smell to our secretions.)* If it's brown? *(No—could be poor hygiene, E. coli or TB.)* What about if it's pink or red? *(Might be normal—menses—but indicates the presence of blood. It only takes a drop of blood, including menstrual blood to put you at risk.)* If the vagina looks red, raw, and "weepy" is that normal? *(No—possibly a non-specific vaginitis or vaginal irritation. I bring up normal vaginal secretions for several reasons. First, I think it is important that you are able to assess yourself: are you intact or are you open? Second, if you're getting ready to go down on a woman, you need to know what "normal" looks and smells like. Third, most of us do not have oral sex with the lights on after an examination. Unfortunately, if you don't realize something is amiss until after you put your mouth on it, it's too late!! And finally, it only takes a mild vaginal infection to increase the risk posed by vaginal secretions. Let's say I'm an HIV-positive woman and I have a mild yeast infection. What cells in the body go to my vagina to try to fight off the infection? White blood cells. And where does HIV live? In white blood cells. So my vaginal secretions could contain more HIV. In fact, instead of taking a quart of my normal vaginal secretions it may now only take a teaspoon to a tablespoon of vaginal secretions to put you at risk. And I make that much.)*

"It's up to you how much risk you are willing to take with vaginal secretions. However, if you want to protect yourself, you need to learn how. *Here I would move to my display of dental dams, safer sex panties, and plastic wrap. I review factors that can interfere with using a barrier for oral sex with a woman such as availability of dental dams, cost, and how to use plastic wrap. Nothing that's available for oral sex with a woman has been tested for HIV prevention (the way that condoms and female condoms have). I believe that more than fifteen years into this epidemic, this is still a statement of the relative value our society places on woman's sexuality. I also discuss the risks of menstrual blood, predicting menses, and overcoming our cultural reluctance to consider women's oral sex desires through the miracles of modern plastic wrap. I then ask for a volunteer to come up and help me demonstrate that you can see, smell, touch, and feel through plastic wrap.*

"Now I want to talk about a woman having oral sex with a man. It takes about a teaspoon to a tablespoon of semen to put you at risk and most men make that much. *(Here I hold up the appropriate measuring spoons to demonstrate amounts.)* It's up to you to decide if that's a risk you want to take. If you want to protect yourself, you need to learn how. *(Now I will talk about scenarios of risk a woman may find herself in, like "trust me," "I won't come in your mouth," and when the woman enjoys oral sex with a man. Using a dildo, an unlubricated condom and another volunteer, I demonstrate how to put a condom on a penis with my mouth. This act is for both safety—when the man is reluctant to use a condom for oral sex—and erotic. It just takes practice. At this point I talk about what I think is one of the most significant barriers to safer sex if not raised to the conscious level. That is that the human body is very wet and the body fluids that put you at risk are also very primal. In order to practice safer sex you have to make a choice to keep these body fluids out of your body. Otherwise, you will continue to be at risk. I chose safety because I care enough about my life to make that my bottom line. But not without some mourning for those body fluids.)*

From this point on I will continue to present vignettes and risk-reduction techniques, and discuss other consensual sexual activities like touching (fingering, fisting), gloves, intercourse, condoms and female condoms, the difference between birth control and safer sex, water sports, douching, bondage, S&M, dressing up, toys, etc.

In closing:

This discussion of safer sex for women and eroticizing safer sex for women evolved as a dialogue about what aspects of our experience of "safer" and "erotic" are unique and which are universal. I find discussion, dialogue, questions and answers, role play and experiential stuff enhances learning. This is particularly useful in helping women imagine and fantasize about things they enjoy and broaching the same with others— safely.

I find it essential to "know my stuff", including current information about AIDS, HIV disease, STDs, and sexual practices. I see it as important to know about, talk about, and explore discussion of sexual activities (even ones you don't personally do yourself) from a risk perspective. I also believe you should have personally tried any safer sex devices or techniques you are talking about and demonstrating.

This dialogue about safer sex is intended to provoke thought; it is intended to provoke change in risky behavior to safer behavior. I liken this to the example of using seat belts. Each time you get in a car you have the choice of using or not using your seat belt. Similarly, each time you participate in a sexual activity, you can practice "safer" or not. Like other risk choices, you will not fly through the windshield each time you drive and fail to use a seat belt. On the other hand, if you fly through the windshield even once, you chances of survival are lessened.

I often tell the story of the first time I came by choice. I was at a spin the bottle party in a closet (literally) dry humping through two pairs of jeans. Every time someone says condoms or saran wrap are too thick, I think of that experience. Of course, I have learned other ways to capture the "big event" since then. And then I learned how to do those things safely. Now I even dream in safer sex. Safety has it's own erotic charm. Safer sex is about an empowered paradigm shift. I would like to share a story with you.

A paradigm is a model or example that explains the world to us and helps us predict behavior. A paradigm is a valid set of expectations based on shared assumptions. It is a scheme for understanding and explaining parts of reality. A paradigm establishes boundaries and tells you how to behave to be successful (a game with boundaries and rules). Paradigm shift is when you change your view, try a new thing a new way. A shift is a new game with new rules. Safer sex is a shift.

A Final Story: The Pig and the Sow

"Once upon a time, there was a man who had a cabin in the mountains and a Porsche to get there. Every Saturday morning, he would drive up to his cabin on a very dangerous road filled with blind curves, unguarded drop-offs, and tricky turns.

But this man was not bothered by danger. After all, he had a great car to drive, he was an excellent driver, and he knew the road like the back of his hand.

One fine Saturday morning, he was driving to his cabin. He was coming up to one of his favorite blind curves. He slowed down, shifted gears, and put on the brakes in preparation for the turn that was about two hundred yards away. All of a sudden, from around that curve, came a car careening almost out of control! The car nearly went off the cliff but, at the last second, its driver pulled the car back onto the road. The car swerved into his lane, then back into its lane, then back into his lane again.

My God, he thought, I am going to be hit! So he slowed almost to a stop.

The car came roaring on toward him, swerving back and forth. Just before it was about to hit him—at the last moment—it swung back into its lane. As it went past him, a beautiful woman stuck her head out of the window of the car and yelled at him at the top of her lungs, "PIG!!"

What? he thought, How dare she call me that! He was incensed by her accusation! Instantly he yelled after her, "SOW!!!" as she continued down the road.

"I was in my lane! She was the one who was all over the place!" he muttered to himself. Then he began to get control of his rage; he smiled and was pleased that at least she didn't get away without his stinging retort. He'd gotten her good, he thought smugly.

And with that, he put the accelerator to the floor, raced around that blind curve . . . and ran into the pig!

This is a paradigm story. He thought the woman was calling him a name. But she was really doing a heroic thing. In spite of the fact that she had almost been killed, she took the time to try to warn him about the pig on the road around the curve. But he had paradigm paralysis. He thought she had called him a name; so he followed "the rule" and called her a name—and thought that was the end of it.

Actually, he had demonstrated the beginnings of some flexibility when he notice that it was she, not he, who was swerving all over the road. If he had paradigm pliancy, he would have responded to her shout by asking himself, What is going on? Then he would have driven around the corner much more cautiously. At the least, he would not have hit the pig. At the most, he could have stopped, picked the pig up, put it in his trunk, an driven away with it.

The moral: During the next decade many people will be coming around blind curves yelling things at you. They will be too busy to stop and explain, so it will be up to you to figure it out.

If you have *paradigm paralysis,* you will be hearing nothing but threats.

If you have *paradigm pliancy,* you will be hearing nothing but opportunity!

I would submit, in light of all that I have said, that safer sex has many contexts.
If I had to develop a "wish list" of things that I think would help women be safer, I
would include:

- *Women-centered information and safer-sex practices*
- *Female-based devices (i.e., female condom)*
- *Assertiveness training to enhance a woman's ability to refuse unsafe and unwanted*
  practices
- *Communication training to improve problem-solving skills and the ability to deal with*
  power relationships and "negotiating."
- *Community education focus that does not ignore the woman's social situation and*
  priorities (i.e., safer sex for a woman who wants to get pregnant is very different than
  one who does not).

"So I hope you learned something this evening. And I hope you enjoyed
yourself. I hope I aroused . . . your curiosity . . . or something. When you
leave tonight, I hope you will think about safer sex, talk about safer sex,
and practice, practice, practice."

23

Gender, Freedom, and Safety: Does the U.S. Have Anything to Learn from Cuban AIDS Policy?

Jennifer L. Manlowe

A long-standing ethical dilemma has preoccupied me ever since I gave a talk recently on Ethics and AIDS to International Health Practitioners from Indonesia and the Philippines at Brown University's International Health Institute. In an epidemic, are health safety and freedom mutually exclusive or interdependent if you live in a country that values collective rights over individual rights? Perhaps the question is so situation-specific that one can only evaluate practices in each sociocultural setting.

When I got a call from *Hermanas* (a nonprofit group of feminist scholars who travel yearly to Cuba) and heard that my fund-raising efforts had made it possible for me to join their delegation's upcoming trip, I was thrilled with the chance to compare U.S. and Cuban policy on HIV "regulation." I had hoped to make this trip for two years now and twice the funding just didn't come through. Now, my goal to travel to Cuba and meet with activists, health practitioners, and people living with HIV and AIDS was realized.

Because I was only going to be visiting Cuba for eleven days, I realized I would only get a surface impression of people's feelings about Cuba's ethics in relation to HIV/AIDS public health policies but, nevertheless, I thought such an impression was worth acquiring. So much of what I did hear about Cuban ethics on AIDS seemed negative. I wanted to see and hear for myself whether people living there felt empowered or imprisoned. As the AIDS Program Coordinator at Brown University, I'd only heard the "incarcerated angle" about Cuba and the mostly Western individualist idea that "individual rights are being held captive to communal rights." I wanted to see for myself.

The people I was able to interview came from the following groups and organizations: the Federation of Cuban Women (the FMC); the Social Organization on Women and the Family; the group of Las Galas (Gay and Lesbian Activists); charter members from Magin: A Feminist Media-Communications Group; workers at the Center for Sexual Education in Havana; family doctors at Pinar del Rio, a male gynecologist at a Polyclinic in Havana, four male doctors and one female psychologist at the sanitorium at Pinar del Rio; and six men and two women living with HIV/AIDS at the AIDS sanitorium in Santiago de Las Vegas (or "Los Cocos," according to locals). To narrow the scope of this essay, I've chosen to focus on my interviews and impressions gathered at Los Cocos.

My thirteen traveling companions (in the Hermanas delegation) and I stayed at the guest house of the Federation of Cuban Women, but only two of the fourteen of us were there to gather information on AIDS. Besides myself, an acupuncturist from Seattle named Shad Reinstein was there to interview health practitioners in the Sanitorium. Shad had not only set up this meeting at Los Cocos but had arranged for a Spanish translator and journalist, Karen Wald, to help us communicate with our contacts there. Karen had become quite friendly with administrators at the sanitorium and told them that Shad and I were AIDS specialists who wanted to compare AIDS care and prevention in Cuba to the United States. The administrators were pleased to accommodate us.

Preliminary Research

Before I traveled to Cuba, I wanted to find how Cuba's public health policy was perceived in Western and European medical journals. In brief, this is the tenor of what I found:

> Cuba represents [a] sort of human and public health nightmare, though a nightmare of hyper-vigilant medical police and of over-observed and over-disciplined bodies: A Foucauldian nightmare of medical "discipline" verging on "punishment." The contrast with Brazil (and with the United States and France) could not be more striking.[1]

This same author, medical anthropologist Nancy Scheper-Hughes, reluctantly finds that

> Cuba is the only nation to have used the "classic" public health tradition—routine testing, contact tracing with partner notification, close medical sur-

veillance and partial isolation of all seropositive individuals—within a national program to contain the spread of the epidemic on the island . . . the
Cuban AIDS program seems to be succeeding.[2]

The ethical ambivalence felt by scholars from the West for the "classic"
tradition also finds expression in the work of public health scholar and
activist Nancy Krieger, who writes,

> Cuba's AIDS program has five key components: (a) protecting the blood
> supply, (b) mass screening of the general population and "high-risk groups"
> (including persons who have worked abroad or had sexual contact with
> foreigners), (c) mass education, (d) isolation of all persons infected by HIV
> (ill or not) and their removal to a sanitorium (with those interned guaranteed
> health care, full salaries, and also social support for their families, and (e)
> clinical research to develop effective treatments. . . . The question we are left
> with is whether Cuba's accomplishments had to be accompanied by the
> coercion of quarantine. The evolving answer fortunately seems to be "no."[3]

I asked a few non-Cubans living in the U.S. what they thought or knew
about sanitoria and AIDS treatment in Cuba. Their responses were often
something along these lines: "Oh, the inhumanity of quarantining HIV
patients who have no choice in the matter!" or "Those people are so poor
that they're giving themselves the virus through self-injecting. Things must
really be desperate there."

Most of my cultural studies searches produced similar notions to the
non-Cuban sentiment articulated above. For instance, professor of women's
studies and medicine Paula Treichler writes in a 1992 article, "In Cuba,
mandatory HIV testing of the general population has identified a small
number of infected people, who have been placed under indefinite quaran-
tine."[4] Also, public health professor and ethicist Ronald Bayer writes,

> The specter of quarantine has haunted all such discussions [on AIDS and
> public health], not because there was any serious consideration in the U.S. of
> the Cuban approach to AIDS—which mandates the isolation of all persons
> infected with HIV—but because of fears that even a more limited recogni-
> tion of the authority to quarantine would lead to egregious intrusions on
> privacy and invidiously imposed deprivations of freedom.[5]

Whenever I would ask a Cuban-American what they thought about
AIDS policy in Cuba,[6] I'd hear, "The sanitoria are very much like country
clubs and are quite a contrast to the average Cuban's living situation,
especially during the U.S. and European Embargo."

Background on the Embargo

A quick overview of the Embargo is in order: The U.S. embargo on Cuba began in 1961 following the 1959 Cuban revolution. The embargo had a limited impact due to Soviet assistance and domestic egalitarian distribution policies. Health and other social indices improved dramatically during the following three decades. Dissolution of the Soviet Union in 1989 greatly weakened the Cuban economy. In 1992 the embargo was made more stringent with the passage of the "Cuban Democracy Act." All U.S. subsidiary trade has since been prohibited, ships from other countries are not allowed to dock at U.S. ports for six months after visiting Cuba, and pressure has been applied to stop other countries from trading with Cuba.[7]

Now that the Berlin Wall has been ground to dust, the Soviet Union dissolved, and the U.S. trade embargo against Vietnam recently eliminated, one would think the Cold War were over. Yet even in the midst of so many global shifts, where U.S.-Cuban relations are concerned, the war is still quite *hot*.[8] For half a decade, since the so-called end of the Cold War, Cuba has confronted what is referred to as its "special period." This describes the severe economic crisis precipitated by the collapse of preferential trade with the former Soviet Union, and exacerbated by the effects of the economic and trade embargo organized by the U.S. government.

The Cubans I interviewed in Havana believe this long-standing economic blockade is about the United States's fury at not being able to make Cuba succumb to U.S. notions of democracy—what many Cubans see as a euphemism for capitalist practices that privilege the powerful few and take advantage of the working and so-called middle classes.[9]

Impressions of the Sanitorium

While riding to the outskirts of Havana to Santiago de Las Vegas (Los Cocos) I wondered how the economic crisis of the "special period" would affect the Cuban government's revolutionary commitment to the health of all.[10] Billboards and signs above the family practitioners continued to promote the Cuban ideal that "Health is the right of all people" (see Figure 1). Upon coming up to the sanitorium, I thought to myself, "Los Cocos looks about as much like a prison as a San Diego health spa!" It was quite palatial, in a Beverly Hills kind of way (see Figure 2). It was made up of several acres

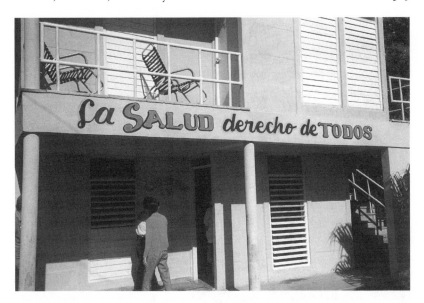

23.1. A family doctor in Pinar del Rio, Cuba, with a banner/motto declaring a common Cuban ideal: "Health is the right of all people."

of modern one- and two-story flats surrounded by lush vegetation, palm trees, and small gardens. The community could be compared to many cohousing projects in Europe and in the U.S.

Because of all the negativity that I had heard (albeit from people who had never been to Cuba) I thought to myself, "Don't be snowed, remember Adolf Hitler's façade during World War II." The German dictator had plucked out the healthiest-appearing survivors among those held in his death camps and promised they would be well-fed and taken care of if they would illustrate to the visiting Red Cross that nothing inhumane was occurring in his camps. They were dressed with faces painted and told to smile. Though the human rights parallels are nil, was this kind of deception happening in Cuba?

The first person I encountered was a man named Marcos who greeted our interpreter with a kiss. They exchanged news briefly. Karen introduced Shad and me to Marcos before asking him to help us unload the hundred pounds of humanitarian aid that we had brought from the U.S.—mostly condoms, birth control, fungal creams, some AIDS videos, and a variety of soaps—many products that are rationed by the Cuban government.[11]

We thanked Marcos and then Shad, Karen, and I walked to the adminis-

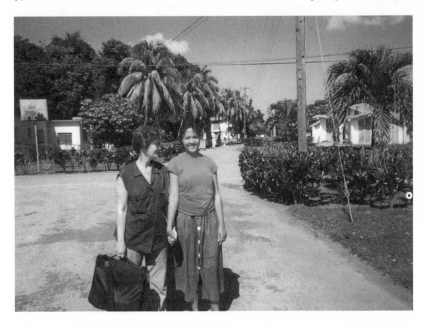

23.2. Karen Wald and young woman with HIV at "Los Cocos" or Santiago de las Vegas in Havana, Cuba.

tration building where the three main sanitorium epidemiologists worked. Their small office was filled with a nicotine fog as they chain-smoked while negotiating with a computer programmer who was updating their database on AIDS/HIV patients.

The head of the epidemiology department invited me to sit down and look over the 1996 statistics on HIV and AIDS as well as the cumulative death toll in Cuba from the virus. In a country of 12 million, only 1,200 people have contracted HIV to date. Two hundred and sixty-two Cubans have died over the past ten years and men outnumber women with the virus a little more than two to one. The epidemiologists printed these statistics on one side of a large piece of paper and I suggested that they use the other side to "save paper," a practice I do in the states. They chuckled and muttered, "You're right, it is the 'special period' after all."

Our translator quickly pulled me away from getting into too deep of a discussion about epidemiology in the U.S. and comparisons between Cuba's notion of AIDS and ours. I learned that in Cuba, they're using a 1987 CDC criteria which doesn't include recent findings of important opportunistic infections that more often affect women: TB, cervical cancer, and pulmonary pneumonia. Karen said, "We don't have much time and it's best if you use it to interview patients." We agreed that it was best to keep moving, and yet I don't regret an ounce of information that I garnered from this group.

A strained relationship between psychosocial surveyors like myself and quantitative analysts like epidemiologists needs to be bridged if we are to complement each others' strengths and weakness. We need to educate each other about cofactors that make HIV and other STDs a real threat to marginalized people (like poor women, especially women of color, and people who are gay, bisexual, lesbian, or who practice the same but do not identify in such a manner). Such a collaboration may help more of us resist further social ignorance as well as further infection.

As Shad, Karen, and I started walking across what felt like an estate, we came upon Marcos again, and this time we asked if he wouldn't mind our taking a look at his living quarters. He was adjusting a water pipe on the roofs, and once it was fixed, he came over to escort us into the house that he shared with five other gay men.

Raul, an active dress designer and drag performer, greeted us with delight. He had worked for Marcos, who I later learned was a famous producer of drag shows in Havana—a popular attraction for both tourists and locals. Raul allowed both Shad and me to take his picture with the dresses that he had most recently designed and performed in (see Figure 3). He was quite pleased with the attention we gave him, and yet he didn't want us to miss the artist behind us who was working on painting his 3-D plates made of terra cotta pottery. The design on his plate was like dancing smurfs on a frog pond (see Figure 4). The artist's name was Sierce, and he had just recently recovered from a serious bout of being bedridden with fever, diarrhea, and other late-stage symptoms that exhaust an AIDS patient. He didn't say much and was concentrating on cultivating the brightest hue of blue with which to work.

Three other men in their late twenties who also lived in the household invited us to sit down in their room. I noticed a colorful poster and asked what it was; one of the men answered, "It's a Gay Pride poster from New York City's 1995 march." To the left of one of the men's beds was a large picture of a pouty-lipped Marilyn Monroe. Shad asked the first man, Miguel, to tell us what it was like living in the sanitorium. He said, "It was my first chance to really 'come out' to myself (and later, my family) about being gay." He went on to describe how much pressure he felt under to

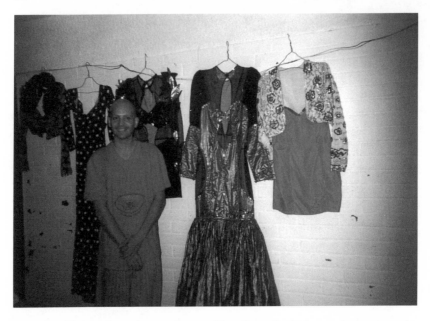

23.3. "Raul" (pseudonym), a patient at "Los Cocos," stands proudly next to the designer dresses he made for his drag show performances in Havana.

stay hidden about his sexual preference as a precollege (equivalent to a U.S. boarding school) history teacher and claimed that being diagnosed with HIV was a far lighter sentence than reconciling his sexual preference to a homophobic world.[12] Miguel told us that when he first arrived at the sanitorium he thought the administrators' probing questions about his sexual preference were going to be punitive and he wasn't sure how he should answer them. After deciding to let them know he was gay, he said he was relieved to find that "they only wanted to know so as to pair him up with the right roommates." He said, "Here in the sanitorium I've made many friends and have found a strong community in which to take pride in my sexual preference." Miguel and his friends have even founded a youth outreach group to other young people in Havana. He claimed, "I never knew I would turn into such an activist."

Both Miguel and his family have come to accept his sexual preference along with his positive diagnosis and have come to assist newcomers to the sanitorium in similar acceptance. It was clear to me that Miguel was the leader in the group of men. The others very much wanted me to take back some poetic writings of Miguel to see if I could have them published.

Because of the 35–year embargo, Miguel's own efforts to publish such an article in the U.S. were futile. And on the island, "writing is truly a heroic act," writes Ruth Behar. Because of the loss of economic support from socialist Europe, there are continual blackouts and food shortages. The once vibrant publishing world, for which Havana was well known, has withered, as even *Granma,* the state newspaper, has been reduced to a single newspaper sheet folded in half.[13] On top of the economic crisis, and because of long-standing homophobia in Cuba, Miguel didn't feel comfortable pursuing such visibility in his own country. It is my understanding that one thing the Revolution of '59 did not do thoroughly is liberate those who are nonprocreative.[14,15]

Our translator, Karen, spotted our next interviewee (an M.D. who was also a newly practicing acupuncturist). She was just outside Marcos's flat and was waiting in a car. Her name was Isis Canceo and she had recently broken her leg, so she needed us to come downstairs to her. Karen jumped up to end the conversation with the men and so did we, but in a fashion that was strangely relaxed. Being at an Ivy League school of medicine, I've never heard of a medical doctor who wasn't in a rush and who wouldn't

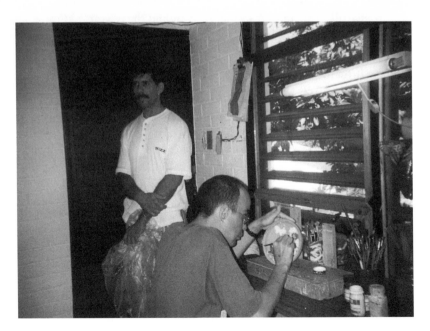

23.4. "Sierce" (pseudonym), a patient at "Los Cocos," paints terra cotta plates as 3-D art.

mind waiting while nondoctors wrapped up a conversation. We gathered addresses and shared more information about HIV in the U.S. and notions on homophobia. We then left their modern home and started walking toward the main building where we would join Dr. Canceo.

Before meeting with her we ran into one of the youngest HIV patients living at the sanitorium. She was a slightly retarded girl named Alicia who had recently turned fifteen—traditionally the cause for a coming of age party called *Quincenieras.*[16] Karen told us that Alicia had contracted HIV just a year ago from a 24–year-old man who claimed to be her boyfriend. He told Alicia that he could prevent her from losing her virginity and from becoming pregnant if they had anal sex. Alicia contracted HIV instead. After questioning me about myself and where I was from Alicia grew silent. The man who gave Alicia the virus is now serving time in prison for statutory rape. When I asked even the most ardent feminists about sexual violence in Cuba, every one of them said, "It rarely happens because our legal system is strong (punitive) against all forms violence, especially violence against women. . . . It's just not tolerated."

Just then Dr. Canceo greeted Shad, and they sat down and began speaking about treating AIDS patients with acupuncturist techniques and "green [herbal] medicine." A Cuban man around thirty years old came up to Karen to say hello, and she introduced him to me. Oscar was very recently diagnosed as seropositive and said he was eager to be of help in acting as a translator if either Shad or I had a need, as he was an English teacher and translator by profession. I brightened at the prospect of having someone to help me translate (even though I have seven years of Spanish, I'm a far cry from being able to conduct an entire interview in Spanish in a timely manner). So I went with Oscar to meet the woman I had hoped to interview, the first woman ever to live in a Cuban sanitorium, Maria Julia Fernandez.

While we were walking I asked Oscar how he was emotionally handling his recent positive diagnosis. He said he was shocked when he received the plea to be tested from the Cuban Health Ministry. The note warned that the man he had slept with a year ago had recently been diagnosed with HIV. Oscar thought one of his friends was playing a joke on him. A few days later, he got a visit, in person, by a few people he had known were living with HIV. As is standard with Cuba's "contact tracing" practices, they implored him, "Please, go get tested." This time he did, and within a few days he found out he was seropositive. At that point, he told me, both he and his parents went in to the sanitorium in Los Cocos for intensive counseling and health advice. Oscar said, "They want to make sure you're not going to do something stupid like kill yourself or go on some kind of destructive rampage." Oscar told me, "They'll keep me here for six months, under health surveillance [which includes confidential contact tracing], hold my job for me and even pay me the same salary while I'm here until I'm able to return to work." I asked him how he felt about being under surveillance and he told me, "I'm not sure yet, it's all so new. I've only been here seven days." Oscar went on to explain to me the logic of why he went to Los Cocos in Havana: because it was the closest sanitorium to his home and work. Each of the thirteen provinces has a sanitorium for exactly this reason of accommodation.

Like some recently diagnosed people I've interviewed in the United States, Oscar seemed to be searching for a bright side to his HIV-positive diagnosis. He said, "I have a chance now not to fritter away life. I want to live the most full life I can, now." When I started to ask Oscar more about his history and family, he said, "That's fine, as long as you tell me about your life too; I want this to be a conversation that is person-to-person, okay?" All my years of feminist research methodology came right up in my face and I realized how right he was. Feminist ethnographers have wrestled for years as to how to do qualitative or in-depth interviews without digging too deeply or one-sidedly. We've tried to avoid exploitation and projection when mediating their story with our own cultural, personal, and political biases. Many of us have worked to analyze without placing Anglo categories of "normal" on cultures that have different notions and historically nuanced versions of their own concepts of "normal."

After telling Oscar a little bit about my work and history of being an advocate through writing the stories of marginalized people (homeless, incarcerated people dealing with addictions, women who've survived domestic and sexual violence, and women living with HIV/AIDS) he seemed eager to share his own story.

The first bit of information Oscar shared related to how much he felt having an absent father contributed to his early initiation into sex. He said, "I only mention it because it may help you understand why I was very sexually active with men since age eleven." He said he later came to realize that he was searching for his father's love and then, only later, started to see women as well. He eventually married the woman he was seeing but the relationship ended after a year. He kept wanting what he termed "a more equal companionship" and felt the woman he was with "wasn't capable of the same." He then met the man who he thinks gave him HIV. "It didn't last," he grimaced and said, "so here I am." When I asked him if he considered himself gay or bisexual he said, "Neither, I'm just a person who looks for certain spiritual and intellectual qualities in others, I don't feel the need to identify myself as gay, as a matter of fact, I can't relate to gay culture at all."

Just then Maria arrived and invited both Oscar and me into her house. After sitting down and chatting briefly, I asked Maria how she found out she was HIV-positive. She told me that it was in 1986, after her husband Reynaldo Morales returned from fighting in Angola (along with 40,000 other Cuban volunteers). Their son had been nine years old and they had both been working for the weekly newspaper *Granma* when Reynaldo had answered the call for internationalist volunteers to serve in Angola in 1984. When he returned two years later, AIDS had just become a reality for Cuba, with one person dead, another HIV-positive, and the beginnings of contact tracing underway.[17] The Health Ministry proposed testing all citizens returning from extended periods abroad, and the military were among the first to be tested.

Maria said, "Reynaldo and many of his comrades returned to Cuba with a strange and mysterious virus." After she found her husband had it, she got tested and discovered she too was seropositive. She told me, "I never thought it could happen to me, after all, I had never been with anyone except my husband Reynaldo (who had died just two months prior to our interview). Now, Maria was living alone at the flat they had shared for ten years in the sanitorium. She, like the other positive women I've interviewed in the U.S., believed her own monogamy would protect her. Maria, like other positive women who have since come to the sanitorium, lives in a single domicile in what appears to me to be very similar to a cooperative or commune—where people have their own room and the opportunity to share meals, laundry, and land if they want to grow food together. They can also opt out of the communal living accommodations if they want, as they appear to have everything they need in their "home." Too, they're given the same pay they had before being diagnosed and coming to the sanitorium. Their jobs are held for them and if they feel unable to return to their jobs after the six months of initial surveillance, education, and nutritional and psychological counseling, they're allowed a prorated income subsidy.

When I asked Maria if she felt mandatory testing was still a good thing she corrected me and told me testing has always been voluntary and it still is. "You see, people give blood here in Cuba in a regular way and their blood is tested unless they refuse and everyone has the option to forego testing."[18]

Maria confirmed my suspicion that health providers in Cuba still assume that it's largely the sexually active man who is at risk and that the only women who are at serious risk are prostitutes and drug users. But Maria, like every other Cuban I'd asked about drug use and prostitution, said, "We really don't have those problems in Cuba, the numbers are quite small." I then told Maria of my experience interviewing a Cuban gynecologist, who told me, "The only women [he] warns of risks of HIV are promiscuous women and prostitutes." He said, "I also recommend that every woman who comes in wanting to get pregnant be tested." I asked the doctor, "Won't you miss a lot of women?" He said, "No, because every woman wants to have a child." I paused and said, "Are there women here in Cuba who don't want a child?" He frowned and said, "Only if they're barren, mentally disturbed, homosexual, or holy women of some sort." I worked to keep my shock to myself, but realized that such a statement might be uttered by many traditionally trained doctors in the U.S., if one just scratched beneath their surfaces a little.

Maria went on to tell me, "We don't rely on doctors for primary sexual education; that's not their specialty. We have the department of sexual education and our media to do much of the HIV/Health and Hygiene instruction as a matter of course for every age group, including the third generation [the elderly]."

According to Karen Wald, Reynaldo and Maria also helped form GPSIDA, the AIDS prevention group, to go out and speak to people in the community about how to protect themselves and others. Until then, most people were not hearing the Health Ministry's attempts at AIDS education. Most people felt they could never get AIDS. It seemed too unreal to them: in Cuba, even as late as 1989—-people thought—almost nobody gets AIDS, and if they do, they're put in a sanitorium. So why worry?

But when women and men, homosexual and heterosexual, old and young, began identifying themselves as HIV-positive at schools, dance clubs, other popular teenage hangouts, and on local and national TV and radio programs, people started getting the message.[19]

Pity for North American Women

As Maria noticed me prepare to close our conversation, a sad look washed over her face. She told me she pitied North American women and girls who couldn't talk about sex with each other and their partners. She said, "I hate to think of how many women will die because of taboos on sex." I asked her how she sought to empower Cuban women to direct their own sexuality and protect their safety and if she had any advice she would want to give North American women. She said, "Tell them to be courageous, to stand strong for their own safety, and not to let the notion of *love* be misunderstood as sex." She ended our interview by saying, "Please carry back home with you my solidarity to seropositive women. I know they are not protected but I hope they will fight and gain their rights and find their worth. I wish I could be with them in this effort."

When I asked Maria to clarify what she meant by "U.S. women are not protected." She said, "They don't have their own safety and health as a right that is governmentally protected." I nodded, thanked Maria for her time, and told her I would take her message back to the U.S. My hope is that we can hear that message and work to realize her wish: that one shouldn't need to be rich to have quality medical care and one shouldn't need to be male to decide when and how to have sex, also that if one is a woman, she shouldn't need to carry a gun to resist unwanted or unsafe sex. Laws should be effective and cultural beliefs should be modified to normalize sexual freedom and health safety regardless of one's social location, race, gender, or sexual preference. To what lengths would we go here in the U.S. to break from our Western, individualist interpretation of human rights that has until very recently dominated the international discourse on AIDS and profoundly influenced public policy? Individual liberty, privacy, free speech, and free choice are cherished values in any democratic society. But they are sometimes invoked to obstruct social policies that favor distributive justice.[20] Could we in the U.S. find cultural capital and national pride through instituting universal access to health care, social welfare, affirmative action, and sexual/physical safety—to facilitate the well-being of those not privileged in the dominant class?

Before traveling to Cuba and meeting with the varieties of people there, I too thought Cuban public health measures there were draconian and hard to palate. After seeing the continuity of care and witnessing the fact that Cuba is providing more support and resources for PWAs—even during this stringent embargo—than many other first world countries, I couldn't as easily answer this question: Does freedom follow safety during an epidemic, or is it so intimately woven into the rhetoric of a socialist ideal that the thought of preserving it individually, rather than collectively, seems unconscionable?

ACKNOWLEDGMENTS

Thanks to all the women and men I interviewed in Cuba, to Shad Rheinstein, my colleague in research at Los Cocos, as well as to the translators Karen Wald and Oscar. Without the support of Janis Strout and the delegation of *Hermanas:* International Network in Central America and the Caribbean, I would not have been able to fly to Cuba as a psychosocial researcher during such a tense political time.

NOTES

1. Nancy Scheper-Hughes, "An Essay: 'AIDS and the Social Body' " *Social Science Medicine* 39, no. 7 (1994): 991–1003.

2. Ibid., 997.

3. Nancy Krieger, "Solidarity and AIDS: Introduction," *International Journal of Health Services* 21, no. 3 (1991): 505–10.

4. Paula Treichler, "AIDS and HIV Infection in the Third World: A First World Chronicle," quoted in *AIDS: The Making of a Chronic Disease,* ed. Elizabeth Fee and Daniel M. Fox (Berkeley: University of California Press, 1992), 392.

5. Ronald Bayer, "Entering the Second Decade: The Politics of Prevention, the Politics of Neglect," quoted in *AIDS: The Making of a Chronic Disease,* ed. Elizabeth Fee and Daniel M. Fox (Berkeley: University of California Press, 1992), 215.

6. An ethical dilemma plagued health authorities: How to protect the rest of the population from unnecessary risk (the responsibility of the Public Health Ministry) without imposing burdensome restrictions on those who carried the virus but were not yet ill? A solution was devised by Dr. Jorge Perez Avila, medical director of the Pedro Kouri Tropical Medicine Institute, when he was named director of the sanitorium in 1989, in consultation with people (living) with AIDS (PWAs), especially those who formed the Grupo Prevencion SIDA (GPSIDA, or AIDS Prevention Group). See Karen Wald, "Cuba's AIDS patient #1 dies," from NY Transfer News Collective. This document is part of the Cuba History section of the documentary collection, World History Archives, and is associated with the world history resource page, Gateway to World History, recorded for World Wide Web on November 21, 1995.

7. M. Frank, *Cuba Looks to the Year 2000* (New York: International Publishers, 1993), quoted in "The Impact of Economic Crisis and Embargo on Health in Cuba," by Richard Garfield et al., paper given on January 16, 1996.

8. Ruth Behar, ed., *Bridges to Cuba* (Ann Arbor: University of Michigan Press, 1995), 5.

9. With the recent (February 24, 1996—Cuba's Independence [from Spain] Day) shooting of two pilots from the Cuban-American exile lobby called Brothers to the Rescue, this fury has increased.

10. World Health Organization Mandate of 1985.

11. As the U.S. embargo mandates, there is a 44–pound limit per traveler en route to Cuba, which is strictly enforced.

12. In 1980 the Mariel boatlift of 125,000 Cubans demanding political asylum had many gay men on board who, along with others, were dubbed "the scum of the revolution" by the Castro regime in a sad effort to save face. See Behar, 8.

13. Behar, 3.

14. Before the revolution came to power in 1959, the situation facing Cuban women was a dismal one. Illiteracy, unemployment, racism, and exploitation all bore down particularly heavily on women. Machismo was in full force, and it was generally believed that a woman's place was in the home. Today, over twenty years later, the status of Cuban women has changed dramatically. Big advances have been made in education, health care, and improving the quality of life. Legal discrimination on the basis of sex has ended and women are playing a more and more important role in society. Hundreds of thousands have joined the work force, occupying many jobs previously reserved for men only. Old ideas and prejudices are being broken down and the question of winning women's full equality is a major topic of discussion. Yet the age-old belief that all women want and are destined to have children still persists.

15. According to Nancy Scheper-Hughes, "Cuba's climate of socialist sexual puritanism led to an early exodus of Gay Cubans from the island." See Scheper-Hughes, 997.

16. "The 15–year-old [bourgeoise] birthday parties are perhaps the only Cuban tradition that Fidel Castro's government couldn't erase by decree. Throughout these 25 years of Revolution, most traditional celebrations have disappeared, but not the 'bourgeois' aspiration represented by *las fiestas de 15*" (Ernesto Jaxier, "Turning Fifteen," in *CUBA Update,* April/June 1995, 32–35.

17. For each seropositive person there is a confidential "sexual contact tree" that traces the spread of the disease through various sexual partners, all of whom are eventually contacted and screened. According to Scheper-Hughes, "Cuban health officials have the most complete record of any nation on the patterns of sexual transmission of HIV/AIDS" (Scheper-Hughes, 998).

18. My colleague Shad told me that the blood supply has always been tested and that that is why only ten people in Cuba have contracted the virus through transfusion.

19. Karen Wald, "Cuba's AIDS patient #1 dies," from NY Transfer News Collective. This document is part of the Cuba History section of the documentary collection, World History Archives, and is associated with the world history resource page, Gateway to World History, recorded for World Wide Web on November 21, 1995.

20. Scheper-Hughes, 1002.

Part IV

Women with AIDS Speak Out

24

Ayisa

Part I: "I don't know anybody with AIDS."

In the beginning, I didn't know anyone with AIDS. Even after all that I had been through—growing up too quickly in high school what with my father and his drugs, my mother dying, my grandmother throwing me out, me sleeping on people's couches for shelter, never really knowing where I was going to live day by day, and never wanting anybody to know how hard life was getting for me—I never knew anybody with AIDS.

I guess what I'm trying to get across is that even though by the tender age of nineteen I thought that I had experienced everything life could throw at me, I was still pretty sheltered. Yes, I could talk a really good game, and I guess I could even be right sometimes (you know how they say that even a broken clock tells the right time *sometimes*), but I had never even seen a person with AIDS (PWA) up close and personal.

Funny isn't it?

And then I was sick with a vaginal disease for a full month. Words like "herpes" and "syphilis" were foreign to me, and so were night sweats and infections. There was lot of talk about STDs (sexually transmitted diseases), and they ran lots of tests, but still the doctors couldn't find anything wrong with me, and my illness remained big mystery. Even though I had all the symptoms, and I asked to be tested for HIV, my doctor wouldn't test me. Said that in his professional opinion, I didn't need to be tested. He thought I was too young.

Fearing for the worst, I went back to a free clinic on the Lower East Side where I had received free medical care and STD testing in the past. Here my age wasn't an issue: they tested right away for the virus. Everything seemed pretty routine and that helped to put my fears to rest. I spoke to a female social worker who advised me to return in three weeks and sent me on my way with a prescription for my vaginal disease. The burning cleared up within a day, the fevers and the night sweats stopped within a week, and I felt fine—ready to resume my life, feeling no pain.

But three to four weeks later, the clinic started to call about my pap smear being irregular. This seemed particularly odd to me because I knew that this clinic had a strict policy about not giving results of any kind over the phone. And then, when I didn't return their calls, the clinic started calling on a daily basis. This lasted for almost a month before a nurse finally got me in instead of my machine. Obviously they weren't going to take no for an answer this time. She said, very tight-lipped:

> "We have an appointment for tomorrow. Can you make it?"
> "What time?"
> "In the morning. Be here."

She hung up the phone.

Part II: "Your Mama is dead. There ain't nobody here for you."

At the clinic, utter hopelessness shot through me like a cannonball. Not two weeks earlier this same women standing before me (the social worker) had said that there was nothing to worry about. Now she was telling me that I was HIV+. I didn't know that there was any difference between being HIV+ and having full-blown AIDS. I just felt like she was telling me that I was going to die!

My first reaction was to want what every little girl wants when something goes wrong: I wanted my mother. I wanted her to come and make it all better. I wanted to crawl in her bed like I had done when I was six and seven to suck my thumb and play in her hair until the monsters went away, until the other little children's teasing no longer mattered, until HIV no longer mattered. Dealing with death and dying—the possibility of *me* dying—I wanted my mother.

This was all too unbelievable. I could have sworn that only a month earlier I'd heard this same social worker tell me not to worry because I was so young and had only had four lovers in my life. I thought I was supposed to be safe because I didn't do drugs and neither did my boyfriend. I thought I was supposed to be safe because I had never had sex with a bisexual, homosexual, or transgendered person—had never had sex with a sex worker.

The social worker broke into my hysteria to remind me that she'd said I was "low risk not no risk"—not exempt. I remember thinking that she couldn't possibly have meant what she'd just told me. Saying "No, no," over and over again, thinking that she was reading the wrong chart, because a chart that said someone had HIV couldn't be mine. That they must have made a mistake at the lab. I'd heard stories of people getting the wrong results, and that's what was happening to me now. By the time I had gotten out of my own head long enough to hear what she was saying, she was babbling something about Western blot and accuracy. I cut her off and shouted, "Take it again!" I told her this doesn't happen to me. To people like me.

Don't get me wrong. I wasn't completely naive about HIV and AIDS. But like a lot of people, I'd been living with two different messages going on in my head: on the one hand, I "knew" that it wasn't like HIV could only happen to certain people or anything; but on the other hand, I thought that I knew who was at risk, and I never thought of myself as one of those people. Being an average African-American teen-age girl growing up in the New York City public school system, and being the daughter of a single parent—my father, no less—I gathered most of my information about HIV and AIDS through public service announcements. I thought that so long as I followed those catchy one-line jingles and little phrases to the best of my ability, I was safe. How hard is it to understand "Get high! Get stupid! Get AIDS"? Well, I didn't get high, and I didn't get stupid. The commercials said, "If you sleep around and have unprotected sex you could be putting yourself at risk for HIV." Well, I didn't sleep around, and I didn't have unprotected sex. My current relationship with "D" was the first one where I had not used a condom throughout because it was serious, because we were serious. We had been in a relationship for over a year, and I felt very protected.

I knew what I was told not to do, and I hadn't done it. And I thought that if you followed the rules—what I thought were the rules—that nothing was going to happen.

But here I was sitting in the social worker's office, a goner. My mother couldn't come fix this or make it go away. And my heart was broken with a wound so deep it went to my core. It wasn't just about my boyfriend and the betrayal that I felt. It was for me, for myself, because I felt like I'd left me, like I had betrayed myself. I felt helpless and stupid sitting there by myself, making all these really important decisions all alone and totally unprepared. For the first time in a long time, being on my own didn't feel so good. I felt like I had screwed up big-time. I had let this man, this virus, this disease into my life, and now there was nothing that I could do about any of it. I couldn't help thinking that it just wasn't worth it. Nothing was worth the conversation that I was having with the social worker, not even love.

That day changed my life forever. Right there in that office in front of that social worker my whole being changed. No longer was I a teen-age girl; I was a person living with HIV. And I had no idea of what that meant.

Part III: "I gotta watch the election returns on TV."

I know I stayed in the clinic till it just about closed. I totally forgot it was election day. I was going to vote; I was definitely going to vote. Voting is very important. It proved that I was an adult, that I could make decisions. It was what our forefathers and -mothers had fought so hard for. But after the talk with the social worker, I couldn't make any more decisions. I didn't want to make any more decisions. Whatever happened, happened. I didn't care.

Returning home that evening felt almost foreign to me. This place that I was looking at didn't even seem like mine anymore. It didn't seem like home. The bed I had shared with my boyfriend didn't seem like our bed anymore, it just seemed like a bed. The laughing, smiling pictures of us all seemed to be looking at me and laughing, teasing. I thought I was losing my mind.

As usual, D wasn't home from work yet. I had time to sit and think. I didn't really want to think, but my brain wouldn't let me do anything else. I only knew that I didn't want to be alone. I called D and told him to make sure to come home this evening because I really needed to speak to him. He asked, "How did it go at the doctor's today?" I knew exactly how it went, but all I said was "We need to talk." D mumbled something about the election and needing to vote, but I shouted, "Fuck the elections, and bring your ass home!" Then I hung up the phone. After that, everything else was a vat of confusion, anger, lots of crying, and finally sleep.

By the time D came home my eyes were puffy and swollen from crying. I remember asking him about his day. Small talk always helped me calm down, and I needed to be calm for this conversation. But by the time I was calm enough to start repeating what the social worker said, I had begun crying hysterically and looking for a way out the room. D heard what I said, stared at me blankly, and reminded me that he needed to watch the elections because if Dinkins—the current mayor of New York city—lost, he was going to lose his job. I looked at him in disbelief, rolled over, asked him not to touch me during the night. I started crying again and then went to sleep. More was thought about our relationship that night than was said. I understood that whatever happened, HIV was my problem and not D's. I was in this boat by myself, and it was up to me whether I was going to sink or swim. The next morning he put the keys on the television and left. Dinkins had lost the election.

Part IV: "I'm always moving forward, HIV+ or not."

Several things have changed since that November day. Certainly I have changed. Although I am not sick, and I thank God for my health, I feel like I'm fighting for my life. My life as a woman. My life as a wife and a mother. I'm fighting because I don't want HIV to have the power to take things away from me.

In the past, I remember wanting lots from my boyfriend: I wanted him to be my husband and to be the father of my children. I wanted us to be together to see our grandchildren grow up. Now *I* want a lot from myself. I want to go to school, to have a good job, and even to have a good man. But I want these things for myself, not so that someone else can be satisfied with me.

As for HIV, I never wanted this. No one wants this.

There is a heated debate going on right know about whether or not HIV+ women should be allowed to have children and about whether or not all pregnant women should be mandatorily tested for the virus. I believe that HIV and AIDS education should be available in every prenatal facility and in every hospital. And I believe that women need to be made more aware that merely becoming pregnant puts them and the fetus at risk for HIV. And I believe that testing and health care should be available to every pregnant woman, to every human being. But although I feel strongly that everyone should have the option of testing for HIV, and although I think that everyone should be able to receive medical care in every form that interests them (whether Western, Eastern, traditional, or nontraditional), I don't believe that anyone should be forced to test, and neither I nor any other woman need to be made to feel like a criminal for having, or wanting to have, a baby.

As for the kinds of HIV/AIDS education that we're offering to people these days, I think that some things need to change. For example, we need to stop using phrases like "high-risk" sex: it only leads people to believe that there's such a thing as "low-risk" sex. Forget it. Sex is sex. The moment you begin exchanging bodily fluids, whether vaginally, orally, or anally, you are at risk.

Finally, I think that women need to be taught that their safety is not only dependent upon their current partner's health, but also upon their past partners' and upon their current partner's past partners. Don't get me wrong: I'm not laying blame or trying to evade responsibility. But I think that people, and women especially, need to be encouraged to watch out for themselves regardless of how much they love or trust their partner. Making that transition from always taking care of others to taking care of ourselves is going to be a difficult one because it goes against everything we've been taught all their lives, but it has got to happen. Women need to lean to practice safe sex as though our lives depend upon it.

25

Carol

When the phone rang for the second time within a ten-minute period, I assumed it was my niece calling about a barbecue we were planning. I quickly snatched the ringing phone and was surprised to hear the doctor I had recently consulted about ongoing health problems introduce herself and politely inquire if I had a moment or two to discuss the results of the blood work she had received from the laboratory. I remember feeling chilled: Even though it was a hot August afternoon, the hairs on my arm were standing straight up. Doctors, in my personal experience, never called with lab results, or any other news for that matter. For the most part, the doctors I had visited over the last three-and-a-half years, in an effort to establish why my health had deteriorated, were inaccessible once office hours were over. I knew instinctively when I heard the doctor's voice that my life would never be the same.

On Friday, August 13, 1993, I learned I had tested positive for the HIV virus. It was the culmination of years of running from one medical specialist to another searching for a reason, an answer, to the increasingly debilitating symptoms that plagued me. At the time of my diagnosis I was afflicted by chronic fatigue, intermittent diarrhea, swollen lymph nodes, headaches and occasional pelvic inflammatory infections, yeast infections, and menstrual irregularities. Starting in 1990 with an unexplained pelvic infection that my gynecologist treated as an aberration rather than as an indication of a disease, I began an odyssey that would entail visiting nine different doctors, undergoing numerous physicals, donating what seemed like a vampirish amount of blood, and submitting myself to a variety of tests with the goal of determining why my once-healthy body was betraying me.

During my almost surrealistic quest for an answer, I encountered more than one practitioner who politely inquired not whether I had marital relations, but did I have problems in my marriage; they then implied a prescription for Xanax or Valium might alleviate the symptoms. I was informed in unctuous tones that women in midlife were prone to depression, and depression often mimicked the symptoms of more serious illnesses. I was told I had a bad attitude because I challenged a doctor's calm assumptions about my disintegrating health. I was probed, poked, and condescended to; I was not taken seriously; I did not get better on Xanax or Valium. As one year became two years, I was confused, increasingly anxious—and of course, well tranquilized.

In 1992, at the age of forty-five, I decided that perhaps my current physician was right: a change in my routine might restore the integrity of my ailing body. My lymph nodes had swollen to the size of lima beans in my neck and beneath my armpits, and I was very frightened but in denial because my most recent physical concluded I was healthy, if somewhat underweight. I was bored with my current job as a personnel administrator and under tremendous stress at home trying to care for the needs of my husband and daughter, who is a special-needs child, while maintaining a spotless home. For years I had contemplated a return to school but always seemed to lack the conviction or necessary time to pursue my nascent dream. I was in most respects an average middle-aged, middle-class woman who was fortunate enough to own her own home and to be able to fulfill a long-suppressed ambition—a change in career, a change in focus. Perhaps a change in health would be forthcoming, or so I rationalized as I announced my plans to my astonished friends and family.

I had decided upon a career in radiation technology and embarked on my undertaking with a zeal and tenacity that alternately amazed and exasperated my family, especially my husband. We rarely had a conversation that provided me with any clues about how he viewed my aspirations, and I was actually grateful that for the most part he seemed to grudgingly accept my newly discovered lust for learning. Meanwhile my lymph nodes were still swollen, my diarrhea worsened, my pelvic complaints increased, and I was always tired. I blamed ill health on the stress and rigors of returning to school in midlife. For six months I prayed that my body would stop betraying me and cooperate with my plans to complete school with a 4.0 average.

August 1992 was a month of serious introspection and old-fashioned cold feet as I weighed the consequences of starting my radiation clinicals, which other students had warned me were physically grueling. My husband's union insurance had temporarily lapsed. I was insured by the institution I was attending but the coverage was minimal, and I was still sick. After much thought I confided in my best friend that my lymph nodes had swollen at the beginning of the school term, and asked if she could recommend a doctor at the clinic where she received her health care. She listened; we cried. Convinced that I had cancer I called a physician who my friend had assured me was caring and sympathetic to women's issues. Interestingly enough my husband, who overheard me making my appointment, questioned me about my dropping weight and asked if my returning to school could have triggered some of the symptoms he had noticed. I reassured him that I was fine, bold liar that I was, and signed on for my fall courses before visiting physician number seven on the quest for health, as I referred to it in my pre-AIDS days.

After yet another physical, more questions about my family's health—both paternal and maternal, which impressed the hell out of me at the time—and of course the mandatory blood work, Doctor Number Seven informed me that based on the lack of any evident pathology, I had chronic fatigue syndrome. When I asked her to clarify what seemed to me to be a facile and ambivalent explanation for my symptoms, I was told that I had an elevated monocyte count, which often is indicative of a past history of mononucleosis. Further discussion revealed that this was a best-guess diagnosis. She expected I would feel better within six months, and my lab tests did not indicate the presence of any virus that would account for my fatigue or swollen lymph nodes. I questioned her about my ability to handle my upcoming school clinicals, the advisability of committing myself to student loans, the possibility of stress worsening my condition; in turn, she advised rest, a good diet, and monthly visits until my condition resolved itself. She conveyed her belief that there was no reason for me to be concerned: "You will be fine within six to twelve months." I was elated that this most recent doctor had not hinted I was a closet neurotic and I began school with a feeling of hope.

Within a week it was clear that my energy level was so low I could barely function on eight hours of sleep, and that to continue clinicals in addition to the required curriculum—anatomy and college math—would be detrimental to both my health and my grade-point average. I advised the dean of students that I had to postpone my clinicals, called my doctor, and cried most of the following weekend. For the next six months I studied with a fury I didn't know I possessed. Somehow, I rationalized, if I could maintain an A average in my classes, there couldn't be anything seriously wrong with me. Meanwhile, my swollen lymph nodes increased in size and number, and I began to have night sweats that left me drenched and weakened even after sleeping eight to ten hours. Once a month I dutifully apprised my doctor of my latest sets of symptoms; once a month I was assured I would feel better; once a month I heard her extend the deadline for my expected recovery from chronic fatigue syndrome; and once a month she performed a new battery of blood tests. I was tested for lupus, toxoplasmosis, and a variety of exotic diseases whose names are unpronounceable. She never discussed with me her intention to test me for other causes for my declining health. Good little anatomy student that I was, I would copy the names of the tests she performed each month and go home and research them in my medical reference books. And I never questioned her about the various blood tests she ordered. She encouraged me to believe in a positive outcome to my situation, and I clung to the tenuous hope she offered, suppressing the intuition that something more insidious was occurring in my body.

In January I began to have nightmares. I would dream my mother was watching me gain weight while she shriveled into a skeleton-shaped wraith, taunting me with our reversal in size. My mother, deceased for the past four years, had been a heavyset woman while I have always been described as petite. There was something jarringly off-key about my repetitive dream. My body, my unconscious, and my very soul were sounding a loud alarm. I realized it was time to press my doctor for some real answers. I was frightened by the vision of myself that my dreams alluded to and that my mirror confirmed. I looked sick and felt terrible.

In February I suggested to the doctor that it seemed reasonable to consider a biopsy of a lymph node since the size of my nodes was still increasing, my weight was still dropping, my diarrhea persisted, and my energy level had plummeted. I was not getting better. In addition, I had recently noticed numbness and pain in my feet and hands. My doctor attributed the pain to possible arthritis compounded by the stress of juggling my responsibilities as a student, wife, and mother. She wrote me yet another prescription for Xanax. I left her office shaky, uncertain, and pissed. Why was I being coddled like a cranky, insecure child? Why didn't she listen to my complaints seriously? Why didn't I feel better? How long was this charade going to continue? Till I died of neglect, keeled over from exhaustion, gave up the search in frustration? Why, after consulting seven doctors in three years, didn't I have a confirmable diagnosis for my very real symptoms? What was wrong with my body, and what was wrong with a medical system that persisted in perpetuating the fallacy that it was all in my mind? What did I have to do to get some intelligent answers to these questions?

Would I ever know what was wrong with me?

I don't know why I refused to acquiesce to her supposedly superior knowledge, why I refused to accept her flimsy diagnosis, especially in light of the fact that her predecessors had alluded to what she now was alluding to — that I was neurotic. Certainly my upbringing had reinforced the belief that doctors know best, doctors are educated professionals, doctors are dedicated to the well-being of their patients. Call it intuition or perhaps an inability to ignore the obvious, but I was more determined than ever to unmask the villainous germ, virus, whatever, that was undermining my health.

My marriage had begun to unravel from the dual strains of school and my continued ill health. My husband, Michael, and I had suffered through other periods of silence and estrangement, most notably when we bought our home. We had gone for counseling to repair our marriage before my illness, and I suggested it now out of a growing sense of impotency. Michael was not acknowledging how ill I was, nor was he lifting a finger to help me cope with the demands school imposed. I was becoming a testy, irritable harridan whom he had decided to ignore. He refused to reenter counseling. I felt betrayed and abandoned by his lack of nurturing, his lack of understanding. My textbooks became my refuge; I was maintaining a 4.0 average despite my ill health and hostile home life. Only my special-needs daughter and my mother-in-law noticed the difference in my behavior. I had become quite skilled at disguising how I felt physically and emotionally, but they saw something my husband was too frightened to see: I looked like hell.

With the exception of my mother-in-law, who vocally expressed her concern and dismay regarding my ill health, and my daughter, who repeatedly questioned me about my appearance, the people I considered my support system tacitly dismissed the obvious signs that I was not the person I had been, even as they reinforced by their silence the growing isolation and frustration I was feeling. Although it was never verbalized, it was evident that friends and family concurred with the doctors I had consulted: I was neurotic.

During March, I was studying the immune system in my anatomy class and time was given to the concerns of the new epidemic in immunology — AIDS. One night I half-jokingly remarked to my husband that maybe I had

AIDS. I began to read off the list of attendant symptoms discussed in my reference notes. Well, that remark certainly captured his attention! He flashed me his most ironic grin and replied, "You must be kidding, Carole!" I dropped the subject and breathed a quiet sigh of relief.

In retrospect I now realize I had harbored suspicions regarding my husband's fidelity since the earlier period when I had coerced Michael into couple's counseling. We had discussed, if infrequently, the threat AIDS posed to sexually active adults who didn't protect themselves. But we never discussed the issues that had prompted me to question him that night. I was terrified to sunder the secrets that lay between our sheets; I buried my doubts along with the opportunity to breathe some honesty into our relationship. If I asked the questions I would have to deal with the answers; I was afraid to jeopardize our marriage further. I loved my husband but resented his inability to empathize with my fears, resented his overt dismissal of my disgust with the medical establishment.

The doctor and I began our duel of wills. I insisted a biopsy was necessary while she vacillated between patronizing good humor—"Wait and see what develops when the school semester ends, maybe your symptoms will abate"—to vague reassurances that she would consider my request if my symptoms warranted a biopsy. At one point she asked me, for the third month in a row, if I had children. I angrily retorted that she had asked me that question before. Didn't she listen to me when I was talking? She apologized and we moved on in our debate, but I had lost all illusion that she cared about my well-being. I was counting the time until my husband's insurance kicked in and actively shopping around for a new physician. I was thoroughly disgusted with clinic care and mortified that so many women had to rely on a system of health care that was neglectful and woefully inadequate in addressing women's concerns.

June rolled around and I entered the examining room for my monthly visit with a belligerent attitude. Enough was enough. I had spent ten months faithfully cataloguing my complaints, which she had alternately acknowledged and dismissed. I challenged her immediately, "Do you have any idea what is wrong with me?" I asked sarcastically.

"No, I don't," she admitted sheepishly, not even meeting my glance, but rather staring at my file as though the answer would rise up from there.

"Will you please refer me to a qualified surgeon to biopsy my nodes?" I asked.

"Yes, I will write a referral for your insurance company." Businesslike demeanor restored, she handed me the name of a local surgeon and coolly inquired if I would like her personally to make the appointment.

"No, I'll make my own appointment, thank you," I replied, my voice betraying my thinly veiled anger.

Without any explanation I got up out of the chair, mumbled a good-bye, and ran out of that clinic, barely registering the astonished stares of the nurses I normally kibitzed with and almost knocking one nurse over in my hasty exit. Fury blazing, tears spilling down my face, I drove home crying hysterically, sunglasses on to disguise my sobbing.

Three years since my first unexplained bout with a pelvic inflammatory infection, and countless visits with a series of physicians, and still, I was lacking a diagnosis; living in mute despair because none of these experts, with their tests and perfunctory examinations, could piece together the pieces of the puzzle.

Pulling into my driveway, I shoved my renegade thoughts aside, raced up the stairs into my kitchen, and grabbed the phone. I dialed the surgeon's number, silently praying that this time I would find the answers, this time someone would connect the dots, someone would listen and care. After explaining what a busy schedule the doctor had, the receptionist, hearing the desperation in my voice, double-booked me for an appointment in three weeks.

The surgeon's waiting room resembled an assembly line: scores of people impatiently thumbed through magazines while others stared at invisible spots on the walls of the graciously appointed reception area. After registering with the receptionist and filling out the necessary insurance and patient information forms, I sat down in one of the few remaining vacant seats, resigned to wait till my name was called. One hour later a nurse ushered me into one of many examining rooms along what seemed an endless corridor, handed me a paper dressing gown, and instructed me to be patient. The doctor was running late. A few minutes later the surgeon came bouncing into the room and introduced himself, apologizing for the delay. Polite civilities exchanged, he proceeded to examine my swollen lymph nodes, commenting on their size and number. Examination completed, he told me to get dressed and meet him in his office down the hall.

Seated in his inner sanctum, I answered his questions regarding my age and general health while he consulted the records Doctor Number Seven had forwarded to his office. He seemed amiable, open, so I was startled when he disingenuously inquired about the anxiety he saw reflected in my eyes: Could it have an emotional component?

He informed me that he had just removed some lymph nodes from a female patient, slightly younger than me, and she was just fine, no sign of malignancy. This last pronouncement was uttered in smooth, silky, supposedly reassuring tones.

"No," I quickly responded, voice quavering, I replied, "What you see in my eyes is fear because I don't know what's wrong with me."

He dropped the question and hastily penciled in a time for me to have two nodes, one in my neck and one beneath my right armpit, removed on an outpatient basis for biopsy. Our verbal exchange lasted perhaps five minutes, his examination perhaps ten minutes; my insurance carrier was billed one hundred and fifty dollars for this initial consultation. I wasn't offended by this latest insinuation that my mind was manufacturing my illness; by now I was accustomed to being dismissed by doctors as a head case. But biopsies didn't lie. Even if my worst fears were realized and the results confirmed my suspicion that a malignancy was present, I would at least know what was ailing me. Science would vindicate me.

In July, one week before my birthday, I was again seated in the surgeon's office waiting for the results of my biopsy. Convinced the news would be bad, I had requested that my best friend come with me in the event I was too upset to drive home alone. After what seemed like an excruciating amount of time, I was escorted by the surgeon himself into the inner sanctum. The news was excellent. I didn't have cancer. Jovially, he exhorted me to resume school, "Be happy and have a wonderful life." My response was obvious relief and puzzlement. Could he clarify for me just what the biopsy did indicate? Clearly exasperated that I hadn't greeted his good news with more enthusiasm, he replied that the biopsy had revealed disphasia of the cell tissues examined. "What does that mean?" I inquired. Impatiently, he explained that disphasia sometimes indicated an autoimmune disorder, such as rheumatoid arthritis, but not to worry, I looked perfectly fine in his professional opinion. Accepting that I was being politely dismissed, I thanked him for his time and left his office, confused and torn between relief that I wasn't suffering from cancer and frustration that I still was missing a diagnosis. Even my friend's evident elation didn't affect my feeling of self-doubt and failure. Once again I had lost the trail of clues en route to the doctor's office.

Once home I called the clinic I had been visiting monthly and badgered one of the nurses I had befriended into giving me the names of three doctors who specialized in treating rheumatoid arthritis. Fortunately I was able to book an appointment for the following week. August was fast approaching, I was scheduled to start my clinicals in September, and the financial aid office at school was pressing me to sign the student loan forms for the coming semester. Lacking solid information to guide me in formulating a decision regarding my future, I gambled that, cancer-free, I could resume my studies, fervently praying that the stress of clinicals and assuming more debt wouldn't aggravate my unknown health situation. I was frantic, disillusioned, and slowly recuperating from my outpatient surgery. My neck, as a result of the removal of a sizable lymph node, was sore, fiery red. I had a raw scar the size of a quarter which throbbed continually.

Subdued and depressed, I was pleasantly surprised when the latest specialist punctually and personally escorted me into an examining room. He was professional but not patronizing, thorough but not redundant, friendly but not obsequious. I liked his quiet, unassuming manner. After some discussion of my symptoms and an examination of my lymph nodes, he looked at me with a penetrating question in his eyes, cleared his throat, and without mincing words asked did I think I could be at risk for the HIV virus. It could be a possibility given my symptoms. Unoffended by the question, I quickly responded, no, I didn't think so, but I didn't follow my husband around twenty-four hours a day. "Well," he replied, "it's pretty clear to me that you definitely do not have rheumatoid arthritis. How do you feel about being tested for HIV? I would like you to consult with the infectious-disease specialist in our practice. Do you have time today to see her? I'll call her now if that is O.K. with you." Smiling, I assured him that would be fine, let's eliminate this as a possibility. Twenty minutes later I was seated across the desk from yet another specialist, nervously fidgeting in my chair while she explained confidential testing. I would pay for the test and my insurance company would not be billed, therefore they would be unaware I was being tested for the HIV virus. Not really comprehending the ramifications of what she was trying to convey, I consented to paying for the test rather than alarming my insurance company, as she delicately paraphrased my choice. Her brief, discreet inquiry concerning my degree of risk suggested she did not consider the white, middle-aged, middle-class suburban wife and mother sitting across from her as someone who was truly at risk for contracting the HIV virus. Clearly uncomfortable, she immediately proceeded to launch into a lengthy inquiry of my travel habits. Could I have contracted some rare virus, germ, some nasty little bug that perhaps had been overlooked in previous health exams? No, I demurred, but still I answered her questions dutifully, diffidently — diligently avoiding, with her complicit but unstated cooperation, any further discussion of the really relevant issues surrounding my HIV test. She did not mention pretest counseling and ended the uncomfortable conversation she had initiated with one quick question: "Do you want to be called with the results of your HIV test or would you like to come back in person?" Startled, I offhandedly replied, "Sure, call me." I was shaking so badly that the nurse, while withdrawing my blood, asked a coworker to get me something sweet. Assessing me with compassion and obvious concern, she whispered soft reassurances, "It's O.K., are you all right, dear?" She physically assisted me into an adjoining office, waiting with me till her coworker returned with a candy bar. I gratefully accepted this rare rendering of grace. To this day I still recall every earthy, careworn wrinkle engraved upon her wise and weary face.

That evening I confronted my husband as he prepared to get ready for bed. "Do you know this new specialist asked me to undergo HIV testing. He thinks there may be a connection between all my symptoms. What do you think?" I challenged, my voice rising one octave, short staccato sighs bridging the silence of our bedroom. "Well, I guess you have nothing to worry about then. I'm tired, let's go to bed." He paused, thoughtfully scrutinizing my reaction. "Are you O.K.?" he asked, real concern reflected in his eyes. "Yes," I murmured, "I am." Catching my tears as they pooled in my eyes, I gratefully received his enveloping hug. We slept cocooned in each other's arms that night, belly to belly, like the lovers we had once been. Feeling foolish that I had ever doubted my husband would protect me, reassured that Michael had not exposed me to the danger of AIDS, I calmly waited for news of my latest blood donations, resigned to the fact that I would more than likely be back where I started in June: lacking a diagnosis.

When the infectious-disease expert informed me that I had tested seropositive for the HIV virus I immediately protested that she must be mistaken. In cool clinical jargon she explained the procedure for verifying a seropositive result, the difference between a Western blot and an Elisa test; severing any hope I still entertained that some terrible mistake had occurred. I slammed the phone receiver down, not bothering to say good-bye, and wailed, screamed, howled my outrage. My daughter, having witnessed my reaction to this phone call, seeing her mother crying, hovered near until, realizing her presence, I gathered her in my arms, mumbling, "Mommy's going to die." I could feel her trembling body as she reacted to my words but I couldn't summon the strength to shield her from my terror. My special-needs daughter, unaware of the content of my conversation with the doctor, confused and frightened by her mother's hysteria, was the one who was forced to deal with the emotional carnage created by the physician's incredible lack of sensitivity. One month later I called this doctor and admonished her that no one should ever be given the option of hearing their test results over the phone. She reminded me that she had given me the choice: I was an intelligent woman; I understood the implications.

By the time of my diagnosis, my T-cell count was 300, my husband's was 220. If I had allowed myself to be persuaded that I was neurotic, I am convinced we would both be dead by now, or at the very least seriously ill from one of the many opportunistic infections associated with a severely depressed immune system. AIDS was not the imminent death sentence I perceived it to be when I was initially diagnosed. My life, my marriage, every aspect of my life was affected by HIV. But the changes in my life have been, for the most part, positive and transformative.

In conclusion, my experience is not, I believe, an isolated incident, a rare occurrence. As an AIDS educator and advocate for better health care I have listened to many stories that confirm this suspicion. Women are frequently dismissed as neurotic or depressed when reporting symptoms that are not easily definable, easily explained. Until our society demands better treatment for all women and implements mandatory health education that empowers women to be savvy consumers, our mothers, daughters, sisters, and friends will continue to suffer and, in some instances, die from the widespread institutional neglect and fiscal disenfranchisement that is epidemic, that is a cancer eroding the foundation of America. HIV is a major public health threat to all women. What are we going to do about it?

26

Yoco

I was born on October 13, 1955, in the Caribbean. I'm the youngest of six children. I left the Caribbean when I was nine years old with my older sisters. My brother died of AIDS four years ago when he was forty-eight; now I have only sisters. We moved to Brooklyn where my sisters raised me with financial help from my parents. Where I come from my parents were poor but they raised me as middle-class (by my country's standards). We always had food and clothing. My father had his own business which he ran with my mother. And because they did well, they sent the kids to the U.S. and sent us money to study and be taken care of by my older sisters.

I just go for men, so I'm heterosexual. I have a sixteen-year-old son and a ten-year-old daughter who both live with me in a small city in Rhode Island. They both have separate fathers to whom I was married at different times in my life. I met my first husband when I was twenty-two, and I had my son when I was twenty-four. My first husband is who I stayed with four years until I realized he wasn't good for me. He wasn't working, and he was never there for me. He used to smoke marijuana and had other girls. That wasn't what I wanted. After breaking up with my first husband, I had a couple of dates and fell in love with another man who was just as bad as my first husband: drugs, girls, etc.

So I decided that going back to where my parents lived might be better for me. I went back to the Caribbean, and that's when I met my second husband. He was ten years older than me, so when he told me he loved me, I believed I could trust him. I didn't love him as much as he loved me; still, I married him and had my daughter. I did it because I wanted someone stable, and he seemed like someone who would always be there for me. He offered security. We eventually moved into separate bedrooms, and after six years I had fallen in love with another man. My husband found out about the affair by following me, so when he came to me and asked if I was seeing someone else, I told him "yes." He accepted it and told me, "I will always love you. I hope this man loves you as much as I love you. I will always be there for you and especially for our daughter, who I love so much." I thought that that settled that. I thought that I would go on like before—in love with this man who was not my husband and taking care of my daughter from my marriage—but I realized that I couldn't once I found out I had HIV.

Right before my diagnosis, life was ideal. My boyfriend and I had such a good life. He was also married and six to eight years older than me. We had known one another since I was eighteen. When I was with him, I was living; I was truly happy. That man offered me everything! I used to see him every Friday, so every Friday was like my birthday. We had six wonderful years together: we traveled on vacation, he gave me jewelry, he gave me all kinds of nice things. And at this time, when life was so good, that's when I found out I had HIV.

I can't believe my boyfriend dumped me as soon as he learned about my diagnosis. I will never forget that day. It was August 28, 1991, and I had a little bump in my face, so I went to see a doctor. The doctor couldn't decide whether it was a big thing or a little thing. She said, "I'll need money." My boyfriend was very supportive at first: that same day he gave me the $900 I needed to invest in medication. But when I collected the money from him he said, "What's that thing on your face?" When I answered, "The doctor said it's nothing—a Zona" (blister), he said, "Well I don't like that." I said, "It's nothing to worry about; I'll be going back to see the doctor in two days." When the day for our appointment came, she asked me to go have an HIV test done. That very night my boyfriend called me and made the same exact request. He had been warned by a friend who said, "Every time you see a Zona, it's a sign of HIV. So tell your girlfriend you both need to get an HIV test." When we both got tested, my results came back positive while his were negative.

My boyfriend became suspicious. He asked "How come you have it and I don't if it has been three years since you've been with your husband?" So I went to see my husband, whom I had not lived with for three years. He was lying down; he was sick. "What's the matter with you?" I asked, but even then I already suspected that he was the one who had infected me. I asked him to get tested, but he refused. Just then, by sheer coincidence his driver told me that he was going to get a test result for my husband. He *had* just been tested, but he hadn't wanted to tell me. When the driver returned I took the envelope from him and opened it to find out that my husband was positive.

Now that I knew the truth and what had happened I went back to see my boyfriend and we cried and cried and cried. He told me, "Don't worry, I will always be there for you." I felt like my life was over. This was in August 1991, and I didn't know the difference between HIV and full-blown AIDS. My boyfriend said, "You must go to the U.S. to see a specialist who deals with AIDS because in the Caribbean, they're not that well informed on the disease and treating it." He gave me money to come to Rhode Island to protect myself from the gossip that would happen if I were to go back to Brooklyn, where people knew me, for AIDS treatment. My sister, four years older than me, lived in Rhode Island so it made sense to go there.

The doctor who I saw in Brooklyn told me to come back in a week after my blood test. During that week I was praying that I would not have HIV. I was hoping that in the Caribbean they had made a mistake. When I saw the doctor in a week she said, "I have good news for you: your T-cells are 890, so you need no medication." That wasn't the good news I had wanted, but by then I knew that I could live for years after my diagnosis. When I told my boyfriend, he said, "Oh that's good news" in a voice that told me he thought I was crazy to be so naive. He's like, "You're gonna die anyway."

After being in Rhode Island a month, I went back to the Caribbean to pack my things and make the big move to the U.S After six months here, my boyfriend from the Caribbean came to visit me. That was when I realized that he was through with me, because he wouldn't touch or hug me when we slept in the same bed. That hurt so much. How could he do that to me? I learned that he already had another girl. When I told him I was going to a Immunology Center here he said, "Why don't you find a new lover there?" I began to get upset and cry. I said, sarcastically, "Oh yes. That's right. An HIV-positive person and an HIV-negative person can't possibly keep going out together." He claimed I didn't understand. When he went back to the Caribbean he used to call me every week, then every month.

A year later I went back to the Caribbean, still remembering that he said he would always be there for me. You know, when we were lovers he would never be late, always prompt. But that time he didn't show up after we had made plans for him to come and see me. I didn't sleep all night that night. I couldn't believe he did that to me. He didn't even call, and that's the worst part. When I called him he said, "I did it on purpose. I have a reason for doing it. . . . We can discuss it Saturday, can I see you Saturday?" That's when I knew he had another girl. That's when I knew I was truly rejected. I said, "No. I want to see you on *Friday*." I hate what he did to me. I mean if *he* rejected me—the one who was supposed to never reject me. . . . That felt so bad. I never felt worse. I felt like a little bird without a branch to hold on to. I went and saw my mother, but I couldn't tell her or anyone close to me in my family because I was afraid that my HIV status would blanket my family in shame, as is often the case in the Caribbean. I could only tell my two closest girlfriends who still live there (we keep in touch by phone still).

I came back to Rhode Island in May 1995. I got a place for myself with my boyfriend's money, and then I got a job at a hospice for people living with AIDS. I give the people there motivation to keep fighting, and they give it to me. They are such fighters. Life is a gamble. You play and I lost. Just hearing that you have HIV takes ten years from your life. No one who doesn't have it can fully understand. It takes so much courage to go public. It's been two years since I was diagnosed, but that rejection from my boyfriend hurt too much: I feel too rejected to go public. I felt safe enough to tell my coworkers at the AIDS Hospice because I could really tell there was love there.

When I look at my two children I feel I have to stand up for them: they're the only ones I have. My son is dealing with my having HIV fairly okay. My daughter's not dealing too well. She thinks a lot about my dying. I tell her, "Don't think about it, I'm fine. Just because I have AIDS doesn't mean I'm gonna die." They never see me when I'm down. I never let them see me down. I go to bed when I'm down. I'm going to see my son through college so he can take care of his sister.

I believe God will help me through this. I believe in God. How could I be here if not for God? If God hadn't helped me, I would have hate for my husband and lover. God is my everything. God is my doctor; God is my everything. When I'm really down I used to talk to friends but now I talk to God. I stay in my room and I don't cry anymore. When I really let my friends know what I feel, they end up crying. So now I just go to my room and talk to God or I go to Church where my pastor knows I have HIV. He treats me like I can handle myself. He says, "You're fine." But I really feel the most love from God. I say to God, "God, I love you very much. Give me strength to accept your will, if it's your will to take me now let me go in peace. But please let me live so I can raise up my two kids." I pray this every day. I thank God every day for being alive. I know I'm not gonna die right now. Not now.

Right now, I'm working on getting back in school. I hope to get a degree in physical therapy at a local college. I'm almost in. I just need money and my one-year transcripts from a college in Brooklyn. Right now I'm a Certified Nursing Assistant (CNA), and I like helping people. I think it's going to be good. To be a full-citizen with my papers all I need is $90, and in three months I would be a citizen. Because I just moved about a month ago, I can't do it right now. So my money's kind of tight. I'm on AFDC and I'm struggling to raise two children. Right now I'm renting a house for $500 and I'm getting $554 and I have to pay light, phone bills, and food. All I get in food stamps is $252 for three people and you can't work more than four hours or they cut you off some. I mean, I can't live a decent life above the board, and I'm not used to that. I would like the people who claim to help me to really help me. They should give me the money and let me work. I mean, give me a chance! I have to take care of my kids, give them shelter, food, health care, and clothing. I can't live like this. I don't like to be dishonest but my kids need clothes, so I work four hours a week under the table. I'm always underneath, never financially stable. For that to happen I would need twice what they give me or for them to let me work without penalizing me. It's degrading to have to go give them a pay-stub every month. If the money's there to help me, why don't they help me? My car's not working.

Thank God that I know I can't waste time—I know I have a fatal illness. Because I need Medicaid to go to a doctor, I know I have too much money, they won't help me. This is no way to live. I would like to live fully because I don't have that much time left. I'm not talking extravagant here. I mean a $3,000 car that works and a son that I can afford to put through college. It's overwhelming so I don't think about it. I try not worry but it's always there. Again, God help me! It hurts!

I would like to be in a support group that could help me understand people with AIDS/HIV more. My experience is that the people that I'm working for have been drug users and prostitutes, so sometimes I wonder if they understand me because I never have been to a group and heard a story like my own. I'm always the only one who acquired HIV through heterosexual transmission. I need peer support. I would like to meet a couple where the woman is HIV-positive and the man is negative. I would like to see how they feel and how he thinks. It would help me believe that it's possible. It's what I want. I want to meet a man who I can tell my status to. But I'm afraid. Because if my beloved boyfriend—the one who had promised to always be there for me—rejected me, who wouldn't?

I'm praying to God that I will find a boyfriend who can accept me with HIV. That's my wish for my birthday.

27

Cliff
Experiences of Transgender HIV

I am a sixty-year-old HIV+ preop female-to-male transgendered person. I got the virus in 1984 from my lover who was using needle
drugs and was also sexual with both men and women. I found out he was
using drugs before I discovered my HIV status and sent him away because I
was afraid of catching AIDS.

Unfortunately, I was too late.

I decided to test for the HIV virus while I was visiting Dusty, my ex-
husband, in Los Angeles one day in October 1987. He mentioned he had
gotten tested for HIV and was negative. I decided I probably should get
tested and be aware of my status too. I thought of the test as a routine
medical test. It turned out to be anything but routine for me.

When I went back to the health department for the results, I thought it
was odd the worker had another man with him as he walked me back to a
room. I thought "Oh no! I must be positive." How easily I changed that
thought to, "The other man probably wants something else and is escorting
us because he'll get it sooner that way." We got inside the room and my
escort closed the door. The worker said, "We got your results back and I'm
sorry to inform you the finding is positive." Shocked, I burst into tears. He
asked if I understood what he had said. I replied through my tears, "Yes.
You said I'm going to die!" He said something comforting—I don't
remember what it was. "What about my friends?" I asked. He said I should
go back five years and notify anyone I had had sex with in that time frame
so they could get tested. He asked me if I was O.K. to drive. I said I
thought I'd be all right and they let me out the back door to the parking
lot so I wouldn't have to run the gauntlet in the waiting room.

At this time, I lived in Tehachapi, a small town in the mountains forty
miles from Bakersfield. Bakersfield was a city of 163,000 residents located
in the central valley of California about 110 miles northeast of Los Angeles.
I got in my car and left the parking lot. Sometime later it came to my
attention that I had passed the same gas station several times. I was driving

in circles around Bakersfield. I pulled into the gas station and called Dusty. I bless his memory as I recall his words. "Can you make it to my place?" I said I thought I could, but I was supposed to go to work at 1 p.m. He told me to call and tell them I couldn't make it to work. I called and told them I had just found out my best friend was dying and I was much too upset to work that evening. I made it to Dusty's place and he held me as I cried. After a couple of hours I was calmer. He came home with me and stayed the weekend to try to keep me together. He even brought me to a drugstore and bought me a fancy vibrator so I could enjoy a new kind of sex.

When Dusty left my house on Monday, he borrowed my motorcycle. Later on during the week, I called and told him if he wanted to make the last few payments, he could keep the motorcycle. He had no transportation and was pleased to accept the bike. I had started to get rid of my possessions so no one would have to do that after my death. They had told me at the health department that after diagnosis my life expectancy was not more than two years. No one was taking into account the fact that most of the people diagnosed at that time had already gotten one of the opportunistic infections and, therefore, were already on death's doorstep by the time they were diagnosed. Shortly after my diagnosis I became depressed and almost suicidal. I had been given the name of a mental health counselor, so I decided to try counseling even though I had never received any before this time and didn't know what to expect. I went to the clinic and asked for the counselor by name. They said she only took people who were drug or alcohol abusers. Did I fit that description? I told them no but she had been recommended to me.

They refused to allow me to see her. Being already under a big strain, I fell apart and sat in the waiting room crying my eyes out. After awhile, a sympathetic man intervened on my behalf.

When I finally saw the counselor, she told me the front desk had not gotten used to her seeing HIV + persons and she would change that. I never had any problem getting in to see her after that. She saved my life by making it possible for me to look ahead a little and make my life better while it lasted. One of the results of her counseling was my enrollment and attendance at the local junior college. (She also started me on antidepressants, but the kind she had prescribed made me feel so strange and hyper that I stopped taking them after a few weeks.)

I moved from Tehachapi to Bakersfield to be closer to school and my

doctors. My new roommate introduced me to a gay man who brought me
into the local support group. Of course, at that time I was the only woman
and I was among several gay men. I met one other woman while in the
group, but she came only once. When I saw her some time later and
inquired her reason for not coming back to the support group, she said she
didn't feel comfortable around the gay men. But I found it very encouraging to be in a group of people who had the same troubles I had, and I
learned some of the ways to cope with my disability.

My medical care has gone through a series of ups and downs. Upon my
diagnoses in 1978, I informed my usual M.D. of my condition. He was
horrified and said he would attempt to treat me if I wished, but instructed
me to tell no one of my condition. He called my attention to the many
problems HIV+ individuals were having with neighbors, schools, jobs, etc.
He said Tehachapi was a very small town with the usual small-town
prejudices and if I let anyone know I would have problems. He also said he
didn't feel qualified to treat my condition because he had not learned
enough about it. He suggested I see a doctor in Bakersfield. About a month
or two later he gave up his private practice to join a care network that I
didn't belong to, so I could no longer get my medical care from him
anyway.

I found the doctor in Bakersfield who was reputed to be an AIDS
specialist and received my care from him for about a year. The first time I
saw him, he was very frank with me. He said the treatment was all based
on gay males and treating me would require some guesswork because there
was no research on women with the disease as yet. He took blood tests,
found I wasn't getting enough protein in my diet, and told me that my T-
cell count was 800. He started me on AZT. It was the only drug available
for HIV+ persons at that time. He was going to give me the usual dose of
60 mg per day. I objected to the dosage saying I had information that studies
had showed the minimum required dosage was 300 mg. He complied with
my request, and I started on 300 mg. I stayed on this dosage for the next
five years. I also took his advice and switched from my vegetarian diet to
one containing meat and fish. I have made sure, since then, to eat protein
with every meal.

I was forced to change doctors once more after a year, and once again it
was because my doctor was switched to a different location and I couldn't
get coverage from my insurance company to continue with him. I tried a
new doctor at a local clinic. He wrote on my chart that I was HIV+ and

ignored my requests for confidentiality. I argued with him but he wouldn't budge from his stance.

I changed doctors again, this time to a doctor recommended by a friend from the support group. I could get free care from this doctor by joining a study he was doing on whether typhoid vaccine would help with HIV. There was a drawback though: The doctor was located east of downtown Los Angeles and this meant that we had to go back ninety miles each way every week for awhile, then every other week. At the end of the study, the typhoid vaccine was found to be a dead end, and shortly after that the doctor moved his practice to the prison at Vacaville, California.

I went to the Hollywood Gay and Lesbian Center for awhile for another study, which petered out and left me again without health care.

At this time, I had been working at the Kern County Housing Authority in their maintenance department. Here, I learned to paint and repair their housing units. I was poorly paid, so I moved into a trailer park. I lived in my mini-motor home with my two dogs. At this time my T-cell count was 500. At the end of a year, I fell into a deep depression and stayed in bed most of the time. I only got up to feed myself and the dogs.

After about a month and a half, I realized what was happening to me and decided to opt out of the situation. I decided to relocate and start my life over. The time was December 1989. I thought for a while and decided I could best help myself by moving to the San Francisco Bay Area. I had considered moving there a year before but friends talked me out of it. I had thought I needed to move there because that was the center of the AIDS epidemic and that meant I could probably access better care there.

I called my friend from the support group who had relocated to Berkeley about six months previously. He said I could use his place while he was out of town for the holidays, so I put my things in storage and gave one of the dogs away. Putting all my necessities in the motor-home, I parked it in front of his place in Berkeley. By the time he returned I had a room and a job as a guard. Later I registered with several temporary agencies for office work. I figured my disability into my career plans and decided I would probably be able to work longer at an office position than by doing physical labor. Of course, this meant I had to wear what my husband calls secretarial bondage; high heels, skirt and makeup. I felt like I was in drag, but I did a good job of it and no one suspected I hadn't worn a dress in twenty years. I made a home for myself in the Bay Area and I still live there.

I looked under AIDS in the phone book and found the AIDS Clinic of the East Bay. I made an appointment and the doctor I visited there was the same one I visited until January 1996. When I obtained a steady position with Alameda County Social Services I picked the insurance company that had his name on their list. That way, when he became too busy to keep his volunteer position at the clinic, I was still able to access his services under my California Care insurance.

He set appointments with me for monthly checkups because at the time I was taking AZT and he wanted to keep an eye on my status. I started getting bouts of diarrhea and had to quit my job in September 1992. I had diarrhea every day until I learned to keep myself on a diarrhea diet which consisted mostly of applesauce and oatmeal and plain white rice. I applied for Social Security Disability income and State Disability, also. I used the services of the AIDS Project of the East Bay, specifically the benefits counselor. I had a lot of trouble gaining access to her help since she was often absent or busy. She told me how to apply for the benefits and read the applications I filled out. I made the changes she told me were needed and filed the applications. It took about two months to finally get them in. One thing she did say that I try to remember was "Always keep copies of anything you send to the government." The state supported me for a year, then the Social Security kicked in. I am now on Social Security and Medicare.

I haven't had any diarrhea since the first part of the year. I went to a seminar in San Francisco given by one of the foremost AIDS practitioners in the city. While there, I got into a conversation with a medical student. Upon finding out I was having a problem with diarrhea, she asked if I took vitamins. I told her I took a lot of vitamins and began naming them. She asked me where I purchased the vitamins and I told her I got them at the drugstore. She told me she had had problems with diarrhea until she changed to health store vitamins, which were pure and didn't have all the fillers.

I thanked her for her concern and said I'd try her solution. Of course, many people had given me solutions. Nothing had worked except the very restrictive diarrhea diet. I took her advice with a grain of salt. After all, upon my insistence, my doctor had put me through all sorts of uncomfortable and lengthy tests, with no resultant increase in knowledge of what was wrong with me. So, I slowly followed her advice by the attrition method. As I ran out of each vitamin, I replaced it with the same vitamin from my local health food store. No results, until I got to the last one. When I replaced that last drugstore vitamin, I got constipated. I was still on the diarrhea diet. I haven't had any problem with diarrhea since that day.

I stopped taking AZT about two years ago. I had been hearing from various people how toxic it is and how if it wasn't doing any good, I probably shouldn't be putting it into a body that was already overworked by the virus. I spoke to my doctor about this and he suggested I stop taking AZT two weeks before my monthly checkup. I did that and when I visited him he asked me how I felt. I said I felt no difference. He told me to stay off it for another month. At that point he took a blood test. Not taking AZT had changed nothing. I haven't taken any since then.

The doctor I went to for free so long now costs me five dollars a visit, and my prescriptions, which used to cost me three to five dollars, are often forty dollars or more. I get $585 monthly from Social Security. They take out forty dollars for my Medicare. After I pay my bills there is nothing left.

Back in 1990 I was still working as a guard and just starting work through the temporary agencies. I attended the First Bisexual Conference and found the man I recently married. He says I walked up to him and told him "I'm HIV+ and I don't have time to waste so give me your phone number." I don't remember that but I know I felt very empowered at the conference, so it may have happened something like that.

When I had some relationship problems with my husband three years ago, we started seeing a counselor who was referred to me through a service for mental health for HIV+ persons. There was no charge for her services. That is a wonderful asset to the community. We went to her for about a year. I have gone back for individual problems since then from time to time. She has never charged me, and is always happy to assist.

The other place I have gotten help is the Center for Aids Resources located on Shattuck Ave. in Oakland. I and my husband, as my caretaker, have received massages. He is allowed a massage once a month and I get one per week. I also get food from the food bank there. Lunches are provided free to all clients every day at noon. If I am there at the time I get to eat free. There is a telephone available for client usage, and I'm sure the washer, dryer, and shower are very helpful for the clients who are without a home or facilities. There is a women's support group there every Thursday and free counseling. The volunteers who staff the Center are always very friendly and helpful.

I've been using their services since 1992. The man who runs the food bank was so nice to me the other day, I stopped in for my groceries (I get two bags full every week), and he asked if it was time to call me by my masculine name. I told him I hadn't changed my identity yet, and I would let him know. He calls me by my name every time I go there, and he remembers what I tell him. His friendliness had enabled me to confide in him, and I was able to tell him about the forthcoming gender change. It felt so good to have someone listen and remember my story.

When I told my gynecologist I was planning to change to a male, he was extremely helpful and offered to help in any way he could. He said he would continue to care for me during and after the transition if I needed his services. My M.D. was shocked and taken aback when I informed him of my decision to change gender. He asked me if I had researched the impact of the change on my health and safety as an HIV+ person. I told him I hadn't found out much yet, but I was looking into it and would let him know what I found out. When I left his office he told me to set my next appointment for two months later. I don't know if he was going to change the length of time between my checkups before I told him my news or if he decided at that point that he'd rather not see me as often, but I'll talk to him about this when I see him next.

I've always been uncomfortable as a woman. Since I was very young I've always dreamed, at night, that I was male. I rescued damsels in distress, swung on vines in the jungle, and led our troops against the foreign invaders. I have always wanted to be male. When I was a child I knew I was going to be a man when I grew up. When my breasts started growing I was resentful because I realized I was going to be a women regardless of how I felt about it. When Christine Jorgenson became a celebrity in the fifties I felt there was a chance I could change my gender. I made inquires and discovered men could become women but women were not able to change their gender.

In May 1995 I found an ad in the *Bay Times* announcing a support group meeting for female-to-male (FTM) transgender people. I called the phone number to ask for the location and time. My call was screened and I was asked to explain why I wanted to attend the meeting before I was given the address and time. My decision to change my gender was made on the way to that meeting. I plan to be careful about the possible impact on my HIV status. I want to start taking testosterone as soon as possible so I will be able to live as long as possible as a male.

My usual doctor said he doesn't know enough about the possible effects and everyone else has said they would have to ask the Gender Clinic. I have applied to the clinic for treatment there. I was told I would have to wait about a month for an appointment. Because of my HIV status, they are putting my case on a faster track. A friend who is not HIV + applied at the same time and was told he will have to wait three months for an appointment. I was originally thinking about having top surgery. One of the older men in our FTM support group advised me to wait for the top surgery at least for a year after starting testosterone. He said my breasts would shrink with the change of hormones. (I am presently taking estrogen replacement therapy for menopausal symptoms.) He said the breasts might shrink enough to make top surgery unnecessary. I would like to avoid the risk of operation and possible complications if I can.

I have heard rumors of HIV + transgendered people, but I have not met any. It is my understanding that Lou Sullivan, the founder of FTM International, died of AIDS. I do not know whether he transitioned before or after becoming HIV +. I hope to have some better information after I talk to a practitioner at the Gender Clinic in about a month. I have recently changed my primary physician because I found a female physician with whom I feel more comfortable discussing my gender issues.

I have discussed my gender change with physicians, nurse practitioners, and nurses. Some have taken it in stride without noticeable reactions. Others have been interested and helpful. A few have reacted with amused condescension. I feel I now have sympathetic and helpful people on my health care team. I realize I now live in an area where the general public is somewhat understanding of gender changes and I feel very good about the resultant freedom to be my real self. Although I have self-esteem problems sometimes, when I am perceived as a man, my esteem for myself and my abilities grows. I felt the same sense of empowerment at the FTM Conference this fall that I felt at the First Bisexual Conference where I found my husband in 1990. A sense that I'm O.K. and whatever I want to do, the world will support me.

28

Noelle

I'm basically a drag queen, a gay man who wears women's clothes. I work in drag, I entertain in drag, and when I go out to party I go in drag. I think of transvestites as mostly being straight men who like to wear women's clothes on weekends. Most of them just want to feel like a woman; they don't care if they really look like a woman. They don't care if they've got a five o'clock shadow and just a little blue eye shadow and some pink lip gloss on. That doesn't bother them. When I go out, I want to look like a woman. I carry myself off as a woman, and I dress so that I don't embarrass myself wherever I happen to find myself. I don't care if people know, but I don't want to throw it in people's faces. If someone comes right out and asks, I'll tell them that I'm a man in a dress. But what bothers me is if someone comes running up to me screaming, "Oh my god, you're a guy!" I used to get very offended, but now I just laugh. It amuses me. Sometimes I say, "Oh, I bet they call you Einstein, don't they? You must be so proud of yourself, you figured that out!"

I had gone for a period in my life where I was living in drag, trying to live as a woman. For then it was fine, but right now I just don't think it's me. When I was doing that it was too much on your mind, "Who knows, who doesn't know, am I getting over?" and it's kind of a lie. I was still pretty much tied into a transgender sort of thing socially. At that time I was also not comfortable with myself. I didn't like myself; I hated myself. I wanted to get a sex change then. Fortunately I ran into a very intelligent woman psychologist who told me that she believed that I could successfully become a woman and lead a very nice life, but that she thought I wanted to get a sex change operation for the wrong reasons: because I wanted to change myself as much as I could possibly change myself because I hated myself. She suggested that I wait until I liked myself and could accept myself for what I was right then before I made that kind of a jump.

I've never really enjoyed being a guy. I think like a woman, I feel like a woman, but I'm not a woman. My feminine side is much more in tune than my masculine side is, and most of my friends are either other transgenders or women. I never liked to limit myself to one specific type of friendship. I'm excited by meeting people of different nationalities, colors, religions: I've always thought of that as an honor. I think there's less tolerance of transgender diversity in the gay community, both male and female, than there is out on the street. It's just getting acceptable for drags to be allowed into the men's bars, into the women's bars.

I found out about my HIV status by a fluke. It was October 1995, and I'd been on vacation with a bunch of friends. One of them got scabies, so when I got back home I went to the local city hospital to get checked out at the Infectious Disease Unit. They give free health care there and the medicine to cure whatever they find, so you don't have to get a prescription and go someplace and pay for it. I don't have health insurance because I've always worked as a bartender and an entertainer in transgender bars; I do a lot of entertaining in straight bars and touristy places too. It's a lifestyle where what you live on you mostly get in cash. I've never had a job that had insurance, and most of the jobs that would come with that I don't think I'd be real happy at anyway. Some bars do offer insurance, most bars could, all bars should. They make enough to cover what it would cost them.

I had never been tested before, and I had no idea that I had the infection. But the people at the Infectious Disease Unit asked me if I'd like to test for HIV. I said, as long as I'm here, I've always meant to do it; I may as well just so I know for the record that everything is fine. I was so sure that my results would be negative that I almost didn't go back for them. After all, I never get sick; I probably hadn't been to a doctor since 1982. Most people that contract HIV have trouble keeping weight on, and I have just the opposite problem. But a few weeks after my checkup, a girlfriend and I were out speed-walking and we passed the hospital, so I decided to stop in and pick up my results. And that's when they told me. When the nurse looked at my file she left the room and came back with another woman who sat down next to me and held my hand without saying anything. And I thought, "Uh-oh."

I used to be an IV drug user, but I haven't touched a needle in ten or eleven years. Everyone I used to share needles with is either dead or real close to it: I think that there's maybe three of us left, and I thought I'd just gotten out by the skin of my teeth. They'd all continued, this little group, but I'd quit. I thought I'd just gotten out in time, but that didn't turn out to be the case: when the hospital gave me my diagnosis and I had a physical, they told me that they thought I'd probably had HIV for ten to twelve years. I'm glad that I found out about it now as opposed to when I must have first contracted it, because there was just so little known about it then; in the early stages I think that what killed most people so quickly was not just the disease but the shame that went along with it, the fear that went along with it, and the ignorance that went along with it.

I was shocked. The room that you're in when they tell you is on the eighth floor, with windows overlooking the river, and when they told me, both women got very close to me as if I was going to run and jump out the window. Later, when I asked them, they told me that people tried to do that before. I told them no, I was going to be fine.

I've been transgendered my whole life. I can remember when I was six years old I had a crush on my cousin Walter who was a motorcycle dude—very Elvis-Presley looking, real handsome. We were at a family reunion at a state park, and I was sitting under a tree picturing myself in the prettiest little party dress getting all of his attention.

I grew up in a little tiny town—a hateful, nasty little town where my family still lives. I go back once a year for Christmas because I'm very close to my mother and my brother—that's all that's left—but I have nothing to do with anyone else. I do not go out while I'm there; I do not socialize. I was so miserable growing up there that I have a very difficult time not hating the people still. I was always different. I grew up effeminate; I was very overweight at the time; I liked to play with girls, not boys; so I was always getting beat up, chased. Grade school wasn't that bad. Elementary school wasn't that bad. Junior high started hell: the gym teachers making fun of me because no one had ever showed me how to do athletic things. I skipped lunch so I wouldn't have to get beat up in the lunch room. We lived two-and-a-half miles outside of town, and I remember walking home by the river in the freezing cold so I didn't have to walk down streets full of people I was afraid of or take the school bus, which was pure hell. At the time, I was also afraid of dogs. I was just basically afraid, and animals could pick up on it, people could pick up on it. When you're afraid, people know, and that's when they'll get you.

Anyway, high school was hell, and when I was sixteen I started college. I'd go to high school in the morning and in the afternoon I'd hitchhike eleven miles up the road to the college where all the hippies were. It was 1969. I made friends up there, friends who wanted to be seen with me. I'd never had friends before. There were kids who would play with me in high school, but then they'd say, "Don't talk to me in school tomorrow. I don't want people to think we're friends." It still hurts. So I just started walking into classes at this college—really, it was primarily an art school—and I was hanging around so much that they all thought I was a student. The basic thing there was pottery, and I did macramé. I set a loom up in a window ledge out in the hallway and made plant holders. It got to the point where I was making five hundred plant holders a week or so, and I was making good bucks selling them to the students. When the teachers who would stop by to talk to me found out that I wasn't actually a student, they encouraged me to put a portfolio together, and I was accepted at the age of sixteen as a part-time student. I could have not finished high school and gone on, but I did finish. I was smart enough that I could basically skip classes, show up for tests, and pass. So I did that and then went on to art school; I was admitted with a scholarship, and I supplemented it with income from doing macramé. I had a 3.5 average.

I did that for two years, and then my graduating class from high school started coming in to the college, and the hell started all over again. I stopped going to class. I just dropped out. This female graduate student I was friends with said to me, "I'm leaving for Santa Cruz. Come with me." So I did. My first friends there were five lesbians who owned a craft shop. They took me in, and I started making crafts for them and selling them, and then they told me I was gay. "No I'm not," I said. "Sure, I have sex with men, but men are for sex; women are for love." I'd heard of homosexuality, but that wasn't what I was doing because, though I'd been having sex with neighborhood kids since I was seven or eight, there was no love involved. Sex was just a release; it was okay to do it with other boys, but you were supposed to save yourself for the woman you loved. When I fell in love with a guy when I was nineteen, that's what really blew my mind. When I finally came out and started going through all these head trips, I called my mother up crying. I told her that I was gay, and she laughed. She thought it was funny. When I started crying, she said, "My God. I thought you knew. I knew." And she apologized. She wasn't thrilled when I started taking hormones and all that stuff.

My conversations with my lesbian friends about whether or not I was gay went on for around a year, and then one of them invited me to a gay bar. And it was just like, this is it, this is what I've been craving all my life. There were men dancing with each other; everyone was dressed nice; it was exciting. It was 1973, and I immediately went to the local pharmacy and pocketed some lipstick and mascara and started using a little bit of makeup and hanging around campus, though I never actually got around to transferring to UC Santa Cruz.

When I had just come out as gay in Santa Cruz, I weighed 285 pounds. I fell in love with this boy and I asked him to go to a movie with me. He said, "If I want to take you to a movie, I'll rent a U-Haul and go to a drive-in." I was crushed—so crushed that I moved to the next town over and went on a crash diet. I went from 285 pounds to 135 pounds in nine months. I ate a bowl of rice and vegetables every other day, and that was it. No fruits, no vitamins. I was very ignorant. My teeth just started breaking off. I had friends who were watching out for me in general, but that generation at that time didn't know much about health and diet. Going to doctors was unheard of; first of all, you've got to pay cash, and who could do that? So I got scurvy. I've had my upper dentures for eleven years, and my lower ones for three. If I'd known then that doing drugs would take the rest of them away, I don't know if it would have changed anything. Now I like to tell people who are still doing drugs that they have nice teeth. I say, "Don't think you're going to keep doing drugs and keep them."

After I left Santa Cruz, I moved to L.A. and started doing drag there. Then I moved to San Francisco where I got involved with a bunch of queens who would go turn tricks and then go home and shoot drugs. And I had a toothache, a horrible, horrible toothache, and I remember one of them saying, "Heroin will take the pain away." And I said, "Okay." For a few months I had other people shoot me up, and then I learned how to do it myself. After four or five months I was shooting just about anything I could put in a needle. I was in my early twenties. I was hustling for money, and I was working part-time as a coat-check girl at one of the gay bars. I was doing shows.

In 1978 I became manager of a gay bathhouse and I did that for eleven years, but I still hustled on the side. The drugs that went on in the bathhouse were just incredible . . . incredible. Anything you could take. I got to the point where I was selling them. Everything was fine until the coke really got to me. I always kept a handle on heroin, downs, valium— even speed I kept a handle on. But coke—I started selling it because it was costing so much money; and then, when I started selling it, I would sell like $1,000 worth a week and still I'd owe the dealer $1,500. I'd be saying to myself, "What's wrong with this picture?" I still do drugs occasionally, but now a quarter of coke can last me two or three days, where I used to think of a gram as a line.

When I look back, I can't remember anything super enjoyable about shooting up. I remember the fear, and I remember the self-destruction. I remember lots of times injecting drugs into me and thinking, "Maybe this is the high I won't live through." I was so mad at the world that I blamed the world for everything that was wrong with me. I don't anymore. It took me until I was thirty-one, thirty-two years old before I started to like myself—before the idea even clicked in my head that I was supposed to, and once I reached that revelation a lot of the anger and the bullshit dropped off of me.

I'm angry at HIV and I'm angry that our government hasn't done more to find a cure for it, but I also have to say that since I've been diagnosed at least I have a direction in my life. It's something I didn't have before. I started like a health kick six months before I found out about my HIV status, and right now I'm in the process of kind of lightening my load. I don't feel like I'm going to die next year or three or four years from now. My first T-cell count was 617; my second T-cell count a month later was 832. I'm not a person who gets sick easily. I walk three to eight miles every other day and I do the Nordic Track machine and stuff like that. I've cut down to half a pack of cigarettes from two-and-a-half packs a day. I'm not taking any medication: just vitamins and acupuncture. I need to stop taking advantage of my body. I'm forty-one.

I told all of my friends about my HIV diagnosis within the first couple of days of finding out. My mother called me the minute I got home from the hospital: That was the hardest thing I ever had to do in my life—telling my mother. At first she said, "No, I don't believe you." Then a few minutes later she said, "What the hell am I talking about? I knew it the minute I heard your voice on the phone." There were a couple of very rough weeks before finding out what my T-cell count was and how far the virus had progressed. Then I immediately started going out and trying to get assistance for this and assistance for that, and finding out that I wasn't entitled to anything because my T-cell count is so high. When I got my diagnosis, I had been unemployed since April 1995 and I was already thinking, "What else is going to go wrong this year?" But then I thought, "Forget it. If you've had it for this long and you're this healthy, you need to think about what else can go right this year." So I went out and found a job that I started January 1, 1996. I'm much happier this way. I'd rather have too many things to get done than not enough. It motivates me.

I haven't gone to any support groups though I have listings for groups for HIV+ transgender people and groups for gay men. I have my own built-in support group with my friends who are transgendered, gay men, and straight people. There were so many people checking up on me during the two weeks between receiving my diagnosis and finding out my T-cell count, telling me, "When you find out what's going on, you can come live at my house. Whatever you need in life, you have it." This isn't true for most transgender people who find out they're HIV+. I'm very fortunate.

I have a friend over at a place where they've just started to work with transgenders as far as giving them medical treatment who got me a doctor who could see me the very next day. I'm too old to qualify as eligible for help by them, but one of the people who ran it knew who I was from seeing my act, and I've also been very big with benefits, so they squeezed me in. I love the doctor they gave me, and I'm still with him. We laugh. He takes the fear out of it for me, and I trust him. He's already worked with a lot of HIV+ people, and he's just starting to learn about transgendered people. He's very curious about it, and very compassionate. A good man. I'm happy with him. And it's free.

HIV education and intervention needs to start happening at the junior high level. That's when kids start learning about their own sexuality—which doesn't mean that they don't already have sex. I mean, it's 1996: this world really needs to get over it. Kids have sex. And if someone wants to reassign their sex, fine: just work with them. If someone wants to cross-dress, what's the big deal? In the days of Marie Antoinette it was the men who wore wigs and high heels. Men were even effeminate until the 1940s; they didn't start getting so butch until the fifties.

I started adjusting my sexual behavior seven or eight years ago in response to watching friends die. Sexually I was always like a promiscuous prude: there were things I would do and things I wouldn't do. Basically all I would do with tricks was oral sex. If I fell in love with someone, then we could start talking about having anal sex. That's completely out of the question now. I never used to use condoms for oral sex, but now I do. It's not so much that I'm afraid of getting anything—I can live with this disease—but I don't know how I would do with dealing about knowing that I gave it to someone.

I think a lot of people in the transgender community are beginning to clean up their act. The camaraderie of drug-taking just disappeared with the introduction of crack. Violence came out more; so did crime. Crack really brings out people's paranoia, both for the person who is doing the crack and for the person whose house they're in who's afraid of being ripped off. Half of these kids would rather sleep in the subway all high on crack than go to someone's house they're so paranoid.

When I came out as a queen, we had role models. And some of them weren't that great. I didn't know I was going to become a prostitute, but I did. I didn't know I was going to be shooting drugs, but I did—because we watched what our elders were doing. Now most of those people, a good 85–90 percent of them, are dead from drugs, from AIDS, from murder. And the ones that are out now have problems of their own trying to get straight, coping with everyday life. So I don't think a lot of the young ones have strong role models, not as strong as we should be. There are some members of the community aiming to be that. I aim to be that. But I'll also say that I'm not going to take these people into my house. I've got enough to do to keep me straight and to keep me going right now. I can't handle the burden of taking on the responsibility for another person's life, and I feel bad about that. People did that for me, and there was a time in my life when I did it for them, but I'm just too old to go through it again now.

Prostitution isn't the great money a lot of people think it is. I had a queen come up to me and say, "How can you bartend? How can you work here and go home with $40-50 a night? I've got to make $300 a night." I said, "It's not what you make, it's what you do with what you make. Getting it's easy. Keeping it's another thing. You're homeless. You live in and out of hotels and friends' houses. That bag with you is the only clothes you own. You make $300 a night, but you spend it all on drugs so you can go out and make $300 a night again. It's not getting you anywhere."

There really needs to be something to help these kids. I would like to see a halfway house for transgenders with HIV. So many of them, once they've got HIV, they think that's it: They think it's a death sentence. There needs to be something for them whether or not they're HIV + — something to give them a sense of self-worth in life other than just being a queen. People need to learn a trade of some sort, to learn how to make money some other way than through prostitution. They need to learn how to contribute something, how to receive something. For so many of them, there's just no place to go but the streets . . .

29

Jeanette

My name is Jeanette, and I am a 31-year-old woman. I was born and raised in New York City by parents who are Jehovah's Witnesses. I had a fairly strict upbringing and usually stayed close to home. Although I dropped out of high school—a decision I eventually came to regret—I did manage to get my GED.

I experimented with marijuana, then started sniffing cocaine. Before I knew it, I was smoking cocaine. I knew I was better than that, so I tried to break the habit at first by getting a decent job in a hospital. But that didn't last for very long because I got involved with a self-destructive guy who was a drug user himself. At first he seemed like any other guy, but being with him put my life in terrible danger because he was abusive: physically, sexually, emotionally—you name it. By the time I realized that, I was in too deep, and it seemed like there was no way out. I had already gone down with him. I'd become a psychologically and physically abused and battered woman with nowhere to run or hide.

I woke up all right, but it was too late to get out unscathed. Here I thought I was so well informed about AIDS and how to get it. I was sure that it couldn't happen to me, not in a million years. Now I know better.

But back then, I thought differently. Since I hadn't been promiscuous, I didn't consider myself to be in any "high-risk group" for AIDS or any other disease. Little did I know that AIDS was living right under my very nose and posing a serious threat to my life. When you are with one partner, you sometimes assume that you're safe from sexually-transmitted diseases (STDs). But really you're not just having sex with your partner; you're also having sex with every other lover they've had for years.

Today I know that this guy had the audacity to infect me with HIV, die of AIDS right in front of me, and still blame me for his predicament. Sometimes I think about how I could have spared myself by doing things differently, but thinking about it doesn't change anything. The plain truth is that once you get yourself into this, there's no turning back.

In 1990 this psychotic bastard was hospitalized with pneumonia. Of course he told me it wasn't AIDS-related. Every time he became ill there was a new excuse for it: emphysema, asthma, bronchitis—you name it. At the same time, his paranoia about AIDS—he was obsessed with the word, with the entire idea of it—meant that he'd constantly bring it up, usually in his usual sadistic fashion. Moments after bragging about the hundreds of conquests he'd had sexually, he'd outright accuse me of sleeping around with any man I could get my hands on and giving him some terrible disease. Pretty funny considering I'd barely been around the block once. Often he'd say things like "I'm taking you with me."

Why did I put up with this? Because the fear I had of this man was so intense that I'd fall into a trancelike state and do whatever he asked of me in the hope of not being physically abused again. And that meant that even when he was hospitalized and would call me up to visit him "or else," I would go. So much for my self-esteem at that time.

One day I finally woke up and said to myself, "If I don't get out now, I may never be able to." I worried about the kind of life I was giving my child (from a previous relationship), who was now six years old and very aware of the situation.

So in 1990, the year that I realized that I was literally in a "dead end" relationship, I got the hell out of New York. I packed up and left for Rhode Island—far away from his miserable surroundings—where I laid low. I thought that I had made the break and could now start over again, safe once more. It was such an illusion.

It wasn't long before my psycho ex called my dear elderly mother from the hospital to tell her that I'd infected him with HIV and had left him to die of AIDS alone in his hospital bed. Of course she was in shock when she called me in tears to me to tell her the truth. It broke my heart to see her in so much pain. How that evil man could get so much pleasure in hurting another human being this way, I will never know. There must be something missing in people like that; they must have no conscience. Luckily I was able to successfully reassure my precious and worried mother of the only truth I knew: that he was telling her those lies only to spite me for leaving him. According to him, if he couldn't have me, no one could. He spooked me when he would get into these dark gloomy moods and ask me if I would die for him.

I have never been so afraid of anyone in my life; he could have been on the other side of the world and still been able to chill me to the bone with a single word.

I decided to go to a clinic and test for HIV. I was fortunate enough to be given my HIV-positive test results from a considerate, caring soul. We still keep in touch today. God bless you Joanne! Even though I suspected it, hearing that I was HIV + stunned me. In that moment I truly realized that evil exists and thrives. I knew that my life would never be the same.

It is still beyond me how a person could purposely endanger another human life. Part of my panic over finding out I was HIV + was because there was this handsome lifeguard I had met over the summer in this new state of Rhode Island. We had been dating for over three months, and the guilt of knowing I might have infected him unintentionally was so overwhelming that I didn't think I could bear it.

I immediately told my lifeguard boyfriend. While he didn't take it too well, he tried to do the right thing by me. He offered to stay with me and see things through, but I felt like that wasn't fair to him when he had his own hang-ups about it to work out on his own. Although we drifted apart, this was a crucial time for me: I could either accept myself as a desirable woman or settle for being "damaged goods." I thought, "I may never be attractive to another man or find myself attracted to another man." I can't say why this was so important to me, but it was at this time. Go figure.

So a couple of weeks after learning my HIV status, and after having resigned myself to thinking that I would never be involved with anyone or be truly loved by anyone again, destiny played a trick on me. I had stopped into a rental center to pick up some electronics stuff when, lo and behold, I noticed that the manager of the store seemed to be staring at me. He was innocently standing behind the counter, looking as fine as a man should be allowed to look. At first I didn't think anything of it, but something kept nagging at me to find out if I was still attractive to men, especially this particular man. After all, it wasn't as though I was wearing a neon HIV/AIDS sign on my forehead, so how would he know? Well it turned out that he was actually interested in me, and I was on cloud nine! But when, within the first few days, the attraction was too strong, I decided to nip this relationship in the bud: I told him my story and my HIV status.

His response was the turning point in my newly acquired HIV + life. He didn't even flinch. It was all right; I was normal. Soon after he sent me a beautiful bouquet of flowers. I had never felt so special. Had he rejected me, things might have been different, the way I look at it. Wherever he is now, I hope he is truly happy, because he will never know what he did for me. Although we are from two totally different worlds and our affair was somewhat brief (two ships that by fate happened to pass in the night), I believe that everything happens for a reason. I needed him to happen in order for me to realize I was full of life and love, and that my HIV-positive status was not primary. First and foremost I was a human being with likes and dislikes and not just someone with an incurable/communicable disease.

Now that my confidence was returning to its rightful place, that special lifeguard I had met the previous summer was coming around. He had gotten the education he needed and had a whole new attitude about everything, namely "us." How ironic. It was the summer of 1991.

We've been together ever since.

Now it's 1995, and we're still going strong. We always practice safer sex as a rule. I could never do to someone what was done to me. It has been almost eight years since I was diagnosed with HIV in 1988, and I thank the Lord that after all these years I have yet to have any symptoms of this disease.

The wicked ex finally died in 1992. No love lost there; more like, "Ding dong, the crackhead is dead." Hell is too good a place for him, if it even exists.

And that's my story . . .

I want to let others know that there are people who don't mind intentionally infecting you. You can prevent that. Being safe means practicing safer sex with everyone, even the ones you least suspect. I was ignorant when I was younger. I couldn't fathom anyone being that cruel, but I've learned that that kind of cruelty does exist, even though no one on earth deserves such treatment. I certainly didn't.

As for me, I'm using this time to achieve my prior goals of going back to school and getting sufficient training for a decent job. I have a good chance of accomplishing some of what I

had planned for my lifetime. Still, I will always know deep down that it did not have to be this way.

May God bless all of you and may you live long, prosperous lives. I know I will to some extent. You will if you simply heed the warnings you're hearing about HIV/AIDS. Practice safer sex, don't share needles, and most importantly, don't be too quick to put your trust into people who "seem" nice. Everything is not always what it seems. I can vouch for that.

30

Cindy

HIV/AIDS has been a part of my life for the past sixteen years, prior to its being labeled as such by the International Committee of the Taxonomy of Viruses. In the community where I played and was known as "The Volunteer Advocate from Hell" in the early eighties, the virus was known as "Muerte de Sangre." Today in the Latino/a community it is known as SIDA.

Prior to this, in the late seventies, I began to notice brief articles in various publications which were describing a very selective virus which was "merely" affecting gay men. Even then my gut instinct told me that there could be no such virus—one that could single out a certain segment of the population and stay within its confines. Sure enough, by 1982 several people in the Latino/a community were describing their affliction of the "Muerte de Sangre," a virus in their blood which would soon cause death.

My first official visit to a person with AIDS (PWA) in the hospital—I went to visit a friend's brother and advocate for him—was reminiscent of a sci-fi movie. Everyone who entered the room had to suit up from head to toe; this caused a great amount of fear for both the visitors and the patients. There were no answers and no protocols or treatment, just uncertainty and fear. After leaving his room I was walking further down the hall when I heard a voice calling out my name. I peeked into the room the voice was coming from and saw what appeared to be an elderly man calling me in, reassuring me not to be afraid. When he identified himself it turned out that he was one of my friends and he was my age—late twenties. As he lay shackled to his bed under 24-hour guard, this gaunt "old" man told me he had AIDS: would I please stop in to talk with him? That was the turning point for me. When I faced my own fear and stepped into the room, my life was changed in that split second. Several weeks later both men had died, leaving many unanswered questions. Both had histories of injection drug use and one had been a recipient of a kidney transplant, but neither was a gay man; nonetheless, they both died from the complications of AIDS.

For the next three years there was little done in the health community as far as any type of prevention or treatment. Once someone was diagnosed, it was a matter of weeks before they would succumb to this virus. Little did I know at a higher level there was a war of egos festering as scientists battled over who could claim credit for isolating the virus with the possible prize of winning the Nobel.

By 1985 there was a test available to detect the HTLVIII/HIV antibody. I enrolled for the test. At that time there were four identified "risk groups" also known as the "four H club": "Haitians, Homos, Hypos and wHores." By the time they were through asking me numerous questions, I qualified for every group. I had recently been medically treated at a clinic in the mountains on the border of the Dominican Republic and Haiti and had been given several intravenous injections while at the clinic.

It was around that time that I was first introduced to a phenomenon that I will refer to in this article as "intentional infection." I have often wondered why this topic is rarely addressed in any forums or publications; my attitude tends to be that the few who do engage in this behavior are exacerbating an already volatile public health threat. At the same time, I think it's important to stop here and say that the anecdotal stories that I am about to tell are the exception to the rule; the vast majority of those who are HIV positive are paragons of the power of example who face major life changes and actually accomplish their goals. Most importantly they take responsibility for themselves and their infection by either always practicing safer sex or informing their partners of their HIV status. In my years of working with those who are HIV-positive, I have seen miracles where men and women would make dramatic changes in their lives; some would say if they had not been diagnosed they would have died as a result of their lifestyle. Many were courageous and dealt with life on life's terms and learned how to truly enjoy life on a daily basis. Still, I think that it's important to address the topic of intentional infection here.

And now, to continue with my story: that same year in Rhode Island (1985) a group had emerged comprising several persons who prior to testing positive for the HIV antibody had been diagnosed with tertiary syphilis. This group became known as the "AIDS Brigade." Anyone affiliated with this group was assumed to be HIV-positive. This was also my first encounter with intentional infection: One HIV-positive male knowingly injected his blind girlfriend with a mixture of his blood and some Dilaudid. She too soon became a member of the "Brigade." Another HIV-positive female sold diabetic syringes only *after* she had used them and managed to infect her brother, her boyfriend, and a score of others. After her death it was determined by anecdotal histories of other HIV-positive injection drug users that she may have infected between thirty and sixty people intentionally. Some of the members of the "Brigade" were forthright: They told you they were infected or would never let you share their works.

By the end of this year there were several pockets of infection within Rhode Island, some among gay men but more among the injection drug users. Among the IDU's there was now the "Spawn Ranch Group" who injected at an isolated farm/salvage shop (or junkyard, how ironic), the "Dumpsters" who shared works next to a dumpster in South Providence, and the "AIDS Brigade," who frequently made trips to New York City to buy heroin and frequent the shooting galleries there. At this time there were not many women infected with the virus. Those who were usually had a history of injection drug use. Within four years that would soon change.

By 1987 I was employed by a state and federally funded substance abuse treatment facility that initiated one of the first outreach programs in Rhode Island. They secured a substantial grant and attempted to train counselors and other professionals around the issues surrounding HIV/AIDS. While I worked there I knew a coworker—someone who belonged to the group of those who engaged in high-risk "behaviors"—who was heavily in denial about his own HIV status. It took him until 1989 to get tested, but in the meantime he had a child, a healthy child, and that incident fed into his denial. When he did test HIV-positive in 1989, he continued unsafe sex with other men. This I felt was another form of intentional infection: He knew he had the virus but because of his fear of rejection and his sexual addiction he could not use condoms or be honest about his status. Prior to his official diagnosis he would often have sex with his clients; later he would often find out that one of them had become HIV-positive. His rationalization was that they were in a high-risk behavior group prior to meeting him, so they were probably already infected.

Only two years prior to his death did he tell the mother of his child his status; one year prior to his death in 1995 he got honest about his status at an NA (Narcotics Anonymous) Meeting and with other men he was involved with. God only knows if he kept frequenting the adult book store's "glory hole" for anonymous sex. (The glory hole, which was used by many men, both infected and noninfected, was a hole in the wall of a private cubicle where a man would place his penis to be fellated or masturbated by another man.) This man was in such denial that he refused to take antiretrovirals such as AZT because he was afraid that if his fingernails became discolored people would know his HIV status. He lived but six years from the time of being diagnosed HIV-positive in August 1989 until his death in March 1995.

From my perspective, intentional infection falls into several groups: the first I've already indicated (people/situations like the man who injected his blind girlfriend and the woman who infected her own brother). The second and third apply to my coworker all which I have mentioned anecdotally. I will do the same for the other types of intentional infection:

1. Intentional infection solely based on intent of spreading and sharing this virus with anyone.

2. Intentional infection based on fear of rejection.

3. Intentional infection that is secondary to an addiction to sex, drugs, or alcohol.

4. Intentional infection where both parties are aware of one partner's HIV positive status but because of either love or delusions of invincibility refuse to take precautions.

Many of my anecdotal reports are a combination of either one or more of the above.

Often injectable drug users who knew of their HIV-positive status would not share this information with their sexual or shooting partners for fear of rejection from the group or person. Sometimes the desire to shoot/inject drugs was so overpowering that there was little or no time for conversations on sterile technique or HIV transmission.

One of my clients who was diagnosed with AIDS in 1991 would purposely mutilate his rectum, for when he was sick he would get a lot of attention, and he feared that if he was well he would be abandoned. This same man would go out on sex binges where he would have anonymous unsafe sex with any man who was willing. He often frequented the adult book store and its "glory hole"; after his sexual escapades, he would call me full of shame and remorse which would only fuel the fires for another round of the same.

One female friend who was diagnosed in 1987 as being HIV-positive was very open and frank about her infection. She had stopped injecting drugs for the most part, with the exception of several relapses. She engaged in safer sex for the most part. She was rediscovering herself, exploring adjunctive therapies in conjunction with the traditional treatments which were available. In short, she began to take fabulous care of herself. She would often visit her partner, who was incarcerated, and tell him of her experiences. They both had prior sexual and IDU histories in common, so when he was released from prison they continued in their usual unsafe mode in both areas. The partner had never been tested and when he did finally test positive for HIV in 1990 it was not a shock for anyone involved: It had been their choice.

Another colleague who also worked as an outreach worker and trainer was married to a man who was HIV-positive. Many of us assumed that with her range of knowledge on the transmission of the virus, she would always practice safer sex. Clinically we all know what needs to be done to try to prevent infection, but when emotions come into play everything may become skewed. Several years into her profession she left work due to gynecological complications. Soon afterward her HIV antibody test came back positive. Was it habit that prevented her from practicing safer sex with her HIV+ partner? After all, prior to her learning of her husband's HIV status they had never used condoms and she had tested HIV-antibody-negative for many years until that one day when everything changed. Did the men and women in the two different scenarios I've just described feel that love would protect the HIV negative woman in each situation, or that they were invincible? Was it low self-esteem, or did they feel that as a couple they should share it all? Does hedonism come into play, or is it a secret death wish?

I would often work with teen-agers, a population that generally suffers an extreme invincibility complex. You know, "It can't happen to me because I am young and strong and will live forever." Today we know that female teen-agers are the most vulnerable group to become infected with HIV; today we know that teen-agers as a whole are one of the fastest-growing groups to become infected with HIV.

And so end my stories. By no means do I wish to portray everyone who is HIV-positive as a group who intentionally infects others. But it does happen and it needs to be addressed, if only for the sake for those who are still putting themselves at risk through behaviors such as sharing injection equipment or engaging in unsafe/unprotected sex. Everyone needs to take the proper precautions: As in the *Rejuvenation of Jeanette,* you cannot judge a book by its cover.

Index